Deep Brain Stimulation for Parkinson's Disease

Deep Brain Stimulation for Parkinson's Disease

edited by

Gordon H. Baltuch

University of Pennsylvania
Philadelphia, Pennsylvania, U.S.A.

Matthew B. Stern

Pennsylvania Hospital
Philadelphia, Pennsylvania, U.S.A.

informa
healthcare

New York   London

Informa Healthcare USA, Inc.
270 Madison Avenue
New York, NY 10016

© 2007 by Informa Healthcare USA, Inc.
Informa Healthcare is an Informa business

No claim to original U.S. Government works
Printed in the United States of America on acid-free paper
10 9 8 7 6 5 4 3 2 1

International Standard Book Number-10: 0-8493-7019-1 (Hardcover)
International Standard Book Number-13: 978-0-8493-7019-9 (Hardcover)

Visit the Informa Web site at
www.informa.com

and the Informa Healthcare Web site at
www.informahealthcare.com

To our patients and their families who inspired us with their courage, trust, and support.

Preface

Parkinson's disease (PD) remains a major cause of neurological disability affecting millions of patients worldwide. While pharmacotherapy remains the primary treatment of PD symptoms, surgical therapies have enjoyed a resurgence in the successful treatment of patients with advanced PD and complications of drug therapy. In carefully selected patients, deep brain stimulation (DBS) is now considered one of the most important advances in PD therapy. Our expanding knowledge of basal gangla physiology and refinements in neurosurgical technique have combined to fuel the development of a procedure that has dramatically improved the lives of numerous patients with severe, advanced PD. As with any novel therapy, enthusiasm must be tempered with the knowledge derived from ongoing research and clinical experience. Costs and surgical risks must be weighed against quality of life and a realistic appraisal of the likelihood of success. Since the very first literature on DBS for treating PD appeared in the late 1980s, there have now been over 30 thousand procedures performed worldwide. While there have been many articles published on DBS in the last five years, the field is continuing to evolve and it is therefore timely to review the current state of DBS therapy in PD. Contributors to this volume have been involved with DBS from a variety of disciplines and have worked to refine the procedure, carefully monitor its effect on motor and non-motor symptoms, and better define both preoperative patient selection and post-operative management. The text should be of interest to those practicing neurology, neurosurgery, rehabilitation medicine as well as to ancillary health professionals working in clinical neuroscience.

Gordon H. Baltuch
Matthew B. Stern

Contents

Contributors

Gordon H. Baltuch Department of Neurosurgery, Hospital of the University of Pennsylvania, Philadelphia, Pennsylvania, U.S.A.

Lisette K. Bunting-Perry Department of Veterans Affairs, Parkinson's Disease Research, Education, and Clinical Center (PADRECC), Philadelphia Veterans Affairs Medical Center, Philadelphia, Pennsylvania, U.S.A.

Kelvin L. Chou Department of Clinical Neurosciences, Brown Medical School, and NeuroHealth Parkinson's Disease and Movement Disorders Center, Warwick, Rhode Island, U.S.A.

Shabbar F. Danish Department of Neurosurgery, Hospital of the University of Pennsylvania, and Department of Bioengineering, University of Pennsylvania, Philadelphia, Pennsylvania, U.S.A.

Santiagio Figuereo Department of Neurosurgery, Hospital of the University of Pennsylvania, Philadelphia, Pennsylvania, U.S.A.

Leif H. Finkel Department of Bioengineering, University of Pennsylvania, Philadelphia, Pennsylvania, U.S.A.

Kenneth A. Follett Department of Neurosurgery, University of Nebraska Medical Center, Omaha, Nebraska, U.S.A.

Paul J. Ford Departments of Bioethics and Neurology, The Cleveland Clinic, Cleveland, Ohio, U.S.A.

Casey H. Halpern Departments of Neurology and Neurosurgery, Penn Neurological Institute at Pennsylvania Hospital, Hospital of the University of Pennsylvania, Philadelphia, Pennsylvania, U.S.A.

Michael Harhay Center for Bioethics, University of Pennsylvania, Philadelphia, Pennsylvania, U.S.A.

Susan L. Heath   Department of Veterans Affairs, Parkinson's Disease Research, Education, and Clinical Center (PADRECC), San Francisco Veterans Affairs Medical Center, San Francisco, California, U.S.A.

Gregory G. Heuer   Department of Neurosurgery, Hospital of the University of Pennsylvania, Philadelphia, Pennsylvania, U.S.A.

David J. Houghton   Department of Neurology, Hospital of the University of Pennsylvania, Philadelphia, Pennsylvania, U.S.A.

Kwan Hur   Cooperative Studies Program Coordinating Center, Hines VA Hospital, Hines, Illinois, U.S.A.

Howard I. Hurtig   Departments of Neurology and Neurosurgery, Penn Neurological Institute at Pennsylvania Hospital, Hospital of the University of Pennsylvania, Philadelphia, Pennsylvania, U.S.A.

Jurg L. Jaggi   Department of Neurosurgery, Hospital of the University of Pennsylvania, Philadelphia, Pennsylvania, U.S.A.

Galit Kleiner-Fisman   Parkinson's Disease Research, Education, and Clinical Center (PADRECC),Veterans Affairs Medical Center, University of Pennsylvania, Philadelphia, Pennsylvania, U.S.A.

Kathryn Kniele   Department of Psychiatry and Behavioral Sciences, Medical University of South Carolina, Charleston, South Carolina, U.S.A.

John Y. K. Lee   Department of Neurosurgery, Hospital of the University of Pennsylvania, Philadelphia, Pennsylvania, U.S.A.

Grace S. Lin Liang   The Parkinson's Institute, Sunnyvale, California, U.S.A.

Paul J. Moberg   Departments of Psychiatry and Neurology, University of Pennsylvania School of Medicine, and Parkinson's Disease Research, Education, and Clinical Center (PADRECC), Philadelphia Veterans Affairs Medical Center, Philadelphia, Pennsylvania, U.S.A.

Jason T. Moyer   Department of Bioengineering, University of Pennsylvania, Philadelphia, Pennsylvania, U.S.A.

Domenic J. Reda   Cooperative Studies Program Coordinating Center, Hines VA Hospital, Hines, Illinois, U.S.A.

Jacqueline H. Rick   Department of Psychiatry, University of Pennsylvania School of Medicine, and Parkinson's Disease Research, Education, and Clinical Center (PADRECC), Philadelphia Veterans Affairs Medical Center, Philadelphia, Pennsylvania, U.S.A.

Keith M. Robinson   Department of Physical Medicine and Rehabilitation, University of Pennsylvania, Philadelphia, Pennsylvania, U.S.A.

Johannes C. Rothlind   Department of Psychiatry, University of California at San Francisco and Parkinson's Disease Research, Education, and Clinical Center (PADRECC), San Francisco Veterans Affairs Medical Center, San Francisco, California, U.S.A.

Uzma Samadani   Department of Neurosurgery, Hospital of the University of Pennsylvania, Philadelphia, Pennsylvania, U.S.A.

Andrew Siderowf   Department of Neurology, University of Pennsylvania School of Medicine, Philadelphia, Pennsylvania, U.S.A.

Tanya Simuni   Parkinson's Disease and Movement Disorders Center, Northwestern University, Feinberg School of Medicine, Chicago, Illinois, U.S.A.

L. Sue Traweek   Department of Physical Medicine and Rehabilitation, University of Pennsylvania, Philadelphia, Pennsylvania, U.S.A.

Atsushi Umemura   Department of Neurosurgery, Nagoya City University Medical School, Nagoya, Japan

Heidi C. Watson   Department of Veterans Affairs, Parkinson's Disease Research, Education, and Clinical Center (PADRECC), Philadelphia Veterans Affairs Medical Center, Philadelphia, Pennsylvania, U.S.A.

Frances M. Weaver   Midwest Center for Health Services Research and Policy Studies and Research, Spinal Cord Injury Quality Enhancement Research Initiative, Hines VA Hospital, and Department of Neurology and Institute for Healthcare Studies, Northwestern University, Chicago, Illinois, U.S.A.

Daniel Weintraub   Departments of Neurology and Psychiatry, University of Pennsylvania, Parkinson's Disease Research, Education, and Clinical Center (PADRECC), and Mental Illness Research, Education, and Clinical Center (MIRECC), Philadelphia Veterans Affairs Medical Center, Philadelphia, Pennsylvania, U.S.A.

Paul Root Wolpe   Departments of Psychiatry, Medical Ethics, and Sociology and Center for Bioethics, University of Pennsylvania, Philadelphia, Pennsylvania, U.S.A.

History of Deep Brain Stimulation

Shabbar F. Danish

*Department of Neurosurgery, Hospital of the University of Pennsylvania, and
Department of Bioengineering, University of Pennsylvania,
Philadelphia, Pennsylvania, U.S.A.*

Gordon H. Baltuch

*Department of Neurosurgery, Hospital of the University of Pennsylvania,
Philadelphia, Pennsylvania, U.S.A.*

INTRODUCTION

The development of deep brain stimulation as a surgical technique has been a culmination of several technologies that have evolved over a period of many centuries. The union of these technologies has occurred through the persistence of dozens of motivated researchers whose contributions have brought the field to where it stands today. This required more than the development of the stimulating electrode—there needed to be a surgical target and an ability to precisely localize that target. Furthermore, advancement in this technique required progressive improvement in our understanding of the functional anatomy of subcortical structures relative to their roles in motor functions. We review the historical development of the surgical targets for movement disorders, the advances in stereotactic localization, and the application of electrical stimulation to these targets.

EVOLUTION OF THE SURGICAL TARGET

Parkinson's disease (PD) was first described by James Parkinson in his famous essay published in 1817 (1). Based on the observations of six patients over time, whom he had never personally examined, his descriptions consisting of tremor, rigidity, postural abnormalities, and bradykinesia were remarkably accurate. Initial medical therapy for PD was not introduced until almost 60 years later, when Jean Martin-Charcot introduced belladonna drops as a treatment for excessive salivation in these patients. However, it would be almost a century before any surgical treatment for PD would be attempted.

Sir Victor Horsley (2) is credited with the first attempts to surgically treat a movement disorder in the late-nineteenth century. Describing athetosis as resulting from abnormal cortical discharges, he performed the first cortical ablation procedure for dyskinesia in 1890 (2). Over the next two decades, there would be little modification to this surgical approach. There would, however, be several other attempted surgical approaches for involuntary movements. The efficacy of posterior rhizotomy for athetoid movements was described in 1912, although the results were never reproduced (3,4). Other procedures included sympathetic ganglionectomy and dorsal cordotomy (5–7). In the time period between 1911 and 1955, 22 different operations had been proposed in the treatment of tremor (8).

It was in the 1920s and 1930s that knowledge of motor function made significant strides. In the early 1920s, careful investigation of cortical stimulation demonstrated two different types of motor responses from the premotor cortex, and that complex movements occurred as a result of interruption between areas 4 and 6 (9,10). As a result, Foerster hypothesized that the effects were produced by a system outside the pyramidal tract, an extrapyramidal system, in which the globus pallidus produced athethoid movements. In 1927, Spatz (11) furthered the concept of the extrapyramidal motor system, into which he integrated the striatum, the pallidum, the subthalamic nucleus, the substantia nigra, the red nucleus, and the dentate nucleus. In addition, he suggested that deficits in this system were responsible for movement disorders, and thought it would be logical to target treatment approaches to this system.

Even though the role of the extrapyramidal system had been introduced, there were still strong proponents for the role of the cortex in producing involuntary movement disorders. P.C. Bucy and Wilson, both emphasized that the destructive lesion must interrupt the underlying mechanism causing the movement disorder, and used this as justification to continue cortical extirpation over the next decade (12–15). The pioneer of the "pyramidal operation," however was Horsley who reported on the extirpation of the anterior central gyrus in a patient with athetosis in 1890 (16). Although this procedure resulted in resolution of athetosis, the patients were left with significant paresis or paralysis in exchange.

Meyers is credited as the first in testing the hypothesis that the extrapyramidal system was involved in the production of movement disorders. He surgically resected the head and anterior segment of the caudate nucleus in a parkinsonian patient via an anterior transventricular approach in which both tremor and rigidity were partially improved. He went on to perform open surgical interventions on various subcortical structures including the caudate, the internal capsule, the putamen, the pallidum, and the ansa lenticularis (17,18). Meyer demonstrated that tremor and rigidity could be improved without the production of paresis or spasticity. Open surgery of subcortical structures was further developed in the 1950s by a number of neurosurgeons, namely Fenelon of Paris, and the issue then became one of accuracy (19–22). Although these neurosurgeons are often credited with the introduction of lesion refinement by electrocoagulation, this technique had been used in the cerebellum for PD in 1935 by Delmas-Marsalet and Van Bogaert (23).

At about the same time as Fenelon, Guiot, and Brion were modifying the approach to the basal ganglia, Dr. Cooper made an accidental discovery that marked a milestone in the surgery for involuntary movement disorders. During a pedunculotomy procedure in a man with tremor and rigidity, the anterior choroidal artery was torn during sharp dissection. The procedure was aborted, and the patient experienced complete relief of tremor and rigidity without the loss of motor strength, confirming findings claimed by Meyer (24,25). Cooper had concluded that ligation of the anterior choroidal artery resulted in infarction of the globus pallidus, its afferent connections, and the thalamus. However, variability in its distribution sometimes led to unpredictable results and eventual abandonment of this technique (26–28).

At this point in time, surgery for involuntary movement disorders had seen the development of over 20 procedures, of which pyramidal tract surgery dominated until the acceptance of the extrapyramidal system and the evidence that lesions in this area could provide benefit without paralysis. However, open surgery of subcortical structures still carried a relatively high morbidity, which necessitated the need for safer and more accurate procedures.

THE STEREOTACTIC METHOD

Although Horsley and Clarke are often credited with the development of the first stereotactic frame, the foundation for this work had been laid down many decades earlier. Paul Broca, best known for his work on cerebral localization, developed a stereographic apparatus in 1868 (29). In 1889, Zernov developed an encephalometer, which was successfully used to drain a post-traumatic cerebral abscess. The Zernov device was the first to employ a system of polar coordinates for determining the spatial localization not only of surface but of certain deep brain structures, and was modified by Rossolimo in the early 1900s by the attachment of an aluminum hemisphere on which there was a map of the cerebral sulci and gyri as well as the subcortical structures. Neither Rossolimo nor Horsley and Clarke had any knowledge of each other's developments (30–32).

The Horsley-Clarke frame itself was invented by Robert Henry Clarke, the neurophysiologist with whom Horsley collaborated on studies of cerebellar functions. It was used for selective stimulation and electrolytic ablation of the deep cerebellar nuclei in animals (33–35). The apparatus was designed to hold an electrode and guide it in a three-dimensional Cartesian coordinate system, and was the first system based on this coordinate system. They were the first to call this methodology "stereotactic" (31).

The first stereotactic frame built specifically for human use was designed by Aubrey Mussen in 1918, a neuroanatomist and neurophysiologist who had worked with Clarke (36,37). Although this frame was never used for a human stereotactic procedure, it was used to develop a human stereotactic atlas similar to Clarke's original animal atlases (37,38). Kirschner developed and used a stereotactic apparatus for the treatment of trigeminal neuralgia in 1933 by targeting the Gasserian ganglion, and achieved high precision (39,40).

Forty years later, Speigel and Wycis modified the Horsley-Clarke frame and developed the stereoencephalotome for use in humans, in 1947 (41). The cardinal difference between this and the Horsley-Clarke frame was the use of intracerebral versus superficial reference points (40,42). This was only possible at this point due to the development and incorporation of ventriculography with the use of the stereotactic frame (31,43). As a result, they were able to develop the first modern stereotactic atlas of the human brain (44).

Several investigators around this time period independently pioneered various stereotactic instruments. J. Talairach, Lars Leksell, T. Reichert and Mundinger, Guiot and Gillingham, Rand and Wells, and Laitinen, among others, all developed stereotactic instruments intended for human intracranial localization, between 1948 and 1952 (32). Both Leksell and T. Riechert developed arc-based stereotactic frames that relied on pneumoencephalography to visualize the third ventricle (45,46).

THE END OF THE PYRAMIDAL TRACT ERA

In 1950, Mackay summarized the status of movement disorder surgery stating that paralysis was an absolute side effect of surgery for involuntary hyperkinesias, and that surgery had little application in this field (47). However, due to the tremendous advancement in intracranial localization, surgical targets could be refined in a well-defined manner with more accurate precision that could previously be achieved. In addition to the development of the modern stereotactic frame and brain atlas, Spiegel and Wycis are credited with the first stereotactic pallidotomy and thalamotomy. Direct lesioning of the globus pallidus was an improvement from the Cooper procedure, as it did not depend on the distribution of the anterior choroidal artery. The clinical benefits, however, were disappointing, and long-term improvement was reported only for rigidity. Tremor and hypokinesia were rarely improved (48,49). At this time, the target was localized in the anterodorsal part of the globus pallidus. The most striking advance in localization of the most effective area within the globus pallidus came from Leksell who after an initial series of anterodorsal pallidotomies progressively moved the target to the posteroventral pallidum. This target gave long-lasting relief of both tremor and rigidity. It is surprising that these remarkable results received very little publicity at the time (50). The pallidum as a target evolved simultaneously with the nucleus ventrolateralis (VL) of the thalamus, which was originally proposed by Hassler. In the years that followed, the VL lesion replaced pallidotomy as a treatment for tremor (51–53).

Thalamotomy was a more effective treatment for tremor than for rigidity, and in this respect the perfect subcortical target had not yet been identified. In 1963, Spiegel and Wycis proposed to destroy the subthalamic area, namely the zona incerta and the prelemniscal radiation—not the subthalamic nucleus as we know it today, based on Meyer's experience with lesions in the Field H of Forel (54,55). Target accuracy, however, was still suboptimal. Hassler found that the lesions they had intended as thalamotomies were situated in the subthalamic area during postmortem histological analysis (56). The original rationale for subthalamotomy was the alleviation of rigidity, but this objective was only partially attained, and it proved to be more efficient against tremor when compared with thalamotomy (57). Early results of subthalamotomy reaffirmed the important conclusion that complete and permanent elimination of tremor could be obtained without damaging the pyramidal tract (57,58).

ELECTRICITY, THE BRAIN, AND STIMULATION

Over the course of a little more than a century, significant advances had been made that allowed deep brain stimulation to develop. The introduction of the extrapyramidal system and the development of stereotactic methods provided a foundation through which deep brain stimulation was born. Until about 1970, the major techniques pertaining to subcortical structures involved ablative methods, and the introduction of deep brain stimulation would come from a different realm of neurological disorders.

It is important to acknowledge the groundwork that has allowed deep brain stimulation to exist in its modern form. Over 200 years ago, Giovanni Aldini published a highly influential book that reported experiments in which the principles of Luigi Galvani and Alessandro Volta were used together for the first time. He actively participated in a series of crucial experiments with frogs' muscles that led to the idea that electricity was the long-sought vital force coursing from the brain to the muscles, and made the connection between electricity and muscular contraction. But even before Aldini, significant observations had been made connecting electricity and medical therapeutics. In 46 AD, Scribonnius Largus introduced the use of the torpedo fish, also known as the electric ray, in the treatment of chronic headaches. Soon after, Discrorides, a Greek physician extended the use of the torpedo fish to the treatment of hemorrhoids (59). In the mid-eighteenth century, Gottlieb used electrical stimulation to treat paralysis, and Benjamin Franklin successfully treated a young girl with seizures using similar principles (60,61). Duchenne, often considered the father of electrotherapy, would apply Aldini's concepts to therapeutic medicine in the mid-nineteenth century (62). But as is often the case, science would rediscover these observations many years later before becoming widely accepted.

Although cortical electrical stimulation can be traced back prior to Aldini in 1801, he is often credited with the first applications of electricity to the human brain. Aldini was able to stimulate the cerebral cortex of one hemisphere and obtain facial muscle contractions on the side opposite to that of the stimulation. This observation, however, had already been made by Hippocrates in 420 BC (63). Aldini's findings remained largely ignored and were rediscovered yet again by Fritsch and Hitzig, who applied electrical microstimulation to the cerebral cortex of dogs in the late 1800s (64). Fritsch had observed that irritation of the brain caused twitching on the opposite side of the body, while dressing a head wound during the Prussian–Danish war (63). In this same time period, several others including Sherrington, Ferrier, Luciani, and Tamburini were performing cortical stimulation experiments in animals, mostly in the context of localizing function and developing a sensorimotor map within the cerebral cortex (63,65,66).

The first formal stimulation studies in humans were performed by R. Bartholow in the 1870s (67). He applied stimulation to the cerebrum of a woman with deep cerebral abscesses and was able to invoke contralateral convulsions. Following this experimentation, the woman died after having several recurrent refractory seizures. As a result, he advocated that such experimentation should not be repeated due to the harm that the intracerebral electrodes could cause the patient.

Cortical stimulation had developed at this point with very little knowledge of the true nature of the electrical impulse, mostly due to a lack of sensitive instruments to measure and display electrical activity (68). Lord Edgar Adrian Douglas and Yngve Zotterman are credited as having been the first to record the electrical responses of single neurons in 1926 (69). This was made possible by the invention of the microelectrode by Ida Henrietta Hyde in 1921, which spurred the age of discovery in neurophysiology from the 1930s to 1950s when the basic principles of nerve and brain function were described (70).

Electrical recordings of the brain can be dated back to Richard Caton in 1875 who applied electrodes to the scalp and directly to the brain surface and noted electrical changes taking place (71). About 60 years later, Hans Berger, who had made the first human electroencephalogram recording, introduced intracerebral depth electrodes for subcortical recordings (72). Subsequently, many groups introduced electrodes deep into the brain to localize epileptic foci and to explore therapeutic avenues in psychotic patients (73–75). Wetzel and Snider published the first report using electrical recordings during movement disorder surgery with the specific purpose of neurophysiologically refining their target location, in 1958 (76). In 1960, Ervin and Mark used evoked potentials to verify the position of their electrode within the sensory thalamus. They stimulated and recorded from the sensory thalamus prior to making a destructive lesion (77). In 1961, Albe-Fessard used a low-impedance, concentric bipolar microelectrode to record from and differentiate various thalamic nuclei. This allowed them to describe a contralateral somatotopic thalamic arrangement (78). Subsequently, "tremor cells" with rhythmic cellular discharges synchronous to the parkinsonian tremor were identified (79–81). As a result, Guiot's group was able to demonstrate that most tremorigenic cells are located in ventralis intermedius (Vim), making it a better target than ventralis oralis posterior (Vop), as was previously advocated by Hassler (56,82,83). By the late 1960s, intraoperative microrecording had become a routine part of stereotactic surgery, the anatomy and physiology of the human thalamus had been extensively explored, and Vim became the optimal target location for tremor (84).

Although microrecordings and preablation stimulation for localization were routinely used, stimulation as a therapeutic tool for movement disorders had still not made their connection. Modern deep brain stimulation was "reinvented" to treat major depression, the same disease entity that was treated when Aldini applied galvanism to treat a 27-year-old farmer (85). In 1948, J. Lawrence Pool considered brain stimulation as an alternative to ablative psychosurgical procedures. Although the patient suffered from advanced PD, the surgery was directed at the depression and anorexia. The electrode was implanted in the caudate nucleus through an open craniotomy and stimulation was carried out via an implanted induction coil (86). At about the same time, Spiegel and Wycis applied their stereotactic technique to the implantation of deep stimulating electrodes to avoid the morbidity associated with open craniotomy (87).

Stimulation further developed as a technique through its utility in pain control. Heath was the first to report pain relief after electrical stimulation of the septal region (88). In 1966, Ervin et al. (89) used stimulation of the caudate nucleus for pain relief. The thalamus was first introduced as a target for pain control by Mazars and White, who successfully used acute stimulation of the ventralposterolateral (VPL) nucleus for the treatment of bodily pain and the ventroposteromedial (VPM) nucleus for facial pain. In 1973, the VPL and VPM were chronically stimulated for the first time both by Mazars and Hosobuchi (90–93). Targeting of the periaqueductal gray matter and periventricular gray matter allowed further refinement of deep brain stimulation techniques when it was introduced in 1977 (94–96).

After the introduction of L-dopa in the late 1960s, there was a sharp decline in interest for the surgical treatment of PD. At that time, the Vim nucleus and the globus pallidus remained the major surgical targets, and ablative procedures of these targets continued. As a result, deep brain stimulation progressed as a technique through its use in psychiatric and pain-control surgery.

CHRONIC STIMULATION FOR MOVEMENT DISORDERS

Although thalamotomy was an established target in the treatment of tremor, and the effects of thalamic stimulation on tremor was well known, the idea to use stimulation as a therapeutic modality did not emerge until Benabid's preliminary report in 1987 on stimulation of the Vim nucleus (97). His follow-up report revealed a long lasting effect from chronic stimulation of Vim, but that it was only effective for tremor and not for other parkinsonian symptoms (98).

An important observation in this regard was that while tremor was significantly reduced with Vim stimulation, dopaminergic medication was unchanged. As a result, the overall quality of life was unchanged due to the lack of effect on the other symptoms of the disease (99,100). Hence, as had been the case for over a century, the search for a better target continued.

Although pallidotomy had been well established as a surgical target, it would not be until Laitinen's report in 1992 that the interest in the globus pallidus would resurface (101). He reported a significant improvement in bradykinesia, rigidity, and drug-induced dyskinesias. The proposal to attempt stimulation of Laitinen's target came from Siegfried and Lippitz, two years later (102). The efficacy of chronic stimulation of the globus pallidus as a therapeutic alternative was reported shortly thereafter by several groups demonstrating the beneficial effects of pallidal stimulation on tremor, bradykinesia, and dyskinesias (103–106). It is interesting to note that the effects of pallidal stimulation in humans were well-documented almost 40 years earlier (107).

How did we get to the subthalamic nucleus as a target? Although thalamic and pallidal targets had been explored before being studied in any animal models, the subthalamic nucleus was only proposed as a target once experimental results revealed its possible clinical efficacy. Barry Kidston, a 23-year-old chemistry graduate student in Maryland, unknowingly synthesized 1-methyl-4-phenyl-4-propionoxypiperidine (MPPP) incorrectly and injected the result. It was contaminated with 1-methyl-4-phynyl-1,2,3,6-tetrahydropyridine (MPTP), and he developed parkinsonian symptoms shortly thereafter. Traces of MPTP were found in his lab, and its effects were eventually discovered after testing the chemical in rats. In 1982, seven people in California were diagnosed with PD after using MPPP contaminated with MPTP, which was tracked down as the cause by J. William Langston (108). As a result, the development of an animal model for PD became possible, and various subcortical structures and their relationships could be explored. Through the perseverance of countless scientists, the pieces of the basal ganglia circuitry puzzle were pieced together. In 1989, Albin et al. (109) related the pathophysiology of movement disorders to the functional anatomy of the basal ganglia. Shortly after, it was shown that lesioning of the subthalamic nucleus in MPTP-treated monkeys could dramatically alleviate all the cardinal motor symptoms of PD (110,111). This allowed a deviation from the traditional belief that subthalamic nucleus (STN) lesions always resulted in disabling hemiballismus. Benabid and the Grenoble group pioneered chronic stimulation of the STN for PD and reported their first patient in 1994, based on the findings from animal experimentation (112,113).

THE LAST TWENTY YEARS

Since the introduction of deep brain stimulation almost 20 years ago, there has been an immense resurgence in interest in the surgical technique. However, we are still asking some of the same questions. How can we improve our targeting? What is the optimal target? In addition, we have started asking some new questions such as how does deep brain stimulation work, and what other disorders can deep brain stimulation be applied to?

As imaging technology has improved, there has been a continued effort to better define subcortical structures. Most recently, it has been found that improved magnetic resonance imaging may allow a greater visualization of STN borders (114). Although the STN has been well established as the ideal target for PD, the search for a better target still continues. Stimulation of the pedunculopontine nucleus has recently demonstrated acute improvements in motor function (115). As a result of the success that PD treatment has enjoyed by deep-brain stimulation, treatments for other disease processes have been attempted. These have included dystonia, obsessive-compulsive disorder, Tourette's syndrome, and refractory depression (116–123).

Although a full discussion of these points is well beyond the scope of this chapter, the intention is to highlight the fact that deep-brain stimulation as a science is still very much in its infancy with enormous potential in the future. Where we are going proves to be just as exciting as where we have already been.

REFERENCES

1. Parkinson J. An Essay on the Shaking Palsy. London: Sherwood, Nelly, and Jones, 1817.
2. Horsley V. Remarks on the surgery of the central nervous system. Br Med J 1890; 2:1286–1292.
3. Putnam T. Treatment of unilateral paralysis agitans by section of the lateral pyramidal tract. Arch Neurol Psychiatry 1940; 44:950–976.
4. Winslow R, Spear I. Section of posterior spinal nerve roots for relief of gastric crises and athetoid and choreiform movements: report of two cases. JAMA 1912; 58:208–210.
5. Gardner W, Williams G. Interruption of the sympathetic nerve supply to the brain: effect on Parkinson's syndrome. Arch Neurol Psychiatry 1949; 61:413–421.
6. Puusepp L. Cordotomia posterior lateralis (fascic Burdachi) on account of trembling and hypertonia of the muscles in the hand. Folia Neuropath Estonia 1930; 10:62–64.
7. Rizzatti E, Moreno G. Cordotomia laterale posteriore nella cura della ipertonie extra-piramidali postencefalitsche. Schizofrenie 1936; 5:117–122.
8. Siegfried J. Neurosurgical treatment of Parkinson's disease. Present indications and value. In: Rinne U, Klinger M, Staum G, eds, Parkinson's Disease: Current Progress, Problems and Management. Amsterdam: Elsevier, 1980:369–376.
9. Foerster O. Analyse und Pathophysiologie der striaren Bewegungsstorungen. Zeitschr f d ges Neurol u Psychiatr 1921; 73:1–169.
10. Gabriel EM, Nashold BS, Jr. Evolution of neuroablative surgery for involuntary movement disorders: an historical review. Neurosurgery 1998; 42:575–590, discussion 590–571.
11. Spatz M. Physiologies des Zentralnervensystems der WirbelTiere. Berlin: Springer, 1927.
12. Bucy P. Cortical extirpation in the treatment of involuntary movements. Res Publ Assoc Res Nerv Ment Dis 1940; 21:551–595.
13. Bucy P, Buchanan D. Athetosis. Brain 1932; 55:479–492.

14. Bucy P, Case T. Athetosis: II-Surgical treatment of unilateral athetosis. Arch Neurol Psychiatry 1937; 37:983–1020.
15. Wilson S. The Croonian Lectures on some disorders of motility and of muscle tone: with special reference to the corpus striatum. Lancet 1925; 2:1–10, 53–62, 169–178, 215–219, 268–276.
16. Tan T, Black P. Sir Victor Horsley (1857–1916): pioneer of neurological surgery. Neurosurgery 2002; 50:607–612.
17. Meyers H. The modifications of alternating tremors, rigidity, and festination by surgery of the basal ganglia. Res Publ Assoc Nerv Ment Dis 1942; 21:602–665.
18. Meyers H. Surgical procedures for postencephalitic tremor with notes of the physiology of the premotor fibers. Arch Neurol Psychiat 1940; 44:455–461.
19. Fenelon F. Neurosurgery of ansa lenticularis in dyskinesias and Parkinson's disease: review of principles and techniques of a personal operation. Sem Hop Paris 1955; 31:1835.
20. Guiot G, Brion S. Traitement des mouvements anormaux par la coagulation pallidale. Technique et resultats. Rev Neurol 1953; 89:578–580.
21. Guiot G, Brion S. Traitement neurochirurgical des syndromes choreo-athetosiques et parkinsonien. Sem Hop Paris 1952; 49:2095–2099.
22. Talairach J, Hecaen H, David M, et al. Recherches sur al coagulation therapeutique des structures sous corticales chez l'homme. Rev Neurol 1949; 81:4–24.
23. Delmas-Marsalet P, Van Bogaert L. Sur un cas de myoclonies rhythmiques continues determines par une intervention chirurgicale sur le tronc cerebral. Rev Neurol 1935; 64:728–740.
24. Cooper I. Ligation of the anterior choroidal artery for involuntary movements: Parkinsonism. Psychiatr Q 1953; 27:317–319.
25. Cooper I. Surgical occlusion of the anterior choroidal artery in parkinsonism. Surg Gynecol Obstet 1954; 99:207–219.
26. Cooper I. An investigation of neurosurgical alleviation of parkinsonism, chorea, athetosis and dystonia. Ann Int Med 1956; 45:381–392.
27. Doshay L. Anterior choroidal surgery and geriatric parkinsonism. Geriatrics 1954; 9:479–483.
28. Merritt H. Evaluation of surgical therapy of disorders of the basal ganglia. Neurology 1956; 6:755–760.
29. Stone J. Paul Broca and the first craniotomy based on cerebral localization J Neurosurg 1991; 75:154–159.
30. Fodstad H, Hariz M, Ljunggren B. History of Clarke's stereotactic instrument. Stereotact Funct Neurosurg 1991; 57:130–140.
31. Kandel EI. Stereotactic method. In: Functional and Stereotactic Neurosurgery. New York: Plenum Press, 1989:67–88.
32. Kandel EI, Schavinsky YV. Stereotaxic apparatus and operations in Russia in the 19th century. J Neurosurg 1972; 37:407–411.
33. Clarke R, Horsley V. On a method of investigating the deep ganglia and tracts of the central nervous system (cerebellum). Br Med J 1906; 2:1799–1800.
34. Clarke R, Horsley V. On the intrinsic fibres of the cerebellum, its nuclei, and its efferent tracts. Brain 1905; 28:13–29.
35. Horsley V, Clarke R. The structure and functions of the cerebellum examined by a new method. Brain 1908; 31:45–124.

36. Olivier A, Bertrand G, Picard C. Discovery of the first human stereotactic instrument. Appl Neurophysiol 1983; 46:84–91.
37. Picard C, Olivier A, Bertrand G. The first human stereotaxic apparatus. The contribution of Aubrey Mussen to the field of stereotaxis. J Neurosurg 1983; 59:673–676.
38. Bullard DE, Nashold BS, Jr. Evolution of principles of stereotactic neurosurgery. Neurosurg Clin N Am 1995; 6:27–41.
39. Richert T. Stereotactic Brain Operations: Methods, Clinical Aspects. Vienna: Burn Huber, 1980.
40. Spiegel E. Methodological and clinical developments in stereotactic surgery: contributions to the physiology of subcortical structures. In: Spiegal E, ed. Guided Brain Operations. New York: Karger, 1982:1–5.
41. Spiegel E, Wycis H, Marks M, et al. Stereotaxic apparatus for operations on human brain. Science 1947; 106:349–350.
42. Redfern RM. History of stereotactic surgery for Parkinson's disease. Br J Neurosurg 1989; 3:271–304.
43. Hayne R, Belinson L, Gibbs F. Electrical activity of subcortical areas in epilepsy. EEG Clin Neurophysiol 1949; 1:437–445.
44. Spiegel E, Wycis H. Stereoencephalotomy. Part I. Methods and Stereotaxic Atlas of Human Brain. New York: Grune and Stratton, 1952.
45. Jensen RL, Stone JL, Hayne RA. Introduction of the human Horsley-Clarke stereotactic frame. Neurosurgery 1996; 38:563–567, discussion 567.
46. Leksell L. A stereotactic apparatus for intracerebral surgery. Acta Chir Scand 1949; 99:229–233.
47. Mackay R. The 1951 Year Book of Neurology and Psychiatry. Chicago: The Year Book Publishers, 1952.
48. Spiegal E, Wycis H. Pallidothalamotomy in chorea. Arch Neurol Psychiatry 1950; 64:295–296.
49. Spiegal E, Wycis H. Thalamotomy and pallidotomy for treatment of choreic movements. Acta Neurochir (Wien) 1951; 2:417–422.
50. Svennilson E, Torvik A, Lowe R, et al. G Treatment of parkinsonism by stereotaxic thermolesions in the pallidal region. Acta Psychiat Neurol Scand 1960; 35:358–377.
51. Hassler R, Riechert T, Mundinger F, et al. Physiological observations in stereotaxic operations in extrapyramidal motor disturbances. Brain 1960; 83:337–350.
52. Laitinen L. Thalamic targets in the stereotaxic treatment of Parkinson's disease. J Neurosurg 1966; 24:82–85.
53. Riechert T. Stereotaxic operations for extrapyramidal motor disturbances with particular regards to age groups. Confin Neurol 1966; 26:213–217.
54. Mundinger F. Stereotaxic interventions on the zona incerta for treatment of extrapyramidal motor disturbances and their results. Confin Neurol 1965; 26:222–230.
55. Spiegal E, Wycis H. Campotomy in various extrapyramidal disorders. J Neurosurg 1963; 20:871–884.
56. Hassler R, Mundinger F, Riechert T. Correlations between clinical and autoptic findings in stereotaxic operations of parkinsonism. Confin Neurol 1965; 26:282–290.
57. Velasco F, Molina-Negro P, Bertrand C, et al. Further definition of the subthalamic target for arrest of tremor. J Neurosurg 1972; 36:184–191.
58. Bertrand C, Martinez S, Hardy J. Stereotactic surgery for parkinsonism. Prog Neurol Surg 1973; 5:79–112.

59. Kellaway P. The part played by electric fish in the early history of bioelectricity and electrotherapy. Bull Hist Med 1946; 20:112–137.
60. Licht S. History of electrotherapy. In: Licht S, ed. Therapeutic Electricity and Ultraviolet Radiation. New Haven: Elizabeth Licht, 1959:1–69.
61. McNeal D. 2000 years of electrical stimulation. In: Hambrecht F, Reswick J, eds. Functional Electrical Stimulation. New York: M Dekker, 1977:3–35.
62. Duchenne G. Physiologie des mouvements. Paris: Bailliere et Fils, 1867.
63. Devinsky O. Electrical and magnetic stimulation of the central nervous system: historical overview. In: Devinsky O, EBeric A, Dogali M, eds. Electrical and Magnetic Stimulaiton of the Brain and Spinal Cord. New York: Raven Press, Ltd., 1993:1–16.
64. Parent A. Giovanni Aldini: from animal electricity to human brain stimulation. Can J Neurol Sci 2004; 31:576–584.
65. Ferrier D. Experimental researches in cerebral physiology and pathology. West Riding Lunatic Asylum Medical Reports 1873; 3:30–96.
66. Sherrington C. On the motor area of the cerebral cortex. In: Denny-Brown D, ed. Selected Writings of Sir Charles Sherrington. London: Hamilton, 1939:397–439.
67. Morgan J. The first reported case of electrical stimulation of the human brain. J Hist Med Allied Sci 1982; 37:51–64.
68. Frank R. The Columbian exchange: American physiologists and neuroscience techniques. Fed Proc 1986; 45:2665–2672.
69. Adrian E, Zotterman Y. The impulses produced by sensory nerve endings: II. The response of a single end-organ. J Physiol (Lond) 1926; 61:151–171.
70. Hyde I. A microelectrode and unicellular stimulation of single cells. Biol Bull 1921; 130–133.
71. Caton R. The electric currents of the brain. BMJ 1875; 2:278.
72. Berger H. Uber das elektrenkephalogram des Menschen. Arch Psychiatr 1931; 94:16–60.
73. Bickford R, Uihlein A, Petersen M. Electrical rhythms recorded from the depth of the frontal lobes during operations on psychotic patients. Proc Staff Meet Mayo Clin 1953; 28:135–143.
74. Delgado J, Hamlin H, Chapman W. Technique of intracranial electrode implacement for recording and stimulation and its possible therapeutic value in psychotic patients. Confin Neurol 1952; 12:315–319.
75. Wada T, Endo K, Marui F. Electrograms immediately recorded from the exposed human brain with description on technique and report of observations. Folia Psychiat Neurol Japon 1950; 4:132–142.
76. Wetzel N, Snider R. Neurophysiological correlates in human stereotaxis. Q Bull Northwestern U Med School 1958; 32:386–392.
77. Ervin F, Mark V. Stereotaxic thalamotomy in the human: II. Physiologic observations on the human thalamus. Arch Neurol (Chic) 1960; 3:368–380.
78. Guiot G, Hardy J, Albe-Fessard D. Delimitation precise des structures sous-coticales et identification de noyaux thalamiques chez l'homme par l'electrophysiolie stereotaxique. Neurochirurgia (Stuttg) 1962; 5:1–18.
79. Albe-Fessard D, Arfel G, Guiot G. Thalamic unit activity in man. Electroencephalogr Clin Neurophysiol suppl 1967; 25:132.
80. Hardy J. Electrophysiological localization and identification. J Neurosurg 1966; 24:410–414.

81. Hardy J, Bertrand C, Martinez N. Activites cellulaires thalamiques liees au tremble-ment parkinsonien. Neuro-Chir (Paris) 1964; 10:449–452.
82. Albe-Fessard D, Arfel G, Guiot G. Derivation d'activites spontanees et evoquees dans des structures cerebrales profondes de l'homme. Rev Neurol (Paris) 1962; 106:89–105.
83. Hassler R, Mundinger F, Riechert T. Pathophysiology of tremor at rest derived from teh correlation of anatomical and clinical data. Confin Neurol 1970; 32:79–87.
84. Tasker R, Organ L, Hawrylshyn P. Sensory organization of the human thalamus. Appl Neurophysiol 1976; 39:139–153.
85. Aldini J. Essai theorique et experimental sur le galvanisme, avec une serie d'experi-ences faites devant des commissaires de l'Institut national de France, et en divers amphitheatres anatomiques de Londres. Paris: Fournier Fils, 1804.
86. Pool J. Psychosurgery in older people. J Am Geriat Soc 1954; 2:456–465.
87. Spiegel E, Wycis H. Chronic implantation of intracerebral electrodes in humans. In: Sheer D, ed. Electrical Stimulation of the Brain. Austin: University of Texas Press, 1961:37–44.
88. Heath R. Studies in Schizophrenia. Cambridge, MA: Harvard University Press, 1954.
89. Ervin F, Brown C, Mark V. Striatal influence on facial pain. Confin Neurol 1966; 27:75–90.
90. Hosobuchi Y, Adams J, Rutkin B. Chronic thalamic stimulation for the control of facial anesthesia dolorosa. Arch Neurol 1973; 29:158–161.
91. Mazars G, Merienne L, Ciolocca C. Intermittent analgesic thalamic stimulation. Pre-liminary note. Rev Neurol (Paris) 1973; 128:273–279.
92. Mazars G, Roge R, Mazars Y. Results of the stimulation of the spinothalamic fasci-culus and their bearing on the physiopathology of pain. Rev Prat 1960; 103:136–138.
93. White J. Pain and the neurosurgeon: a 40 year experience. Springfield, IL: Charles C Thomas, 1969.
94. Hosobuchi Y, Adams JE, Linchitz R. Pain relief by electrical stimulation of the central gray matter in humans and its reversal by naloxone. Science 1997; 197:183–186.
95. Richardson DE, Akil H. Long term results of periventricular gray self-stimulation. Neurosurgery 1977; 1:199–202.
96. Richardson DE, Akil H. Pain reduction by electrical brain stimulation in man. Part 1: Acute administration in periaqueductal and periventricular sites. J Neurosurg 1977; 47:178–183.
97. Benabid AL, Pollak P, Louveau A, et al. Combined (thalamotomy and stimulation) stereotactic surgery of the VIM thalamic nucleus for bilateral Parkinson's disease. Appl Neurophysiol 1987; 50:344–346.
98. Benabid AL, Pollak P, Gervason C, et al. Long-term suppression of tremor by chronic stimulation of the ventral intermediate thalamic nucleus. Lancet 1991; 337:403–406.
99. Kumar K, Kelly M, Toth C. Deep brain stimulation of the ventral intermediate nucleus of the thalamus for control of tremors in Parkinson's disease and essential tremor. Stereotact Funct Neurosurg 1999; 72:47–61.
100. Ondo W, Jankovic J, Schwartz K, et al. Unilateral thalamic deep brain stimulation for refractory essential tremor and Parkinson's disease tremor. Neurology 1998; 51:1063–1069.

101. Laitinen LV, Bergenheim AT, Hariz MI. Leksell's posteroventral pallidotomy in the treatment of Parkinson's disease. J Neurosurg 1992; 76:53–61.
102. Siegfried J, Lippitz B. Bilateral chronic electrostimulation of ventroposterolateral pallidum: a new therapeutic approach for alleviating all parkinsonian symptoms. Neurosurgery 1994; 35:1126–1129, discussion 1129–1130.
103. Ghika J, Villemure JG, Fankhauser H, et al. Efficiency and safety of bilateral contemporaneous pallidal stimulation (deep brain stimulation) in levodopa-responsive patients with Parkinson's disease with severe motor fluctuations: a 2-year follow-up review. J Neurosurg 1998; 89:713–718.
104. Gross C, Rougier A, Guehl D, et al. High-frequency stimulation of the globus pallidus internalis in Parkinson's disease: a study of seven cases. J Neurosurg 1997; 87:491–498.
105. Kumar R, Lang AE, Rodriguez-Oroz MC, et al. Deep brain stimulation of the globus pallidus pars interna in advanced Parkinson's disease. Neurology 2000; 55:S34–S39.
106. Loher TJ, Burgunder JM, Pohle T, et al. Long-term pallidal deep brain stimulation in patients with advanced Parkinson disease: 1-year follow-up study. J Neurosurg 2002; 96:844–853.
107. Toth C, Tomka I. Responses of the human thalamus and pallidum to high frequency stimulations. Confin Neurol 1968; 30:17–40.
108. Langston W. The Case of the Frozen Addicts. Pantheon, 1995.
109. Albin RL, Young AB, Penney JB. The functional anatomy of basal ganglia disorders. Trends Neurosci 1989; 12:366–375.
110. Aziz TZ, Peggs D, Sambrook MA, et al. Lesion of the subthalamic nucleus for the alleviation of 1-methyl-4-phenyl-1,2,3,6-tetrahydropyridine (MPTP)-induced parkinsonism in the primate. Mov Disord 1991; 6:288–292.
111. Bergman H, Wichmann T, DeLong MR. Reversal of experimental parkinsonism by lesions of the subthalamic nucleus. Science 1990; 249:1436–1438.
112. Benabid AL, Pollak P, Gross C, et al. Acute and long-term effects of subthalamic nucleus stimulation in Parkinson's disease. Stereotact Funct Neurosurg 1994; 62:76–84.
113. Pollak P, Benabid AL, Gross C, et al. Effects of the stimulation of the subthalamic nucleus in Parkinson disease. Rev Neurol (Paris) 1993; 149:175–176.
114. Slavin KV, Thulborn KR, Wess C, et al. Direct visualization of the human subthalamic nucleus with 3T MR imaging. AJNR Am J Neuroradiol 2006; 27:80–84.
115. Mazzone P, Lozano A, Stanzione P, et al. Implantation of human pedunculopontine nucleus: a safe and clinically relevant target in Parkinson's disease. Neuroreport 2005; 16:1877–1881.
116. Aouizerate B, Cuny E, Martin-Guehl C, et al. Deep brain stimulation of the ventral caudate nucleus in the treatment of obsessive-compulsive disorder and major depression. Case report. J Neurosurg 2004; 101:682–686.
117. Aouizerate B, Martin-Guehl C, Cuny E, et al. Deep brain stimulation of the ventral striatum in the treatment of obsessive-compulsive disorder and major depression. Med Sci (Paris) 2005; 21:811–813.
118. Aouizerate B, Martin-Guehl C, Cuny E, et al. Deep brain stimulation for OCD and major depression. Am J Psychiatry 2005; 162:2192.
119. Sakas DE, Panourias IG. Rostral cingulate gyrus: a putative target for deep brain stimulation in treatment-refractory depression. Med Hypotheses 2006; 66:491–494.

120. Schlaepfer TE, Lieb K. Deep brain stimulation for treatment of refractory depression. Lancet 2005; 366:1420–1422.

121. Tagliati M, Shils J, Sun C, et al. Deep brain stimulation for dystonia. Expert Rev Med Devices 2004; 1:33–41.

122. Toda H, Hamani C, Lozano A. Deep brain stimulation in the treatment of dyskinesia and dystonia. Neurosurg Focus 2004; 17:E2.

123. Visser-Vandewalle V, Ackermans L, van der Linden C, et al. Deep brain stimulation in Gilles de la Tourette's syndrome. Neurosurgery 2006; 58:E590.

2

Deep Brain Stimulation: Anatomical, Physiological, and Computational Mechanisms

Jason T. Moyer

Department of Bioengineering, University of Pennsylvania, Philadelphia, Pennsylvania, U.S.A.

Shabbar F. Danish

Department of Neurosurgery, Hospital of the University of Pennsylvania, and Department of Bioengineering, University of Pennsylvania, Philadelphia, Pennsylvania, U.S.A.

Leif H. Finkel

Department of Bioengineering, University of Pennsylvania, Philadelphia, Pennsylvania, U.S.A.

INTRODUCTION—THE ALBIN AND DELONG MODEL

Modern understanding of the basal ganglia (BG) dates to the Albin and DeLong model, which proposed a functional relationship between the nuclei of the BG [striatum, pallidum, substantia nigra, and subthalamic nucleus (STN)] (1,2). In this model, the BG controls the initiation and execution of motor programs through the interplay of the direct and indirect projection pathways, both of which originate in the striatum (Fig. 1A). According to the model, activation of the direct pathway results in inhibition of pallidal output and consequent disinhibition of thalamocortical projection neurons. Activation of the indirect pathway results in excitation of the internal segment of the globus pallidus

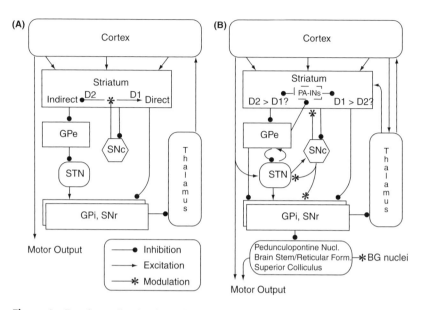

Figure 1   Basal ganglia circuitry. (**A**) The Albin and DeLong model describes the basal ganglia in terms of the direct and indirect pathways. Striatal neurons in the direct pathway express facilitatory D1 receptors and act to increase thalamocortical activity. Striatal neurons in the indirect pathway express inhibitory D2 receptors and act to reduce thalamo-cortical activity. Loss of dopamine, as in Parkinson's disease, leads to decreased direct pathway activity (via reduced D1 facilitation) and increased indirect pathway activity (via reduced D2 inhibition), resulting in impaired movement initiation and execution. (**B**) The existence of the direct and indirect pathways postulated by the Albin and DeLong model is somewhat controversial (122). Nearly all striatal cells coexpress D1 and D2 receptors, although it has been suggested that striatal neurons may predominantly express one type of receptor. Additionally several feedback connections between BG structures have been identified, including the reciprocal connections between STN and GPe, which appear to support low-frequency network oscillations (4,123–125). *Abbreviations*: BG, basal ganglia; GPe, external globus pallidus; GPi, internal globus pallidus; PA-INs, parvalbumin-containing GABAergic striatal interneurons; SNc, substantia nigra pars compacta; SNr, substantia nigra pars reticulata; STN, subthalamic nucleus.

(GPi) and subsequent inhibition of thalamic neurons. The interplay between these two pathways was suggested to selectively enable appropriate actions (via the direct pathway) and suppress inappropriate actions (via the indirect pathway).

Dopamine (DA) was proposed to modulate this interplay. D2 receptors (D2R) were thought to be inhibitory and solely expressed by neurons in the indirect pathway; thus, D2R activation would suppress the indirect pathway. Likewise, D1 receptors (D1R) were believed to be facilitatory and expressed only in the direct pathway: as such, D1R activation would enhance activity in the direct pathway. Loss of DA innervation, as in Parkinson's disease (PD), would result in decreased DA receptor stimulation in both pathways. Thus, activity in the direct pathway would be suppressed and activity in the indirect pathway would be enhanced in PD. Albin and DeLong suggest that this bias of the BG output in favor of the inhibitory indirect pathway leads to deficits in movement initiation and execution. Conversely, over-stimulation of DA receptors (such as following levodopa overdose or D2R blockade) would result in hyperkinesias.

The Albin and DeLong model was a fundamental advance in several respects—it provided a solid foundation for understanding the function of the BG, it accounted for the effects of DA on motor output and, perhaps most importantly, suggested targets (STN and pallidum) for treatment of PD. However, more recent findings at the molecular, cellular, and circuit levels have tested the explanatory limits of the original Albin and DeLong model—especially, findings regarding the effects of pallidotomy and deep brain stimulation (DBS) of BG structures in PD. Although many aspects of the Albin and DeLong model still drive current thinking, it has become clear that interactions within the BG and between the BG and other areas (cortex, thalamus, and brain stem) are complex (Fig. 1B). This complexity is particularly manifest when attempting to understand the mechanisms of DBS for PD—for example, the Albin and DeLong model predicts that PD symptoms would actually worsen with DBS, given the recent finding that DBS of the STN increases STN output.

This chapter will review the ways in which our understanding of the anatomy and functionality of the BG has expanded since the Albin and DeLong model was published. We will do so with an eye toward understanding the mechanisms of DBS of the STN for PD. First, we will describe the anatomy of the STN—its internal organization, its relation to the rest of the BG, and the anatomy of surrounding structures, which may be influenced by DBS. We will also discuss the physiology of the STN and how observations of bursting and oscillatory activity have shown it to be more complicated than originally imagined. Next, we will review several more recent BG models and how these models contribute to our understanding of the BG and the STN. Within this revised context, we will conclude by describing the most current hypotheses of the mechanisms of DBS of the STN.

ANATOMY OF THE SUBTHALAMIC NUCLEUS

The success of STN DBS has contributed to the greatly expanded interest in the STN. With this interest have come findings that the STN communicates with several structures, unlike the Albin and DeLong model. We will discuss the intrinsic anatomy of the STN as presently understood, and then detail the afferent and efferent structures with which the STN is connected.

Intrinsic Anatomy of the Subthalamic Nucleus

The STN is located at the junction of the midbrain and diencephalon as a dense kernel-sized collection of cell bodies. It is surrounded by several nuclei as well as dense bundles of myelinated fibers. Anteriorly and laterally, it is encased by fibers of the internal capsule that separate the STN from the GPi. Superiorly, the fibers of the zona incerta delineate the STN from the thalamus. The lenticular fasciculus, carrying fibers from GPi, lies on top of STN. At its medial border, the nucleus of the Fields of Forel, the Field H of Forel, as well as nigrostriatal fibers run adjacent to STN as STN merges into the lateral hypothalamic area at its rostromedial aspect. Posteromedially, it borders the red nucleus, and its ventral limits are the cerebral peduncle and the substantia nigra pars reticulata (SNr). The ansa lenticularis, which travels from GPi to the ipsilateral ventral anterior/ventral lateral thalamus (VA/VL) (thalamus) also passes STN ventrally. Other nearby fiber tracts include the spinothalamic tract, trigeminothalamic tract, and the medial lemniscus, which passes posteriorly to STN (Fig. 2) (3–5).

The STN was long considered to be a homogeneous structure, consisting solely of projection neurons that were initially thought to be GABAergic but

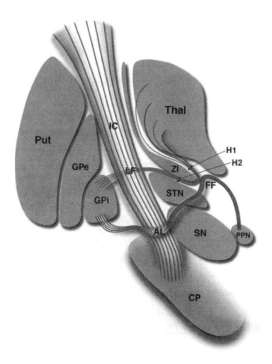

Figure 2 Schematic representation of the major anatomical structures and fiber tracts associated with the subthalamic nucleus. *Abbreviations*: CP, cerebral peduncle; FF, fields of Forel; GPe, globus pallidus externus; GPi, globus pallidus internus; H1, H1 field of Forel (thalamic fasciculus); IC, internal capsule; LF, lenticular fasciculus (H2); PPN, pedunculopontine nucleus; Put, putamen; SN, substantia nigra; STN, subthalamic nucleus; Thal, thalamus; ZI, zona incerta. *Source*: From Ref. 3.

are now known to be glutamatergic (6). Several studies have suggested the presence of GABAergic interneurons in the STN (4,7). The dendritic arbors of STN projection neurons are usually oval with their long axis parallel to the long axis of the nucleus (3,4). The axonal branching patterns of STN neurons vary depending on projection site (8), which may affect their response to DBS. STN neurons interact with each other via intra-STN collateral projections (4).

STN neurons appear to be functionally segregated, with sensorimotor, associative, and limbic areas distinguished by their afferent and efferent connections. The limbic region occupies the medial tip of the STN. The associative section comprises the mid-third of the remaining STN and is located ventral to the sensorimotor region (4,9). All neurons with movement-related activity are located in the sensorimotor region. These neurons appear to be somatotopically arranged, with leg-related neurons located more dorsally, anteriorly, and medially, and arm-related neurons more ventrally and laterally (5,10,11).

Efferent Projections

In-depth investigations of BG circuitry have revealed that the STN projects to several areas in addition to the GPi and the SNr. As mentioned, the STN is segregated into limbic, associative, and sensorimotor areas, which are distinguished by their efferent targets. STN neurons in the limbic region project primarily to the ventral pallidum (VP). STN neurons in the associative and sensorimotor regions project to the external globus pallidus (GPe), GPi/SNr, and substantia nigra pars compacta (SNc). Additional projections to the dorsal striatum (caudate and putamen) have also been described (3,4,9). While the GPi/SNr and GPe still represent the primary projection sites, it is likely that all of these projections will need to be taken into account in order to understand DBS.

Individual subthalamic axons arborize throughout large portions of the pallidum, with a multitude of thin axon collaterals forming a relatively dense meshwork around the dendrites of pallidal neurons (12). As such, single STN neurons can strongly influence a large subpopulation of pallidal neurons in a uniform manner (13). This ability could enable the STN to effectively regulate the gain of the pallidum, as discussed subsequently. Little is known regarding the contribution of the subthalamo-nigral projection to the overall function of the BG. Studies in the rat have suggested that STN neurons might regulate the response of GPi/SNr neurons to subsequent striatal inputs (14). STN–SNc projections may regulate DA release in the striatum (15). Subthalamo-striatal projections are scarce in comparison to those described before. In nonhuman primates, STN-to-caudate projections primarily derive from associative and limbic regions of the STN, whereas efferents to the putamen originate in the sensorimotor region (3,4,13).

Afferent Projections

The STN receives massive projections from the cortex, GPe, and thalamus. Additional, though less numerous, inputs come from the centromedian-parafascicular complex of the thalamus, the substantia nigra, the dorsal raphe nucleus, and the pedunculopontine tegmental nucleus, although the importance of these inputs is largely unknown. We limit our discussion to the cortical and pallidal input pathways.

The existence of a direct cortico-subthalamic projection has been well-documented in animals, whereas the full extent of this projection is still being detailed in humans (12,16). In rodents, the primary motor cortex, cingulate cortex, primary somatosensory cortex, and some areas of the prefrontal cortex are the major cortical sources of inputs to the STN (17). In nonhuman primates, the major projection arises from the primary motor cortex, which terminates in the dorsolateral region of STN. The premotor cortical projections, including the frontal eye field and the supplementary frontal eye field, terminate principally in the ventromedial region (18). Similar anatomical relationships are being explored in humans, as high-frequency stimulation of the STN has been shown to affect the primary sensorimotor cortex, the lateral premotor cortex, midline premotor areas, and the cingulate cortex (19). The cortico-subthalamic afferents seem to respect the subdivisions of the STN into sensorimotor and associative regions.

Understanding of the pallido-subthalamic pathway has largely come about via animal studies. In rodents and in primates, neurons from the lateral portion of GPe target specifically to the lateral two-thirds of the STN, whereas those in the medial part of GPe terminate in the ventromedial STN. In primates, the input from GPe extends over the entire rostrolateral two-thirds of STN (4,20). The GPe projects principally to the region of STN which contains neurons that project back to GPe, and not to the region with GPi-projecting neurons. The projection from GPe is GABAergic and comprises the major inhibitory projection to the STN (3,21).

The GPe-STN projection is an essential component of the indirect pathway of the Albin and DeLong model, allowing striatal inhibition of GPe to be translated into STN excitation of GPi, thus counterbalancing the direct striatal inhibition of GPi. This mechanism would require GPe projections to specifically target STN neurons that project to GPi; however, there is conflicting anatomical evidence as to whether this is the case (4,22). Accordingly, the function of the indirect pathway, if it exists, may be more complicated than suggested by the Albin and DeLong model. For instance, the GPe might interact with other structures to "focus" STN activity—that is, to select cell ensembles for activation (23).

PHYSIOLOGY OF THE SUBTHALAMIC NUCLEUS AND BASAL GANGLIA

The Albin and DeLong model characterizes the interactions between BG structures as unidirectional, and basically either excitatory or inhibitory based on firing rate. Recordings have shown that activity within and between BG structures has additional degrees of complexity. This section will describe these activity patterns, focusing on observations of bursting, synchronization, and oscillations in the STN and BG.

Various types of neuronal discharges have been distinguished in the STN, including irregular, tonic, and bursting activity. It is estimated that 55% to 65% of the STN neurons fire irregularly, whereas 15% to 25% fire tonically and 15% to 50% present bursting activity in primates (24). Neurons responding to movement are either irregular or tonic and are found in the dorsolateral STN. Bursting neurons do not respond to movement and are located in the ventral STN (5). In patients with PD, STN neurons exhibit large amplitude spikes with an irregular firing pattern (25). These have a mean firing rate of 37 ± 17 Hz. The effect of dopaminergic medication on the firing rate of STN neurons has been variable, but generally leads to an increase in the percentage of spikes occurring in bursts or irregular discharge patterns (26,27). Accordingly, DA does not lead to a simple reduction in STN activity, as anticipated in the Albin and DeLong model. STN cells with periodic behavior have been identified and further characterized in the same patient population, being classified as either tremor cells (2–6 Hz), cells with high (>10 Hz) frequency periodic activity, or as cells with both tremor and high-frequency components (10). Synchronization of the high-frequency periodic activity has been closely linked to limb tremor in parkinsonian patients (10,28), and termination of high-frequency periodic behavior is observed with dopaminergic treatment (27).

Synchronous activity has been shown to exist not only within STN, but also between STN and other BG structures. One study demonstrated that high-frequency stimulation of the motor cortex resulted in a normalization of mean firing rate in the STN and GPi, and reduced synchronized periodic neuronal activities between these two structures (29). This is supported in humans by the observation that transcranial magnetic stimulation of motor areas results in the excitation of subthalamic neurons and that responsive neurons were somatotopically organized (30). More recently, there has been increased evidence for anatomical segregation of processing streams between the cortex and STN, due to the finding of multiple functional subloops distinguished by their frequency, cortical topography, and temporal relationships (31).

Oscillations in the Basal Ganglia

Four major categories of oscillations in the local field potential (LFP) have been observed in the BG: alpha (7–13 Hz), beta (11–30 Hz), high gamma (~70 Hz), and very high-frequency oscillations (~300 Hz). Alpha frequencies develop in the GPi and STN of monkeys treated with MPTP and are highly prevalent in human PD patients (32,33). These oscillations correlate well with the appearance, the cycle-to-cycle activity, and the termination of physical tremor, so it is believed that activity in this band underlies parkinsonian tremor. In vitro work has suggested that these low-frequency oscillations are the result of changes in STN-GPe connectivity following DA loss (34). In agreement with this hypothesis, a computational model of a simple GPe and STN network is shifted between uncorrelated spiking and correlated periodic bursting modes when the synaptic strengths were adjusted to model DA loss (35).

Likewise, LFP oscillations and increased cell synchronization in the 11 to 30 Hz beta band have been observed in STN and GPi of PD patients and MPTP-treated monkeys. These oscillations desynchronize with movement initiation and dopaminergic medication (27,33,36) and are weaker in both healthy monkeys (37) and dystonic patients without PD symptoms (38). In striatum, oscillations in this range are present in healthy monkeys at rest, but desynchronize with movement (39). These authors suggest that beta oscillations represent baseline activity of the striatum and that this activity becomes desynchronized as multiple patches of striatum are activated in order to initiate movements. By extension, it may be that 11 to 30 Hz oscillations throughout the BG represent a resting state of activity. The loss of DA in PD might inhibit the ability of cell ensembles to separate from this activity and shift into a "prokinetic" state for movement initiation and control.

Brown's group suggests that the prokinetic state is characterized by oscillations of approximately 70 Hz. Oscillations at this frequency increase with movement initiation and levodopa treatment (36). This activity is coherent with activity in motor cortical areas (33) and is only rarely seen in PD patients off of medication. These studies suggest that approximately 70 Hz activity is important for movement and is contingent upon a reduction in beta-band activity (38). The same could also be true for 300 Hz rhythms, which have been observed during self-paced movements in human PD patients on levodopa treatment but not off of levodopa (40).

REVISED UNDERSTANDING OF THE BASAL GANGLIA

Beginning with the Albin and DeLong description, a number of models have attempted to characterize the function of the BG. The idea that the BG carries out "action selection" remains a central theme and is consistent with the akinesia and bradykinesia in PD. In this section, we give an overview of other functions that have been ascribed to BG [additional models are presented in Refs. (41) and (42)].

Resource Allocation

One proposed role of the BG is regulating the allocation of motor resources between competing systems (e.g., sensory, affective, and cognitive systems) (43). This is essentially action selection, but it helps to explain at least two characteristics of BG function: the BGs use of disinhibition versus direct excitation, and the closed loop architecture of the BG. If all systems had direct excitatory access to the motor output, overload situations (in which all systems are competing for the motor output) would result in the selection of all actions with potentially disastrous results. The Redgrave group suggests that tonic inhibition of all but one action avoids this problem. In rest situations, the maintenance of tonic inhibition might be accomplished by the regular spiking of STN neurons, which are tonically active in the absence of synaptic input (44). The Redgrave group also suggests that the looped architecture of the BG provides it with negative feedback to the source system, preventing the BG from becoming overloaded. Robot models which select between competing desires (hide out of fear vs. forage out of hunger) based on this concept have validated several aspects of this theory (45).

Sequential Learning

Several models have explored the role of the BG in sequential learning. The learning process consists of the conversion of a series of sequential movements to a motor program that can be executed automatically. One of these models, the Beiser and Houk model (46), described the BG as a collection of modules working in parallel to encode a motor program in response to a series of environmental cues. In this model, the BG are described as a collection of parallel modules linking cortex, striatum, GPi, and thalamus, based on anatomical descriptions of "parallel loops" in the BG (47,48). Each module represented an independent loop through these structures. Striatal medium spiny projection neurons (MSNs) responded to specific spatial patterns of cortical input and established functional ensembles via inhibitory collaterals with other MSNs. The looped architecture of the model permitted activity to be sustained and modified while new environmental cues were presented, enabling several different action sequences to be stored as unique patterns of BG activity.

Though this model used a very simplified representation of the BG, it was able to capture two critical elements of BG function, which have subsequently received support. The first of these was to cast striatal MSNs as pattern detectors (49). An MSN can fire in response to activity in a small subset of its 10,000 to 15,000 inputs coming from a diverse set of input structures and integrate inputs over a relatively long (50 msec) time scale (50,51)—making MSNs ideal for such a role (46). The second critical aspect was ensemble activity in the striatum—several experiments have indicated that the striatum is composed of ensembles of neurons that respond selectively and independently (52–55).

The model of Berns and Sejnowski (56) focused more on the role of the indirect pathway in supporting sequential learning. Interestingly, this model relied on the feedback loop between GPe and STN to store patterns, indicating a potential role for the oscillatory activity frequently observed in these structures during recordings. Activity in the STN lagged activity in the GP, allowing the network to string together individual "actions" into a sequence. Dopamine reinforcement guided this process in a role similar to that of the temporal difference (TD) models described below. After learning, this sequence could be recalled solely by cuing the first action in the sequence. A strongpoint of this model was its ability to reproduce sequential learning deficits similar to those in PD, ability to correct this deficit with pallidal lesion (STN lesion was not modeled), and inclusion of oscillatory activity in the BG.

Dimensionality Reduction

Based on the massive convergence in the cortico-striato-pallidal pathway, Bar-Gad et al. (56a) suggest that the BG perform a dimensionality reduction operation in order to optimize action selection—it is estimated that there are four orders of magnitude fewer neurons in the output nucleus (GPi) than in the input (cortex) (57). In this model, the BG still select actions and do so in a way reminiscent of Redgrave's framework of resource allocation (the BG represent a central relay station through which all actions are selected). However, the emphasis is on the compression and prioritization of incoming information via principal component analysis, so that potential actions can be more effectively sampled and selected. Dopamine optimizes the dimensionality reduction and data storage process by sending a reinforcement signal to the BG. Accordingly, loss of DA, as in PD, results in a network with limited storage capacity and suboptimal action selection.

Dynamically Modulated Interactions Among Ensembles

Consideration of the ventral regions of the BG (nucleus accumbens, ventral STN, and ventral pallidum) suggests a potential role for the oscillatory activity observed in the BG. Recent studies have shown that during periods of awake behavior, cells in PFC and striatum fire phase-locked to the hippocampal theta rhythm. Along the longitudinal axis of the hippocampus, cells are organized into functional ensembles, with each ensemble selectively firing during specific behavioral components of a task. For example, as a rat navigates a maze, different ensembles respond to specific locations, turns, and proximity to reward (58). Similar ensembles have been identified in ventral striatum (54). Several studies have suggested that during a perceptual or behavioral task, striatal cells or ensembles temporarily lock to the ongoing theta rhythm, and these phase-locked ensembles then contribute to the ongoing computation—whereas those ensembles whose firing is not phase-locked to theta do not contribute (59,60). Thus, a common theta rhythm, established by the hippocampus, but entraining cells in cortex and striatum, seems to facilitate the coordination of cell groups across structures. Similar mechanisms, potentially in other frequency bands (such as high gamma), may direct the integration of information in the dorsal striatum. Action selection could then be achieved via the phase-locking of cell ensembles to dynamic modulation in the afferent input.

What Does Dopamine Do? Modulation and Reinforcement Properties

Dopamine seems to play two roles in BG function—reinforcement and modulation. As a first approximation, it is convenient to partition these roles between the two activity modes that DA neurons exhibit—with the regular spiking mode controlling modulation and the phasic bursting mode controlling reinforcement. Since regular spiking has been shown to control tonic DA levels, it can be further reasoned that spiking controls modulation via tonic DA, whereas bursting controls reinforcement via phasic DA [61]. Most models focus on one or the other of these roles—for instance, the Berns and Sejnowski and dimensionality reduction models discussed previously use dopamine solely as a training signal, which controls synaptic plasticity. Alternatively, the Albin and DeLong model posits DA as a modulatory signal, controlling the relative strengths of the direct and indirect pathways. There is strong experimental evidence that DA plays both roles, and recent findings indicate how these two separate roles may be integrated into a single cohesive model of DA function.

The concept of DA as a reinforcement signal is partially based on analogies between DA neuron firing during instrumental learning and the computed prediction error in TD reinforcement learning algorithms (62,63). In these algorithms, an "actor" (the BG) and a "critic" (DA neurons) work together in order to learn actions which will maximize reward—not only immediate reward but also long-term reward (64). For a given action, the critic weighs immediate consequences with the probability of future reward and sends a reinforcement signal to the actor, which makes decisions based on maximizing this reinforcement signal. DA neurons share several characteristics with the critic in TD algorithms— they encode reward prediction errors, respond progressively earlier as learning proceeds, stop signaling when learning is complete, and pause when reward is withheld after learning has been completed (64–67). Importantly, DA has been shown to affect synaptic plasticity (both potentiation and depression) in the striatum (68–73).

However, the physical deficits in PD might seem to be more closely related to problems with modulation rather than learning, especially given that levodopa affects primarily the tonic DA levels postulated to control modulation (74). Dopamine modulates several properties of MSNs—both intrinsic properties (sodium, calcium, and potassium channels) and synaptic properties—though the reported effects are complex and often inconsistent (75). In general, D1R activation enhances MSN activity, whereas D2R activation decreases MSN activity, as in the Albin and DeLong model. However, these effects may be voltage-dependent, calcium-dependent, or both (76,77). Further complicating matters is the finding that most MSNs coexpress both D1Rs and D2Rs (78–80). Synaptically, however, a clearer picture is emerging. In vivo experiments in the ventral striatum have shown that D1Rs and D2Rs differentially control hippocampal and cortical inputs to the nucleus accumbens (81). In this study, D1R activation facilitates hippocampal inputs without affecting cortical inputs. Similarly, D2 affects only cortical inputs, with increased D2R activation suppressing cortical inputs, and decreased D2R activation facilitating cortical inputs.

Although the functional correlates of these findings need to be researched in dorsal striatum, they do suggest that DA's effects are primarily synaptic rather than intrinsic. Ongoing modeling studies in our lab support this conclusion, and suggest that the intrinsic effects of DA on MSNs are not primarily intended to change the response properties of MSNs. Instead, DA's intrinsic effects may control calcium influx into spines in order to control synaptic plasticity (82), in agreement with previous suggestions (83,84). This places the focus of DA on regulating synaptic plasticity, with the modulatory effects of DA on MSN intrinsic properties being the means to this end. Clearly, further research is needed to fully explore this concept.

Current Understanding of the Basal Ganglia and Subthalamic Nucleus

In summary, the BG are important for action selection as well as other functions—including but not limited to resource allocation, sequential learning, and dimensionality reduction. Given the complexity of the BG, most models focus on one aspect of BG function, out of necessity. Likewise, the role of the STN is complicated, and proposals regarding STN function usually depend on which BG function is being discussed. The STN may regulate the gain of the BG, scaling the output as input levels increase or decrease (45), or it may regulate the gain of the indirect pathway, as in the Albin and DeLong model (1,2). STN neurons might regulate the response of GP and SN neurons to subsequent striatal inputs (14). The ability of STN cells to spike regularly without synaptic input may underlie movement inhibition during resting conditions (44). STN–SNc projections may regulate DA release in the striatum (15). The STN may select ensembles in the GPi through interactions with striatal inputs (23). With the GPe, it may form a pacemaker that controls the timing of BG activity (34). Or, the STN may support sequential learning by associating sequential steps in cooperation with the GPe (56).

HOW DOES DEEP BRAIN STIMULATION WORK?

Inhibition or Excitation?

Based on the observation that STN DBS has similar clinical effects as STN lesions, it was initially assumed that DBS must silence STN activity (85). Within the context of the Albin and DeLong model, reduced STN activity would reduce activation of GPi, which would disinhibit the thalamic projection neurons. Thus, suppressing STN should increase movement. Several mechanisms were proposed for how stimulation might inhibit the STN [reviewed in Ref. (86)]. Among these were the depolarization blockade hypothesis, which suggested that repetitive stimulation of STN cells sufficiently depolarized the cell membrane to inactivate sodium channels and prevent cell firing (87). Another influential idea was the synaptic inhibition hypothesis, which proposed that stimulation preferentially activates afferents to STN rather than the neurons themselves (88). Since the majority of these afferents are inhibitory, the resulting effect would be a suppression of activity (89).

Several studies provided results supporting the hypothesis that DBS silenced STN neurons. Extracellular stimulation of rat STN slices produced a long-lasting (seconds to minutes) suppression of single-cell activity following cessation of the stimulation (87). Later experiments showed a similar, though shorter duration suppression of firing following high-frequency microstimulation in human STN (90). These results agreed with similar experiments in human thalamus (86) and GPi (88). Observations of activity during STN stimulation (using artifact removal) did not reveal any spiking (90,91). In vitro studies of STN neurons revealed that they express sodium currents that inactivate slowly during prolonged stimulation, supporting the depolarization blockade hypothesis (92). Decreased mRNA expression of cytochrome oxidase (a catalyst for aerobic respiration) indicated that STN cell activity decreased during prolonged (45 minutes) stimulation (91).

Downstream recordings, however, painted a more complicated picture. Since the STN is excitatory, suppression of STN neurons should reduce activity in efferent structures such as the GPi and SNr. Although some studies found that downstream activity was reduced (91,93), several others found it to be increased (94–96). Similar experiments in GPi also suggested that DBS activates the target structure (97). Microdialysis experiments in rats indicated that effective STN stimulation increased glutamate concentration in downstream structures, indicating that DBS increases activity in the STN (98). Positron emission tomography (PET) and functional magnetic resonance imaging (fMRI) studies in humans during STN stimulation found increased blood flow in downstream structures, again suggesting that STN activity is increased by DBS (99–101).

Accordingly, recordings within the STN suggested that DBS worked by inhibiting STN neurons, whereas downstream recordings indicated that the STN was actually activated by DBS. A modeling study by McIntyre et al. (2004) showed how these apparently mutually exclusive findings might be reconciled. By creating a detailed computational model of a thalamocortical relay cell and exposing it to realistic stimulation patterns, this group was able to show that a cell's axon and soma can become decoupled during DBS. In other words, DBS can drive the axon to fire at high frequencies independently of somatic activities—so somatic recordings might suggest that the cell is being inhibited when in fact the output is increased (Fig. 3). Stimulation of inhibitory synapses by DBS, as suggested by the synaptic inhibition hypothesis, enhanced this effect by inhibiting the soma but not the axon. Depolarization blockade did not occur below 200 Hz in the model—as with in vitro STN cells (102). Further studies have indicated that this effect (activation of the axon regardless of somatic activity) is achieved in STN and GP cells as well (103).

It must be emphasized that axonal activation is dependent on the cell's location relative to the electrode—cell axons within 2 mm of the electrode are activated, whereas axons further away are suppressed (Fig. 3) (104). Accordingly the net effect of DBS on the targeted structure is a complex pattern of activation and inhibition. In the human STN, which is not much larger than the stimulating electrode, it seems likely that the primary effect is activation of axonal projections

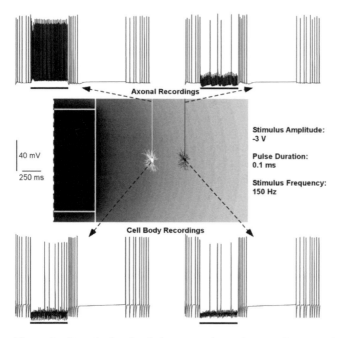

Figure 3 Deep brain stimulation can activate the axonal output of a model thalamocortical cell independently of somatic activity. The axon of the white cell is driven at or near the stimulation frequency (*top left*, stimulation duration indicated by the black bar underneath the spike recordings), even though somatic recordings suggest that the cell is being inhibited (*bottom left*). This effect depends on distance from the stimulating electrode (*the large black rectangle at left*)—the axon of the black cell is not decoupled from the soma and this cell is actually inhibited by the stimulation (*top and bottom right*). The net result is a complex pattern of activation and inhibition, although given the small size of the subthalamic nucleus (STN) compared to a stimulating electrode, it seems likely that the primary effect is activation of STN output. *Source*: From Ref. 103.

at or near the stimulation frequency. It is not clear what effect the inhibition of cells further removed from the electrode plays in the mechanisms of DBS.

"Information Lesion" and Other Current Theories

If DBS activates STN output, the clinical benefits of DBS cannot be explained within the context of the Albin and DeLong model, and more complicated descriptions of BG activity such as those discussed earlier must be invoked. The most current idea is that DBS induces an "information lesion" of the STN. This theory relies on the concept that the bursts and low-frequency (alpha and beta) oscillations characteristic of the parkinsonian STN contribute to the physical symptoms of tremor and akinesia. DBS is thought to force STN axons to spike at highly regular intervals, rather than in irregular bursts. Using an analogy with information theory (105), it seems reasonable to conclude that regular spiking carries less information than bursting and is, therefore, easier to ignore by downstream structures.

Several computational models have asked what effect replacing bursting with regular spiking has on BG function, and whether regular spiking carries less information than bursting. A simple network model suggested that irregular activity in one neuron deleteriously affected information transfer between two other neurons, whereas regular, high-frequency driving of the neuron restored information transfer (106). Similarly, a reduced mathematical model of the STN, GPe, GPi, and thalamus implied that regular spiking in the GPi (as opposed to periodic bursting) improved the relay ability of thalamic cells (107). A single cell model was able to link the frequency dependence of DBS to increasingly regular spiking—effective frequencies led to regular spiking, ineffective frequencies did not—supporting the information lesion hypothesis (108).

Physiologically, few studies have been performed to investigate the meaning of an information lesion. A potential effect of repetitive high-frequency stimulation with no information content might be downstream synaptic depression resulting in an effective lesion of the STN or its efferent structures (103), although this would be inconsistent with the findings of downstream activation mentioned before (94,98). To this end, one study researched the induction of synaptic plasticity following high-frequency (100 Hz) stimulation of the STN; the results showed that relatively few (13/46) neurons exhibited any long-term synaptic plasticity (109). However, studying downstream synaptic plasticity might be an interesting way to quantify the information content of regular spiking versus pathological bursting, as it has been shown that natural stimulation patterns (presumably containing physiologically relevant information) induce significant, highly variable changes in synaptic strength (110).

Recent research has suggested that the regular firing imposed by DBS may be beneficial to BG function beyond simply canceling out pathological PD activity. Optimal stimulation frequencies (120–180 Hz) are first harmonics of the high gamma rhythms (~70 Hz) suggested to be essential for proper BG function (111). Effective stimulation frequencies may induce synchronization (either in STN axons or in downstream structures) at 70 Hz (112). This idea appears to agree with experimental observations in monkeys (94) and rats (96), in which downstream cells responded to stimulation with regular firing but at lower frequencies. This also suggests a common mechanism by which levodopa and DBS might alleviate parkinsonian symptoms—the attenuation of pathological oscillations (15–30 Hz) in favor of high gamma (60–80 Hz) oscillations (113). Similarly, DBS might mimic ~300 Hz oscillatory activity in downstream neurons at roughly twice the stimulation frequency.

An alternative, though related, hypothesis is that the desynchronization of pathological oscillations (rather than the replacement with higher frequency oscillations) is the primary mechanism of DBS. The main support from this argument derives from computer modeling experiments using coupled oscillators (114) and a reductionist network model of the STN (115). A stimulation protocol based on this technique, in which multiple electrodes are used to deliver out-of-phase stimulation signals (consisting of the filtered local field potential) throughout the target structure, has shown some promise in preliminary clinical trials (115). A study finding decreased correlations between multiple STN cells as well as decreased oscillatory bursting in single STN cells (116), during DBS in primates adds some support to this hypothesis (although the results are difficult to interpret given that STN somatic recordings do not necessarily reflect STN axonal output during DBS, as discussed earlier).

It is also possible that DBS of the STN might activate the remaining (<20–50%) dopaminergic neurons in SNc (or their efferent axons, which course near the STN on the way to the rest of the BG). STN stimulation at low (20 Hz) frequencies has been shown to increase DA cell firing rates and facilitate burst firing after an initial (up to 30 minutes) pause (15). This study did not examine the effects of higher frequency, clinically effective stimulation. Activation of SNc-DA neurons or their efferent projections could explain why levodopa treatment can be reduced with STN stimulation but not GPi or thalamic stimulation. It might also explain why DBS is indicated only for patients with good response to levodopa—since levodopa is broken down in the synaptic cleft of DA neurons, a levodopa response suggests that at least some SNc neurons remain intact. The few experiments performed to examine this hypothesis have been mostly positive. DBS in rat STN has been shown to increase DA breakdown products (HVA, DOPAC) and tyrosine hydroxylase (the rate-limiting enzyme in DA synthesis), but not DA in 6-OHDA lesioned rats (117). A similar study measured a significant increase in DA but not DOPAC (118). An in vitro rat slice study found that stimulating the STN increased the firing rate of SNc neurons (119). Stimulation of the entopeduncular nucleus (the rat GPi equivalent) does not increase metabolites or DA, as would be expected given that levodopa cannot generally be decreased with GPi DBS (117). Studies using PET in humans have not been able to find increased striatal DA with STN DBS (120,121), though the authors note that the changes in concentration may be too small to detect with this method.

In summary, it seems most likely that STN DBS works through a combination of mechanisms. It is generally believed that one of the primary mechanisms of DBS is the overriding of pathological BG activity, specifically bursting and low-frequency oscillations in the STN–GP network. The replacement of these activities with higher frequency regular spiking may represent an information lesion or may enhance "prokinetic" oscillations normally present in the healthy BG. Additional mechanisms through which DBS might achieve its beneficial effects might be via desynchronization of low-frequency "antikinetic" oscillations or stimulation of dopamine-releasing cells in the SNc. It is also quite possible that DBS activates other structures or fibers not considered previously, given the complex anatomy of the STN and its nearby structures.

The success of DBS for PD has lead to consideration of its use for a number of disorders: depression, obsessive-compulsive disorder, cluster headaches, and epilepsy are a few examples. For the most part, these disorders are less well-understood than PD, and the procedures are certainly less-established and less available for research. Accordingly, if the technique of DBS is to be further honed for clinical use, the brunt of work must be borne by research into its application in PD. Progress in understanding the mechanisms of DBS in PD will continue to have broad impact on our understanding of BG function and the role of these nuclei in coordinated action.

REFERENCES

1. Albin R, Young A, Penney J. The functional anatomy of basal ganglia disorders. Trends Neurosci 1989; 12(10):366–375.
2. Delong M. Primate models of movement disorders of basal ganglia origin. Trends Neurosci 1990; 13(7):281–285.
3. Hamani C, Saint-Cyr J, Fraser J, Kaplitt M, Lozano A. The subthalamic nucleus in the context of movement disorders. Brain 2004; 127:4–20.
4. Parent A, Hazrati L. Functional anatomy of the basal ganglia II. The place of the subthalamic nucleus and external pallidum in basal ganglia circuitry. Brain Res Rev 1995; 20:128–154.
5. Rodriguez-Oroz MC, Rodriguez M, Guridi J, et al. The subthalamic nucleus in Parkinson's disease: somatotopic organization and physiological characteristics. Brain 2001; 124:1777–1790.
6. Rafols JA, Fox CA. The neurons in the primate subthalamic nucleus: a Golgi and electron microscopic study. J Comp Neurol 1976; 168:75–112.
7. Levesque JC, Parent A. GABAergic interneurons in human subthalamic nucleus. Mov Disord 2005; 20(5):574–584.
8. Sato F, Parent M, Levesque M, Parent A. Axonal branching pattern of neurons of the subthalamic nucleus in primates. J Comp Neurol 2000; 424:142–152.
9. Temel Y, Blokland A, Steinbusch HW, Visser-Vandewalle V. The functional role of the subthalamic nucleus in cognitive and limbic circuits. Prog Neurobiol 2005; 76(6):393–413.
10. Levy R, Hutchison WD, Lozano AM, Dostrovsky JO. High-frequency synchronization of neuronal activity in the subthalamic nucleus of Parkinsonian patients with limb tremor. J Neurosci 2000; 20(20):7766–7775.
11. Romanelli P, Heit G, Hill BC, Kraus A, Hastie T, Bronte-Stewart HM. Microelectrode recording revealing a somatotopic body map in the subthalamic nucleus in humans with Parkinson disease. J Neurosurg 2004; 100:611–618.
12. Carpenter MB, Carleton SC, Keller JT, Conte P. Connections of the subthalamic nucleus in the monkey. Brain Res 1981; 224:1–29.
13. Smith Y, Hazrati LN, Parent A. Efferent projections of the subthalamic nucleus in the squirrel monkey as studied by the PHA-L anterograde tracing method. J Comp Neurol 1990; 294:306–323.
14. Kita H, Kitai ST. Intracellular study of rat globus pallidus neurons: membrane properties and responses to neostriatal, subthalamic and nigral stimulation. Brain Res 1991; 564:296–305.
15. Smith ID, Grace AA. Role of the subthalamic nucleus in the regulation of nigral dopamine neuron activity. Synapse 1992; 12(4):287–303.

16. Afsharpour S. Topographical projections of the cerebral cortex to the subthalamic nucleus. J Comp Neurol 1985; 236:14–28.
17. Kitai ST, Deniau JM. Cortical inputs to the subthalamus: intracellular analysis. Brain Res 1981; 214:411–415.
18. Stanton GB, Goldberg ME, Bruce CJ. Frontal eye field efferents in the macaque monkey: II. Topography of terminal fields in midbrain and pons. J Comp Neurol 1988; 271:493–506.
19. Payoux P, Remy P, Damier P, et al. Subthalamic nucleus stimulation reduces abnormal motor cortical overactivity in Parkinson disease. Arch Neurol 2004; 61:1307–1313.
20. Carpenter MB, Batton RR, Carleton SC, Keller JT. Interconnections and organization of pallidal and subthalamic nucleus neurons in the monkey. J Comp Neurol 1981; 197:579–603.
21. Smith Y, Parent A. Neurons of the subthalamic nucleus in primates display glutamate but not GABA immunoreactivity. Brain Res 1988; 453:353–356.
22. Smith Y, Charara A, Hanson JE, Hubert WG, Kuwajima M. Chemical anatomy and synaptic connectivity of the globus pallidus and subthalamic nucleus. In: Kultas-Ilinsky K, Ilinsky I, eds. Basal Ganglia and Thalamus in Movement Disorders. New York: Kluwer Academic/Plenum Publishers, 2001:119–134.
23. Mink JW. The basal ganglia: focused selection and inhibition of competing motor programs. Prog Neurobiol 1996; 50(4):381–425.
24. Wichmann T, Bergman H, DeLong MR. The primate subthalamic nucleus. I. Functional properties in intact animals. J Neurophysiol 1994; 72(2):494–506.
25. Hutchison WD, Allan RJ, Opitz H, et al. Neurophysiological identification of the subthalamic nucleus in surgery for Parkinson's disease. Annals of Neurology 1998; 44(4):622–628.
26. Levy R, Dostrovsky JO, Lang AE, Sime E, Hutchison WD, Lozano AM. Effects of apomorphine on subthalamic nucleus and globus pallidus internus neurons in patients with Parkinson's disease. J Neurophysiol 2001; 86(1):249–260.
27. Levy R, Ashby P, Hutchison WD, Lang AE, Lozano AM, Dostrovsky JO. Dependence of subthalamic nucleus oscillations on movement and dopamine in Parkinson's disease. Brain 2002; 125:1196–1209.
28. Krack P, Benazzouz A, Pollak P, et al. Treatment of tremor in Parkinson's disease by subthalamic nucleus stimulation. Mov Disord 1998; 13:907–914.
29. Drouot X, Oshino S, Jarraya B, et al. Functional recovery in a primate model of Parkinson's disease following motor cortex stimulation. Neuron 2004; 44:769–778.
30. Strafella AP, Vanderwerf Y, Sadikot AF. Transcranial magnetic stimulation of the human motor cortex influences the neuronal activity of subthalamic nucleus. Eur J Neurosci 2004; 20:2245–2249.
31. Fogelson N, Williams D, Tijssen M, vanBruggen G, Speelman H, Brown P. Different functional loops between cerebral cortex and the subthalamic area in Parkinson's disease. Cerebral Cortex 2006; 16(1):1664–1675.
32. Hurtado JM, Gray CM, Tamas LB, Sigvardt KA. Dynamics of tremor-related oscillations in the human globus pallidus: a single case study. Proc Natl Acad Sci USA 1999; 96(4):1674–1679.
33. Williams D, Tijssen M, Van Bruggen G, et al. Dopamine-dependent changes in the functional connectivity between basal ganglia and cerebral cortex in humans. Brain 2002; 125(Pt 7):1558–1569.

34. Plenz D, Kital ST. A basal ganglia pacemaker formed by the subthalamic nucleus and external globus pallidus. Nature 1999; 400(6745):677–682.
35. Terman D, Rubin JE, Yew AC, Wilson CJ. Activity patterns in a model for the sub-thalamopallidal network of the basal ganglia. J Neurosci 2002; 22(7):2963–2976.
36. Brown P, Oliviero A, Mazzone P, Insola A, Tonali P, Di Lazzaro V. Dopamine dependency of oscillations between subthalamic nucleus and pallidum in Parkinson's disease. J Neurosci 2001; 21(3):1033–1038.
37. Nini A, Feingold A, Slovin H, Bergman H. Neurons in the globus pallidus do not show correlated activity in the normal monkey, but phase-locked oscillations appear in the MPTP model of parkinsonism. J Neurophysiol 1995; 74(4):1800–1805.
38. Silberstein P, Kuhn AA, Kupsch A, et al. Patterning of globus pallidus local field potentials differs between Parkinson's disease and dystonia. Brain 2003; 126(Pt 12): 2597–2608.
39. Courtemanche R, Fujii N, Graybiel AM. Synchronous, focally modulated beta-band oscillations characterize local field potential activity in the striatum of awake behaving monkeys. J Neurosci 2003; 23(37):11741–11752.
40. Foffani G, Priori A, Egidi M, et al. 300-Hz subthalamic oscillations in Parkinson's disease. Brain 2003; 126(Pt 10):2153–2163.
41. Houk JC, Davis JL, Beiser DG, eds. Models of Information Processing in the Basal Ganglia. Cambridge, MA: The MIT Press, 1995.
42. Gillies A, Arbuthnott G. Computational models of the basal ganglia. Mov Disord 2000; 15(5):762–770.
43. McHaffie J, Stanford T, Stein B, Coizet V, Redgrave P. Subcortical loops through the basal ganglia. Trends Neurosci 2005; 28(8):401–407.
44. Bevan MD, Wilson CJ. Mechanisms underlying spontaneous oscillation and rhythmic firing in rat subthalamic neurons. J Neurosci 1999; 19(17):7617–7628.
45. Gurney K, Prescott T, Wickens J, Redgrave P. Computational models of the basal ganglia: from robots to membranes. Trends in Neurosciences 2004; 27(8):453–459.
46. Beiser D, Houk J. Model of cortical-basal ganglionic processing: encoding the serial order of sensory events. J Neurophysiol 1998; 79:3168–3188.
47. Alexander GE, DeLong MR, Strick PL. Parallel organization of functionally segregated circuits linking basal ganglia and cortex. Annu Rev Neurosci 1986; 9:357–381.
48. Houk JC. Information processing in modular circuits linking basal ganglia and cerebral cortex. In: Houk JC, Davis JL, Beiser DG, eds. Models of Information Processing in the Basal Ganglia. Cambridge, MA: The MIT Press, 1995:3–9.
49. Zheng T, Wilson CJ. Corticostriatal combinatorics: the implications of corticostriatal axonal arborizations. J Neurophysiol 2002; 87(2):1007–1017.
50. Wolf JA, Moyer JT, Lazarewicz MT, et al. NMDA/AMPA ratio impacts state transitions and entrainment to oscillations in a computational model of the nucleus accumbens medium spiny projection neuron. J Neurosci 2005; 25(40):9080–9095.
51. Blackwell KT, Czubayko U, Plenz D. Quantitative estimate of synaptic inputs to striatal neurons during up and down states in vitro. J Neurosci 2003; 23(27):9123–9132.
52. Pennartz CM, Groenewegen HJ, Lopes da Silva FH. The nucleus accumbens as a complex of functionally distinct neuronal ensembles: an integration of behavioural, electrophysiological and anatomical data. Prog Neurobiol 1994; 42(6):719–761.

53. Pennartz CM, Lee E, Verheul J, Lipa P, Barnes CA, McNaughton BL. The ventral striatum in off-line processing: ensemble reactivation during sleep and modulation by hippocampal ripples. J Neurosci 2004; 24(29):6446–6456.
54. Deadwyler SA, Hayashizaki S, Cheer J, Hampson RE. Reward, memory and substance abuse: functional neuronal circuits in the nucleus accumbens. Neurosci Biobehav Rev 2004; 27(8):703–711.
55. Cromwell HC, Hassani OK, Schultz W. Relative reward processing in primate striatum. Exp Brain Res 2005; 162(4):520–525.
56. Berns G, Sejnowski T. A computational model of how the basal ganglia produce sequences. Journal of Cognitive Neuroscience 1998; 10(1):108–121.
56a. Bar-Gad I, Morris G, Bergman H. Information processing, dimensionality reduction and reinforcement learning in the basal ganglia. Prog Neurobiol 2003; 71:439–473.
57. Bergman H, Feingold A, Nini A, et al. Physiological aspects of information processing in the basal ganglia of normal and parkinsonian primates. Trends Neurosci 1998; 21(1):32–38.
58. Hampson RE, Simeral JD, Deadwyler SA. Distribution of spatial and nonspatial information in dorsal hippocampus. Nature 1999; 402(6762):610–614.
59. Lee H, Simpson GV, Logothetis NK, Rainer G. Phase locking of single neuron activity to theta oscillations during working memory in monkey extrastriate visual cortex. Neuron 2005; 45(1):147–156.
60. Jones MW, Wilson MA. Theta rhythms coordinate hippocampal-prefrontal interactions in a spatial memory task. PLoS Biol 2005; 3(12):e402.
61. Floresco SB, West AR, Ash B, Moore H, Grace AA. Afferent modulation of dopamine neuron firing differentially regulates tonic and phasic dopamine transmission. Nat Neurosci 2003; 6(9):968–973.
62. Barto AG. Adaptive critics and the basal ganglia. In: Houk JC, Davis JL, Beiser DG, eds. Models of Information Processing in the Basal Ganglia. Cambridge, MA: MIT Press, 1995:215–232.
63. Sutton RS. Learning to predict by the method of temporal differences. Machine Learning 1988; 3:9–44.
64. Montague PR, Hyman SE, Cohen JD. Computational roles for dopamine in behavioural control. Nature 2004; 431(7010):760–767.
65. Ljungberg T, Apicella P, Schultz W. Responses of monkey dopamine neurons during learning of behavioral reactions. J Neurophysiol 1992; 67(1):145–163.
66. Hollerman JR, Schultz W. Dopamine neurons report an error in the temporal prediction of reward during learning. Nat Neurosci 1998; 1(4):304–309.
67. Schultz W, Apicella P, Ljungberg T. Responses of monkey dopamine neurons to reward and conditioned stimuli during successive steps of learning a delayed response task. J Neurosci 1993; 13(3):900–913.
68. Pennartz CM, Ameerun RF, Groenewegen HJ, Lopes da Silva FH. Synaptic plasticity in an in vitro slice preparation of the rat nucleus accumbens. Eur J Neurosci 1993; 5(2):107–117.
69. Arbuthnott GW, Ingham CA, Wickens JR. Dopamine and synaptic plasticity in the neostriatum. J Anat 2000; 196 (Pt 4):587–596.
70. Thomas MJ, Beurrier C, Bonci A, Malenka RC. Long-term depression in the nucleus accumbens: a neural correlate of behavioral sensitization to cocaine. Nat Neurosci 2001; 4(12):1217–1223.

71. Centonze D, Picconi B, Gubellini P, Bernardi G, Calabresi P. Dopaminergic control of synaptic plasticity in the dorsal striatum. Eur J Neurosci 2001; 13(6):1071–1077.
72. Wickens JR, Reynolds JN, Hyland BI. Neural mechanisms of reward-related motor learning. Curr Opin Neurobiol 2003; 13(6):685–690.
73. Goto Y, Grace AA. Dopamine-dependent interactions between limbic and prefrontal cortical plasticity in the nucleus accumbens: disruption by cocaine sensitization. Neuron 2005; 47(2):255–266.
74. Hefti F, Melamed E. Dopamine release in rat striatum after administration of L-dope as studied with in vivo electrochemistry. Brain Res 1981; 225(2):333–346.
75. Nicola SM, Surmeier J, Malenka RC. Dopaminergic modulation of neuronal excitability in the striatum and nucleus accumbens. Annu Rev Neurosci 2000; 23:185–215.
76. Hernandez-Lopez S, Bargas J, Surmeier DJ, Reyes A, Galarraga E. D1 receptor activation enhances evoked discharge in neostriatal medium spiny neurons by modulating an L-type Ca2+ conductance. J Neurosci 1997; 17(9):3334–3342.
77. Hernandez-Lopez S, Tkatch T, Perez-Garci E, et al. D2 dopamine receptors in striatal medium spiny neurons reduce L-type Ca2+ currents and excitability via a novel PLC[beta]1-IP3-calcineurin-signaling cascade. J Neurosci 2000; 20(24):8987–8995.
78. Surmeier DJ, Eberwine J, Wilson CJ, Cao Y, Stefani A, Kitai ST. Dopamine receptor subtypes colocalize in rat striatonigral neurons. Proc Natl Acad Sci USA 1992; 89(21):10178–10182.
79. Aizman O, Brismar H, Uhlen P, et al. Anatomical and physiological evidence for D1 and D2 dopamine receptor colocalization in neostriatal neurons. Nat Neurosci 2000; 3(3):226–230.
80. Hopf FW, Cascini MG, Gordon AS, Diamond I, Bonci A. Cooperative activation of dopamine D1 and D2 receptors increases spike firing of nucleus accumbens neurons via G-protein betagamma subunits. J Neurosci 2003; 23(12):5079–5087.
81. Goto Y, Grace AA. Dopaminergic modulation of limbic and cortical drive of nucleus accumbens in goal-directed behavior. Nat Neurosci 2005; 8(6):805–812.
82. Moyer JT, Wolf JA, Contreras D, Finkel LH. Dopaminergic modulation and afferent input integration in a computational model of the nucleus accumbens medium spiny neuron. In: Society for Neuroscience. Washington, DC, 2005.
83. Kotter R. Postsynaptic integration of glutamatergic and dopaminergic signals in the striatum. Prog Neurobiol 1994; 44(2):163–196.
84. Wickens JR, Kotter R. Cellular models of reinforcement. In: Houk JC, Davis JL, Beiser DG, eds. Models of Information Processing in the Basal Ganglia. Cambridge, MA: MIT Press, 1995:187–214.
85. Limousin P, Pollak P, Benazzouz A, et al. Effect of parkinsonian signs and symptoms of bilateral subthalamic nucleus stimulation. Lancet 1995; 345(8942):91–95.
86. Dostrovsky JO, Lozano AM. Mechanisms of deep brain stimulation. Mov Disord 2002; 17(suppl 3): S63–S68.
87. Beurrier C, Bioulac B, Audin J, Hammond C. High-frequency stimulation produces a transient blockade of voltage-gated currents in subthalamic neurons. J Neurophysiol 2001; 85(4):1351–1356.
88. Dostrovsky JO, Levy R, Wu JP, Hutchison WD, Tasker RR, Lozano AM. Microstimulation-induced inhibition of neuronal firing in human globus pallidus. J Neurophysiol 2000; 84(1):570–574.

89. Shink E, Smith Y. Differential synaptic innervation of neurons in the internal and external segments of the globus pallidus by the GABA- and glutamate-containing terminals in the squirrel monkey. J Comp Neurol 1995; 358(1):119–141.

90. Filali M, Hutchison WD, Palter VN, Lozano AM, Dostrovsky JO. Stimulation-induced inhibition of neuronal firing in human subthalamic nucleus. Exp Brain Res 2004; 156(3):274–281.

91. Tai CH, Boraud T, Bezard E, Bioulac B, Gross C, Benazzouz A. Electrophysiological and metabolic evidence that high-frequency stimulation of the subthalamic nucleus bridles neuronal activity in the subthalamic nucleus and the substantia nigra reticulata. Faseb J 2003; 17(13):1820–1830.

92. Do MT, Bean BP. Subthreshold sodium currents and pacemaking of subthalamic neurons: modulation by slow inactivation. Neuron 2003; 39(1):109–120.

93. Benazzouz A, Gao DM, Ni ZG, Piallat B, Bouali-Benazzouz R, Benabid AL. Effect of high-frequency stimulation of the subthalamic nucleus on the neuronal activities of the substantia nigra pars reticulata and ventrolateral nucleus of the thalamus in the rat. Neuroscience 2000; 99(2):289–295.

94. Hashimoto T, Elder CM, Okun MS, Patrick SK, Vitek JL. Stimulation of the subthalamic nucleus changes the firing pattern of pallidal neurons. J Neurosci 2003; 23(5):1916–1923.

95. Garcia L, Audin J, D'Alessandro G, Bioulac B, Hammond C. Dual effect of high-frequency stimulation on subthalamic neuron activity. J Neurosci 2003; 23(25): 8743–8751.

96. Maurice N, Thierry AM, Glowinski J, Deniau JM. Spontaneous and evoked activity of substantia nigra pars reticulata neurons during high-frequency stimulation of the subthalamic nucleus. J Neurosci 2003; 23(30):9929–9936.

97. Anderson ME, Postupna N, Ruffo M. Effects of high-frequency stimulation in the internal globus pallidus on the activity of thalamic neurons in the awake monkey. J Neurophysiol 2003; 89(2):1150–1160.

98. Windels F, Bruet N, Poupard A, et al. Effects of high frequency stimulation of subthalamic nucleus on extracellular glutamate and GABA in substantia nigra and globus pallidus in the normal rat. Eur J Neurosci 2000; 12(11):4141–4146.

99. Ceballos-Baumann AO, Boecker H, Bartenstein P, et al. A positron emission tomographic study of subthalamic nucleus stimulation in Parkinson disease: enhanced movement-related activity of motor-association cortex and decreased motor cortex resting activity. Arch Neurol 1999; 56(8):997–1003.

100. Jech R, Urgosik D, Tintera J, et al. Functional magnetic resonance imaging during deep brain stimulation: a pilot study in four patients with Parkinson's disease. Mov Disord 2001; 16(6):1126–1132.

101. Hershey T, Revilla FJ, Wernle AR, et al. Cortical and subcortical blood flow effects of subthalamic nucleus stimulation in PD. Neurology 2003; 61(6):816–821.

102. Hallworth NE, Wilson CJ, Bevan MD. Apamin-sensitive small conductance calcium-activated potassium channels, through their selective coupling to voltage-gated calcium channels, are critical determinants of the precision, pace, and pattern of action potential generation in rat subthalamic nucleus neurons in vitro. J Neurosci 2003; 23(20):7525–7542.

103. McIntyre CC, Savasta M, Walter BL, Vitek JL. How does deep brain stimulation work? Present understanding and future questions. J Clin Neurophysiol 2004; 21(1):40–50.

104. McIntyre CC, Grill WM, Sherman DL, Thakor NV. Cellular effects of deep brain stimulation: model-based analysis of activation and inhibition. J Neurophysiol 2004; 91(4):1457–1469.
105. Shannon CE. A mathematical theory of communication. Bell System Technical Journal 1948; 27:379–423.
106. Montgomery EB Jr, Baker KB. Mechanisms of deep brain stimulation and future technical developments. Neurol Res 2000; 22(3):259–266.
107. Rubin JE, Terman D. High frequency stimulation of the subthalamic nucleus eliminates pathological thalamic rhythmicity in a computational model. J Comput Neurosci 2004; 16(3):211–235.
108. Grill WM, Snyder AN, Miocinovic S. Deep brain stimulation creates an informational lesion of the stimulated nucleus. Neuroreport 2004; 15(7):1137–1140.
109. Shen K, Zhu Z, Munhall A, Johnson S. Synaptic plasticity in rat subthalamic nucleus induced by high-frequency stimulation. Synapse 2003; 50:314–319.
110. Dobrunz LE, Stevens CF. Response of hippocampal synapses to natural stimulation patterns. Neuron 1999; 22(1):157–166.
111. Brown P. Oscillatory nature of human basal ganglia activity: relationship to the pathophysiology of Parkinson's disease. Mov Disord 2003; 18(4):357–363.
112. Garcia L, D'Alessandro G, Bioulac B, Hammond C. High-frequency stimulation in Parkinson's disease: more or less? Trends Neurosci 2005; 28(4):209–216.
113. Brown P, Mazzone P, Oliviero A, et al. Effects of stimulation of the subthalamic area on oscillatory pallidal activity in Parkinson's disease. Exp Neurol 2004; 188(2):480–490.
114. Tass PA. Desynchronization of brain rhythms with soft phase-resetting techniques. Biol Cybern 2002; 87(2):102–115.
115. Hauptmann C, Popovych O, Tass P. Effectively desynchronizing deep brain stimulation based on a coordinated delayed feedback stimulation via several sites: a computational study. Biol Cybern 2005; 93:463–470.
116. Meissner W, Leblois A, Hansel D, et al. Subthalamic high frequency stimulation resets subthalamic firing and reduces abnormal oscillations. Brain 2005; 128:2372–2382.
117. Meissner W, Harnack D, Reese R, et al. High-frequency stimulation of the subthalamic nucleus enhances striatal dopamine release and metabolism in rats. J Neurochem 2003; 85(3):601–609.
118. Bruet N, Windels F, Bertrand A, Feuerstein C, Poupard A, Savasta M. High frequency stimulation of the subthalamic nucleus increases the extracellular contents of striatal dopamine in normal and partially dopaminergic denervated rats. J Neuropathol Exp Neurol 2001; 60(1):15–24.
119. Lee KH, Chang SY, Roberts DW, Kim U. Neurotransmitter release from high-frequency stimulation of the subthalamic nucleus. J Neurosurg 2004; 101(3):511–517.
120. Hilker R, Voges J, Ghaemi M, et al. Deep brain stimulation of the subthalamic nucleus does not increase the striatal dopamine concentration in parkinsonian humans. Mov Disord 2003; 18(1):41–48.
121. Abosch A, Kapur S, Lang AE, et al. Stimulation of the subthalamic nucleus in Parkinson's disease does not produce striatal dopamine release. Neurosurgery 2003; 53(5):1095–1102; discussion 102–105.
122. Bar-Gad I, Bergman H. Stepping out of the box: information processing in the neural networks of the basal ganglia. Current Opinion in Neurobiology 2001; 11:689–695.

123. Parent A, Hazrati LN. Functional anatomy of the basal ganglia I. The cortico-basal ganglia-thalamo-cortical loop. Brain Res Rev 1995; 20:91–127.
124. Bolam JP, Hanley JJ, Booth PA, Bevan MD. Synaptic organisation of the basal ganglia. J Anat 2000; 196 (Pt 4):527–542.
125. Wichmann T, DeLong MR. Pathophysiology of Parkinson's disease: the MPTP primate model of the human disorder. Ann NY Acad Sci 2003; 991:199–213.

3

Indications for Subthalamic Nucleus Deep Brain Stimulation Surgery

Kelvin L. Chou

*Department of Clinical Neurosciences, Brown Medical School,
and NeuroHealth Parkinson's Disease and Movement Disorders Center,
Warwick, Rhode Island, U.S.A.*

INTRODUCTION

Parkinson's disease (PD) is a progressive neurodegenerative disease that is estimated to affect between 100 and 200 per 100,000 people over 40 years of age, and over one million people in North America alone (1,2). Although first described by James Parkinson in 1817 in his "Essay on the Shaking Palsy," (3) an effective medical treatment was not discovered until 1967, when levodopa was introduced. Prior to that, the main treatments for PD were surgical. The number of surgeries on PD patients peated after Spiegel and Wycis introduced stereotaxis in 1947 (4), allowing for more precise localization of surgical lesions in the basal ganglia. But with the widespread use of levodopa, surgery for PD almost disappeared. Despite the effectiveness of levodopa on motor symptoms in PD, long-term use of this drug was associated with disabling side effects, such as dyskinesias and wearing-off, which were difficult to manage medically. Interest in surgical procedures for PD resumed with the success of pallidotomy in the early 1990s (5) and continued when Benabid and his colleagues published their findings on high frequency deep brain stimulation (DBS) for the treatment of motor symptoms in PD (6). DBS of the subthalamic nucleus (STN) is now an FDA-approved treatment for medically refractory PD.

Over the last decade, the number of centers offering DBS worldwide has increased, and more PD patients in the future will be faced with the decision of whether or not to undergo this procedure. Critical to the success of DBS for the treatment of PD is the proper selection of surgical candidates. There now exists a significant amount of data that allow us to predict, in general, which patients will derive the greatest benefit from this procedure, as well as which patients tend to maintain the benefit from DBS long-term. This chapter will discuss the major considerations that go into determining appropriate STN DBS candidates.

PATIENT SELECTION FOR SUBTHALAMIC NUCLEUS DEEP BRAIN-STIMULATION: CORE CRITERIA

In 1992, the Core Assessment Program for Intracerebral Transplantations (CAPIT) was published (7). The main purpose of this publication was to establish a common diagnostic and methodologic evaluation program that could be used by surgical centers to evaluate patients for transplantation procedures. However, as ablation techniques such as pallidotomy gained more prominence, and as DBS techniques became more refined, a need to publish core evaluation guidelines for all surgical therapies was recognized. This resulted in a working committee that eventually published their recommendations as the Core Assessment Program for Surgical Interventional Therapies in Parkinson's Disease (CAPSIT-PD), in 1999 (8). In their guidelines, a set of clinical diagnostic criteria for PD was established including definitions for levodopa responsiveness. In addition, exclusionary cognitive and behavioral criteria were proposed, "off" and "on" states were formally defined, and clinical rating scales for evaluation of parkinsonian symptoms and dyskinesias were recommended.

While there is no standard screening for patients considering DBS surgery, many surgical centers have adopted their own protocols that generally follow these guidelines, especially with regard to the diagnosis of PD, responsiveness to dopaminergic therapies, when to consider surgical options, and making sure that there are no significant cognitive or behavioral deficits that preclude surgery. These five points form the basis for the selection of DBS candidates, and will be discussed individually.

Diagnosis of Parkinson's Disease

A diagnosis of idiopathic PD is crucial to a successful outcome from STN DBS surgery. Patients with atypical parkinsonian syndromes such as multiple system atrophy (MSA) and progressive supranuclear palsy (PSP) are often referred for consideration of DBS because there often are no other treatment options. However, such patients tend not to respond well to DBS. Visser-Vandewalle et al. (9) implanted STN electrodes in four patients with levodopa-unresponsive MSA. While there were improvements in the Unified PD Rating Scale (UPDRS) motor scores at one month postoperatively, the improvements in motor function declined over the next two years. The diagnosis in these cases was not confirmed pathologically, but even if they were correct, the results suggest that the improvements in motor function are not as sustained as they are in patients with PD. Tarsy et al. (10) reported a patient with a clinical diagnosis of MSA whose parkinsonism did not improve with bilateral STN stimulation. Bilateral STN DBS was also unhelpful in a patient with post-anoxic parkinsonism (11).

Okun et al. (12) recently reviewed the records of 41 patients who had been referred to their center as deep brain stimulation failures. Twelve percent of these patients had diagnoses that would not be expected to respond to DBS, suggesting that many clinicians still need education regarding appropriate DBS candidates. These diagnoses included MSA (2 patients), corticobasal degeneration (1 patient), PSP (1 patient), and myoclonus (1 patient).

Two patients have been reported where the clinical picture was typical for PD, but did not respond to STN DBS and were later discovered to have MSA, at autopsy (13,14). These latter two cases underscore the fact that pathologically proven atypical parkinsonian syndromes show little response to DBS, and emphasize the difficulty that can sometimes occur in making an accurate diagnosis of PD.

Early studies demonstrated that the accuracy of a clinical diagnosis of idiopathic PD was 76% when compared to postmortem findings (15,16). A later study found that the accuracy could be improved to approximately 90% with the application of more stringent diagnostic criteria (17). Movement disorder specialists also have a high accuracy for the diagnosis of idiopathic PD, with a sensitivity of 91.1% and a specificity of 98.4% (18). A variety of clinical diagnostic criteria exist for diagnosing PD, including the criteria adopted by CAPSIT-PD (7,8,15,19). While there are subtle variations between the different criteria, all agree that the diagnosis requires the presence of two of the three cardinal motor features (rest tremor, bradykinesia, or rigidity), with at least one feature being bradykinesia. Another feature necessary for diagnosis is a clear-cut response to dopaminergic therapies. Such a response is highly typical of idiopathic PD—a poor response suggests an atypical parkinsonian syndrome. Finally, patients should not have any features in their medical history or neurological examination that suggest any of the syndromes listed in Table 1.

The CAPSIT-PD committee also recommended that patients have disease duration of at least five years before considering surgery. Such a requirement improves the accuracy of diagnosing idiopathic PD, because the defining features of some of the atypical parkinsonian syndromes, such as eye movement abnormalities in PSP and autonomic dysfunction in MSA, may not appear until later in the course of the disease (20,21).

Dopaminergic Responsiveness

Dopaminergic responsiveness is not only typical of PD but is one of the best indicators of a good outcome from STN DBS. Charles et al. (22) evaluated 56

Table 1 Differential Diagnosis of Parkinson's Disease

Corticobasal degeneration
Dementia with Lewy bodies
Dentatorubral-pallidoluysian atrophy
Drug-induced parkinsonism due to antipsychotics, antiemetics,
 or other dopamine blockers
Huntington's disease
Hydrocephalus
Multiple system atrophy
Neoplasm
Neurodegeneration with brain iron accumulation
Parkinsonism-dementia-ALS complex of Guam
Postinfectious parkinsonism
Post-traumatic parkinsonism
Progressive supranuclear palsy
Spinocerebellar ataxia
Toxins, such as carbon monoxide or manganese poisoning
Vascular parkinsonism
Wilson's disease

consecutive PD patients three months after undergoing bilateral STN stimulation, and found that improvement in motor symptoms from levodopa preoperatively correlated with improvement from stimulation. Among individual motor symptoms, responsiveness of rigidity seemed to be the strongest predictor. Welter et al. (23) studied 41 patients with bilateral STN electrodes placed for PD and evaluated them postoperatively at six months. They demonstrated that the lower the preoperative UPDRS motor score in the "on" drug state, the better the effect from STN stimulation, again confirming that dopaminergic response is a strong predictor of success from stimulation.

As would be expected, dopaminergic-resistant features are generally unresponsive to STN stimulation. Several long-term studies have shown that axial symptoms such as speech, gait, and postural instability continue to progress despite changes in stimulation parameters and improvement of other motor symptoms (24–27). In addition, Welter et al. (23) demonstrated that the severity of the axial motor score in the "on" state was predictive of a poor outcome from DBS. Axial symptoms in PD may be partly due to the progressive development of nondopaminergic lesions in the brain (28), which may explain why DBS is not effective for these symptoms. The one exception to the "dopaminergic responsiveness" rule is parkinsonian tremor, which may be refractory to anti-PD medications but responds nicely to stimulation (24–27,29,30).

Thus, it is essential to carefully test dopaminergic responsiveness when evaluating a patient for DBS surgery. Several DBS centers use a suprathreshold levodopa challenge dose for this purpose (22,23,27,30). However, assessment of dopaminergic response can be performed in other ways as well. Two recent studies used the patient's usual dose of anti-parkinsonian medications for preoperative motor assessments and found that the preoperative improvement in UPDRS motor scores with this method also predicted a good response from bilateral STN DBS (31,32). Pinter et al. (33) reported similar results using an apomorphine challenge as a predictor of response to STN DBS. This may be a useful alternative to test patients who for some reason are unable to tolerate levodopa.

The evaluation of dopamine response should begin with an examination using the UPDRS in the "off" medication state, defined as the condition after a patient has not received anti-parkinsonian medication for at least 12 hours (7). The proposed surgical candidate should then be given their challenge dose, and when the patient has noticed a good response, an examination should be performed using the UPDRS. At the very minimum, acceptable surgical candidates should have a 33% reduction in their UPDRS scores (8).

When to Consider Surgical Evaluation

Because DBS surgery is not a benign procedure, it should be offered to patients only when the risk to benefit ratio is favorable. At this point, surgery should be considered only when PD patients continue to suffer from levodopa motor complications despite optimal medical management. These complications can include dyskinesias, wearing off, and on-off phenomena. As DBS has regularly been shown to be effective in improving these motor complications even as long as five years after surgery (24,25,34), patients with such advanced disease stand to benefit most from this procedure. Other situations that may warrant an evaluation for STN DBS include patients with disabling tremor and PD patients who are intolerant of anti-parkinsonian medications because of severe nausea or vomiting. Of course, many patients can delay the need for surgery with adjustments in their medications, so a concerted effort should be made to alter the timing and doses of dopaminergic medications before sending patients for surgery. A minority of patients will choose not to have surgery after medication optimization.

Patients should be tried on maximally tolerated doses of carbidopa/levodopa, dopamine agonists, and catechol-O-methyltransferase (COMT) inhibitors prior to surgery. Other strategies for medication adjustments include:

1. A trial of amantadine for patients with dyskinesias.
2. Anticholinergics such as trihexyphenidyl or high dose levodopa (up to 1500 mg/day) for patients with medication refractory tremor. Clozapine may also be attempted (35).
3. For patients with wearing off between medication doses, switching to regular release carbidopa/levodopa and shortening intervals between doses. Apomorphine should be considered for patients with sudden "offs."
4. For dyskinesias and on-off fluctuations, switching to regular release carbidopa/levodopa, decreasing the dose and moving medication intervals closer together may help. Low dose dopamine agonists and COMT inhibitors may also be helpful.

5. For patients with severe nausea, adding extra carbidopa (25–100 mg) or domperidone (not available in US).

It has been proposed that STN DBS could be potentially neuroprotective, that is, slow down the progression of PD. The mechanistic theory is that STN DBS, by suppressing the excitatory glutamatergic outflow of the STN, could reduce glutamate-mediated excitotoxicity of the substantia nigra (36,37). If this were true, then patients should obviously be offered DBS at an early stage of their disease in order to prevent progression. However, while there is considerable evidence in the rat model of PD that lesioning the STN protects nigral cells (38,39), there is no convincing evidence in humans that high frequency STN DBS is neuroprotective in PD. A recent study demonstrated that PD still progressed after bilateral STN DBS surgery in 30 patients using ^{18}F-fluorodopa (F-dopa) positron emission tomography (PET) (40). The striatal uptake of F-dopa decreased at a rate of 9.5% to 12.9% in this study, a number consistent with the normal disease progression rate reported in other F-dopa PET studies (41,42). Thus, there is no justification at this time to send patients for STN DBS because of possible "neuroprotective" effects. Similarly, there is no evidence that operating on early PD patients delays or prevents levodopa motor complications.

Cognitive Criteria

The presence of dementia or significant cognitive impairment is considered a contraindication for STN DBS. Some centers may use cognitive screening tools such as the Mini-Mental State Examination (43) or the Mattis Dementia Rating Scale (44) to exclude patients from surgery. Most DBS centers use detailed neuropsychological testing and determine the presence of dementia using DSM-IV criteria, defined as the "development of multiple cognitive deficits that include memory impairment and at least one of the following cognitive disturbances: aphasia, apraxia, agnosia, or a disturbance in executive functioning. The cognitive impairments must be sufficiently severe to cause impairment in occupational and social functioning and represent a decline from a previously higher level of functioning (45)." The exact neuropsychological tests used may vary from center to center and are discussed in more detail in chapter 15.

Preoperative screening for dementia is mandatory. Demented patients may be unable to provide appropriate feedback both intraoperatively and postoperatively. This may affect the ability of the surgical team to place the DBS electrode optimally and would likely interfere with the effectiveness of postoperative programming. More importantly, however, cognition in PD patients may worsen irreversibly after DBS surgery, especially in more elderly patients (46) and those with preexisting cognitive impairment (12,47,48). Long-term studies in patients with PD undergoing STN stimulation have shown that cognitive decline post surgery is not infrequent, ranging from 7% to 22% (24,26,49). In the study by Funkiewiez et al. (49), the postoperative mental decline was thought to be related to the surgical procedure. The timing of the cognitive decline to surgery is unclear in the other two long-term studies.

The exact changes underlying permanent cognitive deterioration due to STN DBS are unclear, but may be due to a number of factors. Surgical trauma, especially with a higher number of electrode passes, is a likely contributor. Chronic stimulation, by itself, may cause downstream changes in neurotransmitter activity, affecting thinking and memory. The stimulation may spread to adjacent structures involved in thought processes. Finally, a reduced cognitive reserve due to advancing age is possible.

Behavioral Criteria

There are reports of patients becoming severely depressed after DBS surgery, to the point where some even attempt suicide (24,30,50–52). It is of particular interest that these adverse psychiatric results have been reported more often after bilateral STN DBS surgery than after pallidotomy or globus pallidus (GPi) stimulation. The reasons for this are unclear. Perhaps the electrical stimulation field spreads to limbic fibers near the STN and results in depression (53). Some investigators have argued that these patients have a past psychiatric history that may predispose them to postsurgical depression (50,54,55). Whatever the underlying cause, there is not enough data to know which patients pose the greatest risk. Until we discover which preoperative clinical factors are predictive of postoperative depression, it is reasonable to exclude patients with uncontrolled psychiatric illness from having DBS surgery.

Another reason to exclude unstable psychiatric patients is that they may be unable to provide the feedback needed postoperatively in order achieve optimal results. Furthermore, depression may confound interpretation of motor symptoms in PD. There is one case report of a woman with medication refractory depression after STN DBS surgery who needed electroconvulsive therapy (ECT) (55). Ultimately, ECT was effective for her depression, but increasing the stimulator parameters did not improve her motor symptoms until her depression resolved. Depression can also cause significant impairment of attention, memory, and executive function, resulting in a neuropsychological evaluation consistent with dementia. Such a "pseudo-dementia" disappears when the depression is controlled. Thus, if mood is not assessed or improperly evaluated, it may result in the exclusion of a candidate who might otherwise be appropriate.

OTHER CONSIDERATIONS

Age

Younger age has been reported to be predictive of a good outcome from DBS surgery. In general, many surgical centers have been using 70 years of age as a cutoff, because early studies looking at predictive factors demonstrated that patients under age 70 tended to show greater motor improvement than patients over 70 (22,23). Why younger patients have better DBS motor outcomes is not entirely clear, but makes some intuitive sense, as older patients have more comorbidities and may take longer to recover from surgery. Older patients are also more likely to have cognitive impairment. Saint-Cyr et al. (46) demonstrated that patients undergoing STN DBS over the age of 69 were more likely to have cognitive decline postoperatively, even if they did not have signs of dementia on preoperative neuropsychological testing. Levodopa tends to lose its efficacy with age—suggested possibilities for this phenomenon include the presence of increased non-dopaminergic, vascular, or other degenerative lesions in the brain (56). Since DBS helps only levodopa responsive symptoms in PD, it too may lose its effectiveness in older patients for similar reasons.

Russmann et al. (57) recently studied the effects of STN DBS in 13 patients over age 70 and compared their results to 39 patients under the age of 70. Overall, the patients over age 70 had their levodopa dosages reduced by 49% compared with a 74% medication reduction in younger patients. In addition, the UPDRS "off" motor scores postoperatively, were less improved in the older group than in the younger group. Finally, postoperative gait and postural instability scores while "on" medication worsened in patients over age 70, while in patients under 70, they did not change. While these findings support an age-based cutoff for surgery, the investigators pointed out that their older cohort was not uniform in their response to DBS. Five of these 13 patients did not require any dopaminergic medications after surgery. Thus, it appears that a strict age requirement for DBS may exclude some good candidates. When looking at possible differences between these five patients and the eight who had a less robust response, the patients with better results had better preoperative axial scores "off" medication.

At this point, potential surgical cases over the age of 70 should be evaluated on an individual basis. It will be important to identify factors that can predict who will do well over age 70, although preoperative axial signs may turn out to be a predictor of outcome in this age group.

General Health

The entire DBS implantation procedure is an arduous and lengthy process. From the initial surgical planning, to microelectrode recording, to electrode and battery implantation bilaterally, some patients can be in the operating room for eight hours or more. The surgery is physically demanding, not only because of the length of the procedure, but also because patients may be "off" of their routine PD medications during much of the procedure. Furthermore, patients are awake for a significant portion of the surgery, and must be able to provide appropriate feedback in the operating room. In order to tolerate this procedure, it is essential that patients be in good general health. The presence of significant comorbid medical illnesses, such as uncontrolled hypertension or diabetes, severe cardiopulmonary disease, or poor renal or hepatic function are relative contraindications to DBS surgery.

In addition to being in good physical health, patients should also have strong emotional support from their families or caregivers. The immediate postoperative period, as the neurologist increases stimulation parameters while simultaneously decreasing medications, is a time of constant change and can sometimes be frustrating, especially when patients expect to be better immediately after surgery. Patients may also need a significant amount of aid, as frequent visits to the physician or nurse practitioner are often necessary for DBS programming. Some patients and many caregivers will have difficulty coping with the transition to a more independent and less physically dependent condition. Family members need to be understanding of the entire experience, and a lack of support can undermine an otherwise successful outcome.

Expectations of Outcome

Although selection of appropriate candidates is critical to the success of STN DBS, a surgery may not be considered successful by the patient if their expectations are not met. Therefore, it is important to make certain that patients have a realistic expectation of the surgical results. The results of the dopaminergic challenge can be a valuable tool in educating patients about the degree of benefit that can be reasonably expected from surgery. For example, studies have shown that STN DBS does not improve PD symptoms significantly beyond their best preoperative "on" condition (24–27). Thus, if the patient still needs to use an assistive device to ambulate when the medications are "on," then surgery will be unlikely to improve their gait. Surgery should not be offered until the expectations of outcome are clearly understood by the patient.

SCREENING TOOL FOR SURGICAL CANDIDATES

The proper selection of candidates for STN DBS is best accomplished by an experienced surgical center with a multi-disciplinary team that includes movement disorders neurologists, neurosurgeons, neuropsychologists, neurophysiologists, psychiatrists, nurse practitioners, and nurses. Nevertheless, while many PD patients evaluated for DBS surgery qualify for the procedure a significant proportion do not. General neurologists and general practitioners provide much of the routine care for PD patients in the United States, and are a major referral source for potential DBS candidates, yet many are unclear on the inclusion and exclusion criteria for DBS. A retrospective analysis of 98 PD patients referred to a single PD center for DBS evaluation found that approximately 30% of the patients evaluated were not suitable candidates for the procedure (58). The most common cause for exclusion was the presence of cognitive or psychiatric disorders, while mild symptoms were the second most common cause.

Table 2 Characteristics of Appropriate Subthalamic Nucleus
Deep Brain Stimulation Candidates

The patient has a diagnosis of idiopathic PD without evidence of an atypical
  parkinsonian syndrome.
Sustained response to levodopa.
Presence of complications from chronic levodopa therapy such as dyskinesias,
  wearing off, and on-off phenomena or, alternatively, a tremor predominant
  presentation.
Absence of dementia or active psychiatric illnesses.

Okun et al. (59) specifically developed a screening tool for the evaluation of
DBS candidates that was targeted to aid community practitioners in identifying
the proper PD patients. The resulting questionnaire, entitled the Florida Surgical
Questionnaire for Parkinson's Disease (FLASQ-PD), has five parts: (*i*) criteria
for diagnosing idiopathic PD, (*ii*) potential contraindications to PD surgery,
(*iii*) general patient characteristics such as age, duration of disease, and frequency
of dyskinesias, (*iv*) favorable/unfavorable characteristics such as cognitive function, and (*v*) medication trial information. This survey can be filled out in a few
minutes, and allows for a simple score that will assess the appropriateness of pur-
suing a full multidisciplinary PD surgical work-up. In general, the best candidates
have a score greater than 25, while patients with scores less than or equal to 15 are
unsuitable for surgery. The FLASQ-PD still needs to be validated prospectively,
but may turn out to be a useful triage tool in the future.

SUMMARY

STN deep brain stimulation is now a safe and effective treatment option for
patients with PD. In order to ensure a successful outcome, however, it is important to select the appropriate candidates for the procedure. The appropriate surgical candidate for STN DBS (Table 2) has a diagnosis of idiopathic PD with a clear
and sustained response to levodopa and suffers from complications of chronic
levodopa therapy or has a disabling tremor despite optimal medical management.
Furthermore, the potential candidate should have no dementia or active psychiatric issues. Ideally, the patient should also be young (i.e., less than 70 years of
age), although well-selected older patients can also respond favorably. Future
studies are necessary to clearly establish both positive and negative predictive
factors of surgical outcomes. Until that point, however, selection of patients is
best accomplished at experienced surgical centers.

REFERENCES

1. Marras C, Tanner CM. Epidemiology of Parkinson's disease. In: Watts RL, Koller WC,
   eds. Movement Disorders: Neurologic Principles and Practice. 2nd ed. New York: The
   McGraw-Hill Companies, Inc., 2004:177–195.

2. Lang AE, Lozano AM. Parkinson's disease. First of two parts. N Engl J Med 1998; 339(15):1044–1053.
3. Parkinson J. An Essay on the Shaking Palsy. London: Sherwood, Neely, and Jones, 1817.
4. Speigel EA, Wycis HT, Marks M, et al. Stereotaxic apparatus for operations on the human brain. Science 1947; 106:349–350.
5. Laitinen LV, Bergenheim AT, Hariz MI. Leksell's posteroventral pallidotomy in the treatment of Parkinson's disease. J Neurosurg 1992; 76(1):53–61.
6. Limousin P, Pollak P, Benazzouz A, et al. Effect of parkinsonian signs and symptoms of bilateral subthalamic nucleus stimulation. Lancet 1995; 345(8942): 91–95.
7. Langston JW, Widner H, Goetz CG, et al. Core assessment program for intracerebral transplantations (CAPIT). Mov Disord 1992; 7(1):2–13.
8. Defer GL, Widner H, Marie RM, et al. Core assessment program for surgical interventional therapies in Parkinson's disease (CAPSIT-PD). Mov Disord 1999; 14(4):572–584.
9. Visser-Vandewalle V, Temel Y, Colle H, et al. Bilateral high-frequency stimulation of the subthalamic nucleus in patients with multiple system atrophy—parkinsonism. Report of four cases. J Neurosurg 2003; 98(4):882–887.
10. Tarsy D, Apetauerova D, Ryan P, et al. Adverse effects of subthalamic nucleus DBS in a patient with multiple system atrophy. Neurology 2003; 61(2):247–249.
11. Krack P, Dowsey PL, Benabid AL, et al. Ineffective subthalamic nucleus stimulation in levodopa-resistant postischemic parkinsonism. Neurology 2000; 54(11): 2182–2184.
12. Okun MS, Tagliati M, Pourfar M, et al. Management of referred deep brain stimulation failures: a retrospective analysis from 2 movement disorders centers. Arch Neurol 2005; 62(8): 1250–1255.
13. Chou KL, Forman MS, Trojanowski JQ, et al. Subthalamic nucleus deep brain stimulation in a patient with levodopa-responsive multiple system atrophy. Case report. J Neurosurg 2004; 100(3): 553–556.
14. Lezcano E, Gomez-Esteban JC, Zarranz JJ, et al. Parkinson's disease-like presentation of multiple system atrophy with poor response to STN stimulation: a clinicopathological case report. Mov Disord 2004; 19(8):973–977.
15. Hughes AJ, Daniel SE, Kilford L, et al. Accuracy of clinical diagnosis of idiopathic Parkinson's disease: a clinico-pathological study of 100 cases. J Neurol Neurosurg Psychiatry 1992; 55(3):181–184.
16. Rajput AH, Rozdilsky B, Rajput A. Accuracy of clinical diagnosis in parkinsonism—a prospective study. Can J Neurol Sci 1991; 18(3):275–278.
17. Hughes AJ, Daniel SE, Lees AJ. Improved accuracy of clinical diagnosis of Lewy body Parkinson's disease. Neurology 2001; 57(8):1497–1499.
18. Hughes AJ, Daniel SE, Ben-Shlomo Y, et al. The accuracy of diagnosis of parkinsonian syndromes in a specialist movement disorder service. Brain 2002; 125(Pt 4):861–870.
19. Gelb DJ, Oliver E, Gilman S. Diagnostic criteria for Parkinson disease. Arch Neurol 1999; 56(1):33–39.
20. Quinn NP. How to diagnose multiple system atrophy. Mov Disord 2005; 20 (suppl 12):S5–S10.
21. Scaravilli T, Tolosa E, Ferrer I. Progressive supranuclear palsy and corticobasal degeneration: lumping versus splitting. Mov Disord 2005; 20(suppl 12):S21–S28.

22. Charles PD, Van Blercom N, Krack P, et al. Predictors of effective bilateral subthalamic nucleus stimulation for PD. Neurology 2002; 59(6):932–934.

23. Welter ML, Houeto JL, Tezenas du Montcel S, et al. Clinical predictive factors of subthalamic stimulation in Parkinson's disease. Brain 2002; 125(Pt 3):575–583.

24. Kleiner-Fisman G, Fisman DN, Sime E, et al. Long-term follow up of bilateral deep brain stimulation of the subthalamic nucleus in patients with advanced Parkinson disease. J Neurosurg 2003; 99(3):489–495.

25. Krack P, Batir A, Van Blercom N, et al. Five-year follow-up of bilateral stimulation of the subthalamic nucleus in advanced Parkinson's disease. N Engl J Med 2003; 349(20):1925–1934.

26. Schupbach WM, Chastan N, Welter ML, et al. Stimulation of the subthalamic nucleus in Parkinson's disease: a 5 year follow up. J Neurol Neurosurg Psychiatry 2005; 76(12):1640–1644.

27. Rodriguez-Oroz MC, Obeso JA, Lang AE, et al. Bilateral deep brain stimulation in Parkinson's disease: a multicentre study with 4 years follow-up. Brain 2005; 128(Pt 10):2240–2249.

28. Agid Y. Parkinson's disease: pathophysiology. Lancet 1991; 337(8753):1321–1324.

29. Krack P, Benazzouz A, Pollak P, et al. Treatment of tremor in Parkinson's disease by subthalamic nucleus stimulation. Mov Disord 1998; 13(6):907–914.

30. Herzog J, Volkmann J, Krack P, et al. Two-year follow-up of subthalamic deep brain stimulation in Parkinson's disease. Mov Disord 2003; 18(11):1332–1337.

31. Pahwa R, Wilkinson SB, Overman J, et al. Preoperative clinical predictors of response to bilateral subthalamic stimulation in patients with Parkinson's disease. Stereotact Funct Neurosurg 2005; 83(2-3):80–83.

32. Jaggi JL, Umemura A, Hurtig HI, et al. Bilateral stimulation of the subthalamic nucleus in Parkinson's disease: surgical efficacy and prediction of outcome. Stereotact Funct Neurosurg 2004; 82(2-3):104–114.

33. Pinter MM, Alesch F, Murg M, et al. Apomorphine test: a predictor for motor responsiveness to deep brain stimulation of the subthalamic nucleus. J Neurol 1999; 246(10): 907–913.

34. Deep Brain Stimulation for Parkinson's Disease Study Group. Deep-brain stimulation of the subthalamic nucleus or the pars interna of the globus pallidus in Parkinson's disease. N Engl J Med 2001; 345(13):956–963.

35. Friedman JH, Lannon MC. Clozapine-responsive tremor in Parkinson's disease. Mov Disord 1990; 5(3):225–229.

36. Benazzouz A, Gao DM, Ni ZG, et al. Effect of high-frequency stimulation of the subthalamic nucleus on the neuronal activities of the substantia nigra pars reticulata and ventrolateral nucleus of the thalamus in the rat. Neuroscience 2000; 99(2):289–295.

37. Rodriguez MC, Obeso JA, Olanow CW. Subthalamic nucleus-mediated excitotoxicity in Parkinson's disease: a target for neuroprotection. Ann Neurol 1998; 44(3 suppl 1): S175–S188.

38. Nakao N, Nakai E, Nakai K, et al. Ablation of the subthalamic nucleus supports the survival of nigral dopaminergic neurons after nigrostriatal lesions induced by the mitochondrial toxin 3-nitropropionic acid. Ann Neurol 1999; 45(5):640–651.

39. Piallat B, Benazzouz A, Benabid AL. Neuroprotective effect of chronic inactivation of the subthalamic nucleus in a rat model of Parkinson's disease. J Neural Transm Suppl 1999; 55: 71–77.

40. Hilker R, Portman AT, Voges J, et al. Disease progression continues in patients with advanced Parkinson's disease and effective subthalamic nucleus stimulation. J Neurol Neurosurg Psychiatry 2005; 76(9):1217–1221.

41. Morrish PK, Rakshi JS, Bailey DL, et al. Measuring the rate of progression and estimating the preclinical period of Parkinson's disease with (18F)dopa PET. J Neurol Neurosurg Psychiatry 1998; 64(3):314–319.

42. Morrish PK, Sawle GV, Brooks DJ. An (18F)dopa-PET and clinical study of the rate of progression in Parkinson's disease. Brain 1996; 119(Pt 2):585–591.

43. Folstein MF, Folstein SE, McHugh PR. "Mini-mental state". A practical method for grading the cognitive state of patients for the clinician. J Psychiatr Res 1975; 12(3):189–198.

44. Mattis S. Dementia Rating Scale Professonal Manual. Odessa, FL: Psychological Assessment Resources, 1988.

45. Diagnostic and Statistical Manual of Mental Disorders. 4th ed. Washington, DC: American Psychiatric Association, 1994.

46. Saint-Cyr JA, Trepanier LL, Kumar R, et al. Neuropsychological consequences of chronic bilateral stimulation of the subthalamic nucleus in Parkinson's disease. Brain 2000; 123(Pt 10):2091–2108.

47. Hariz MI, Johansson F, Shamsgovara P, et al. Bilateral subthalamic nucleus stimulation in a parkinsonian patient with preoperative deficits in speech and cognition: persistent improvement in mobility but increased dependency: a case study. Mov Disord 2000; 15(1):136–139.

48. Limousin P, Krack P, Pollak P, et al. Electrical stimulation of the subthalamic nucleus in advanced Parkinson's disease. N Engl J Med 1998; 339(16):1105–1111.

49. Funkiewiez A, Ardouin C, Caputo E, et al. Long term effects of bilateral subthalamic nucleus stimulation on cognitive function, mood, and behaviour in Parkinson's disease. J Neurol Neurosurg Psychiatry 2004; 75(6):834–839.

50. Berney A, Vingerhoets F, Perrin A, et al. Effect on mood of subthalamic DBS for Parkinson's disease: a consecutive series of 24 patients. Neurology 2002; 59(9): 1427–1429.

51. Doshi PK, Chhaya N, Bhatt MH. Depression leading to attempted suicide after bilateral subthalamic nucleus stimulation for Parkinson's disease. Mov Disord 2002; 17(5):1084–1085.

52. Krack P, Limousin P, Benabid AL, et al. Chronic stimulation of subthalamic nucleus improves levodopa-induced dyskinesias in Parkinson's disease. Lancet 1997; 350(9092):1676.

53. Bejjani BP, Damier P, Arnulf I, et al. Transient acute depression induced by high-frequency deep-brain stimulation. N Engl J Med 1999; 340(19):1476–1480.

54. Houeto JL, Mesnage V, Mallet L, et al. Behavioural disorders, Parkinson's disease and subthalamic stimulation. J Neurol Neurosurg Psychiatry 2002; 72(6):701–707.

55. Chou KL, Hurtig HI, Jaggi JL, et al. Electroconvulsive therapy for depression in a Parkinson's disease patient with bilateral subthalamic nucleus deep brain stimulators. Parkinsonism Relat Disord 2005; 11(6):403–406.

56. Blin J, Dubois B, Bonnet AM, et al. Does ageing aggravate parkinsonian disability? J Neurol Neurosurg Psychiatry 1991; 54(9):780–782.

57. Russmann H, Ghika J, Villemure JG, et al. Subthalamic nucleus deep brain stimulation in Parkinson's disease patients over age 70 years. Neurology 2004; 63(10): 1952–1954.

58. Lopiano L, Rizzone M, Bergamasco B, et al. Deep brain stimulation of the subthalamic nucleus in PD: an analysis of the exclusion causes. J Neurol Sci 2002; 195(2):167–170.

59. Okun MS, Fernandez HH, Pedraza O, et al. Development and initial validation of a screening tool for Parkinson disease surgical candidates. Neurology 2004; 63(1): 161–163.

4

Deep Brain Stimulation Preop Assessment and Teaching

Heidi C. Watson and Lisette K. Bunting-Perry

Department of Veterans Affairs, Parkinson's Disease Research, Education, and Clinical Center (PADRECC), Philadelphia Veterans Affairs Medical Center, Philadelphia, Pennsylvania, U.S.A.

Susan L. Heath

Department of Veterans Affairs, Parkinson's Disease Research, Education, and Clinical Center (PADRECC), San Francisco Veterans Affairs Medical Center, San Francisco, California, U.S.A.

INTRODUCTION

Preparing the patient with Parkinson's disease (PD) and their family for deep brain stimulation (DBS) surgery is both an art and a science. It is imperative that the patient and his/her family have confidence in the treatment team to gain successful surgical outcomes and confidence in living with DBS technology. The surgery itself is only one part in the journey of living with PD technology. Realistic expectations, education, and interdisciplinary care planning will provide the patient/family with the knowledge they need in the preoperative, interoperative, and postoperative stages. This involves teaching the patient about surgical risks and what to expect before, during, and after surgery. DBS education and teaching should be considered a process that spans from the first day of evaluation and continues through to follow-up, after the surgery.

The purpose of this chapter is to guide the reader through the key aspects of patient education as it relates to DBS surgery for PD. This chapter will provide the reader with methods to enhance patient/family education. Tables and figures have been designed to assist the health care provider in preoperative and postoperative teaching. The chapter concludes with web-based DBS resources for health care professionals, patients, and family members.

ASSESSMENT

The previous chapter discussed the method by which to ascertain the appropriateness of a patient as a surgical candidate. The thoughtful selection of candidates to be referred to the surgical team is essential to good clinical outcomes. Once a patient presents to the surgical team the assessment for surgical candidacy continues. In the beginning stages of DBS candidacy, the provider should have a discussion with the potential candidate and perform a thorough assessment of a patient's learning method, decision making style, and knowledge base. Establishing a baseline of the patients' education needs is done prior to proceeding with DBS surgery plans.

Assessing a patient's learning method is the first step. Often health care providers assume that all patients would like information delivered in a factual straightforward method. However, adult learners differ in how they process information. Learning is mediated by the anxiety of anticipating the DBS procedure. Assessing the patient for anxiety and learning needs can be difficult under this emotionally changed situation. Next, assess the patient's decision making style. Ask the patient, "Who helps you make decision about your health care?" This question is the key to involving an identified health care proxy in the DBS education process. Thus, there will be a third party who will receive education on the procedure and can clarify information for the patient. Assess the level of knowledge regarding PD and the expectation of surgical procedure. Patients should be able to describe that the surgery will provide them with their "best on" time and that DBS surgery is a treatment for PD, much like medication has been a treatment. Furthermore, the patient/family should articulate that DBS surgery is not a cure for PD. Patients and their families often view the DBS surgical procedure as the answer to their prayers. Educating a patient/family is essential in preparing the patient/family for realistic expectations for DBS surgery.

Psychosocial Assessment

The successful DBS candidate has an intact psychosocial support system. The ability of the patient to be supported emotionally, spiritually, and physically through the DBS procedure is essential. Throughout this text we will use the term family to describe the support system for the patient. Family care can be defined as "anyone who shows up when illness strikes . . . and stays on to help" (1).

Education Procedure: Preoperative

The patient/family should be educated in the process of preoperative assessment. The assessment may take several weeks to complete and the patient/family may be anxious and voice concerns regarding "failing" the evaluation. Educating the patient/family in the need for thorough evaluation will diminish their apprehension. The patient/family should understand that DBS surgery is not appropriate for every patient and good clinical outcomes are predicted by careful preoperative assessment (2). Keeping in mind that patients who do not meet the criteria for DBS surgery often express feelings of disappointment and anger at being denied the procedure. Patients and families should be given the opportunity to discuss their feelings and maintain hope in living with a chronic progressive neurologic disease.

The patients sent for preoperative assessment have been selected by criteria presented in chapter 3. In summary the neurologist has evaluated the patient by confirmation of the diagnosis of idiopathic PD, degree of disability, optimization of pharmacological therapeutics, cognitive status, surgical risk, medical stability, and age. The preoperative testing further deduces the projected efficacy of DBS technology through diagnostic, psychological, motor testing, and diary reporting.

On/Off Motor Testing

The most significant test of efficacy for treatment of motor symptoms by DBS surgery is "on/off" motor testing. The patient will be well served through education on this procedure. The primary goal of motor testing is to objectively observe the patient in the "off" medication state and in the "on" medication state (2).

The procedure for on/off testing is as follows. The patient is instructed to withhold dopaminergic medications for up to 12 hours. The patient typically takes the last dose of dopaminergic medication at 8 PM and plans to arrive at the clinic for an 8 AM appointment. Some patients are not able to comply with this request related to akinesia in the "off" state. Assessing the patients' ability to tolerate an "off" state examination and evaluating the families' ability to transport a PD patient in the "off" state is important. If this request is unduly a burden on the patient and family, the medication evaluation may be modified or omitted.

Once the patient arrives to the clinic in the "off" state, he/she will be rated for motor function as defined by section III of the Unified Parkinson's disease rating scale (UPDRS). After "off" testing is performed, the patient is instructed to take his/her usual dopaminergic medications and wait until he/she feels in a good "on" state. Then the motor testing is repeated for comparison. The on/off scores should demonstrate a 30% improvement from "off" to "on" state to consider the patient for DBS surgery (3).

Efficacy of DBS surgery in PD is predicted by good motor functioning in the "on" state. The presence of dyskinesias in the "on" state should not be a concern, as dyskinesias are a side effect of dopaminergic therapeutics. Educating the patient that dyskinesias often resolve after surgery, as the stimulation is optimized and PD medications are reduced, is helpful in their establishing realistic expectations. Several clinicians have reported the value of videotaping patient during the preoperative on/off testing. The videotapes are beneficial in educating the patient/family in the postoperative period to demonstrate the efficacy of the procedure (4,5).

Motor Diary

The goal of the motor diary is to have 48 hours of recorded on/off and dyskinetic activity for the patient. Educating the patient/family in the completion of the motor diary can improve the collection of accurate objective data. Patients are instructed by a training video on the diary completion (4).

The patient will be instructed to complete 24-hour diaries, which are divided into 30-minute time slots. Thus the patient will record measures of percentage of (*i*) "on" time, (*ii*) "off" time, and (*iii*) "on" time with troublesome dyskinesias. Each measure should be explained to the patient. The general rule is to historically report four hours of "off" time and/or four hours of disabling dyskinesia within a 24-hour period to be eligible for DBS surgery. The diaries are also helpful in determining if current dopaminergic therapeutics has been optimized (5).

Neuropsychiatric Testing

Baseline cognitive functioning is critical in determining the capacity of the patient to benefit from DBS technology. Patients/families should be educated that this extensive testing is lengthy and can take up to four hours to complete. This testing provides the patent/family/team with a baseline measure of cognitive function. The ability of the patient to reason, concentrate, and interpret abstract concepts will guide the treatment team in determining the viability of DBS surgery. Furthermore, neuropsychological testing performed at follow-up visit with help determines effects of DBS on cognition (6).

Medical Clearance

The patient should be medically cleared for the surgical procedure. Typically medical clearance is provided by internal medicine. Patients should have optimized treatment for other medical conditions prior to the surgery to prevent decompensation postoperatively. Patients with comorbid conditions should receive additional clearance to determine risk of surgery and anesthesia. A noncontrast MRI of the brain should be completed and reviewed, prior to surgery, to assess for anomalies, which would be a contraindication to DBS surgery.

History

A careful history of medications, allergies, and medical problems will help guide the team in preoperative and postoperative care.

Medication History

A thorough history of all over the counter, herbal, and prescription medications should be recorded. Patients should be screened for substances that prolong coagulation. Many common medications, vitamins, and herbals can result in increased clotting time.

Allergies

A careful record of allergies is essential in preventing complications. Often patients will minimize allergic experiences and not discuss them with the treatment team. Specific questions should be asked regarding allergic reactions to betadine, antibiotics, tape, and latex. Medical records should be flagged with identified allergies.

History of Comorbid Conditions

PD is a complex disease with both motor and nonmotor symptoms. Anxiety is a common nonmotor symptom of PD and many patients are prescribed antianxiety agents (7). Alerting the surgical team to the need for anxiety management in the surgical suite can assist in providing comfort for the patient during a long surgical day. Pain is reported in 50% of patients with PD and may improve with DBS surgery. Evaluation of pain and pain management during the operative day will enhance the comfort of the patients and improve recovery (8).

Advanced Directives

Advanced directives are standard for a patient who is preparing to have major surgery. An advanced directive is a process of planning for health care. The two documents to be prepared by the patient, prior to surgery, include the Durable Power of Attorney for Health Care (DPAHC) and the living will. The DPAHC is essential because the patient identifies a health-care proxy to speak for them in the event that they cannot communicate any health care desires (9). The DPAHC and living will should be entered in the medical record and should be reviewed with the patient prior to surgery. Guidelines and paperwork for the DPAHC and living will can be found on the World Wide Web.

EDUCATION OF DEEP BRAIN STIMULATION MODEL EQUIPMENT

The internal equipment shown in Figure 1 is reviewed with the patient. If a model of equipment is available, allow the patient to see the lead wires, connection wires, and the neurostimulator. The location of the dual channel neurostimulator should be discussed with the patient/family and the neurosurgeon. The neurostimulator is usually placed in the upper chest on the right side, in an effort to preserve the left side for a cardiac pacemaker, should one be necessary. However, this may not be the ideal location for all patients. Special consideration may be taken to place the neurostimulator elsewhere, dependent on the patients' life style and activities.

Preserving Self-Image

As DBS surgery is a treatment to improve quality of life, preserving a patient's body image is paramount. Surgical scars and skull changes relating to the placement of hardware should be reviewed. On top of the head, the patient will typically have two bilaterally placed scars and two quarter sized bumps that protrude

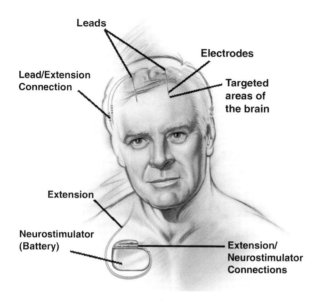

Figure 1 Deep brain stimulation (DBS) Medtronic model. *Source*: Courtesy of Medtronic.

from the normal shaped skull. The patient will have a scar about three inches across where the neurostimulator is placed and an inch long scar behind the ear, from the connection wire. The use of a wig or hats may be discussed if the patient is uncomfortable with the scars shown on the head. The skin over the connection wire can be irritated if rubbed by the glasses. The placement of the glasses against the skin should be assessed in order to prevent skin break-down behind the ear.

Risk of Infection

Teaching the patient about the risk of infection is important for prevention and early identification. Infection can occur up to 12 months post surgery (10). If the infection is identified immediately, it is possible to treat with antibiotics and avoid removal of hardware. In general, if the infection migrates to the hardware, it may be necessary to remove the equipment (10). The neurosurgeon will evaluate the extent of equipment removal. If the device has been removed due to infection, it is possible to reschedule the patient for DBS after the infection has resolved (11).

Skin Preparation

To reduce the occurrence of infection patients can prepare the skin for surgery using a surgical scrub, such as dynahex. The patient/family should be instructed to use the surgical scrub on the top of the head and around the area identified for implantation of the neurostimulator, for three days prior to surgery. Patients should avoid contact of the surgical scrub solution around the eyes. Shaving the head prior to surgery is discouraged, as there is not evidence to suggest that infections are reduced (10). However, the patient may choose a short hair cut prior to DBS surgery to assist in managing the care of the incisions in the postoperative stage.

Complications of Surgery

The complications associated with the surgery are listed in a Table subsequently. These include infection, intracranial hemorrhage (ICH), stroke, deep vein thrombosis (DVT), cardiac complications, anesthesia complication, seizures, and others (Table 1). These risks should be given considerable thought, as some complications can cause permanent damage. The patient/family should weigh these complications against the potential benefits. The patient should form an advanced directive before undergoing surgery (11).

Day of Surgery

Patients typically arrive for surgery early in the morning on the day of surgery. Orders have been given to the patient/family regarding nothing by mouth (NPO) status and what medications they may take with a sip of water prior to arriving at the hospital. Patients will be off Parkinson's medications for the surgical day. The rationale for being "off" medications is two-fold: (*i*) Dyskinesias can interfere

Table 1 Risks/Complications of Surgery

Infection—may result in device explantation
Pulmonary embolism, DVT
Subcortical hemorrhage
Stroke—loss of vision, weakness, paralysis, dysphagia, aphasia, and sensation loss
Seizure
Cerebrospinal fluid leak
Skin erosion
Memory loss or confusion
Personality change
Coma
Death
Anesthesia complications
Pneumonia
Heart attack
Pneumocephalus

Note: As with any major surgery, there is a risk of complications. Likelihood of complications is less than 10%, very serious complications is 3% to 4%.
Abbreviation: DVT, deep vein thrombosis.

with keeping the patient positioned correctly during the preparation for surgery and (*ii*) testing of the stimulator interoperatively should be done without influence of medications (see chap. 6). The patient should consult with neurosurgery regarding instructions for non-PD medications that are currently prescribed. Likewise, patients should be educated in the rare adverse reaction of neuroleptic malignant syndrome (NMS) related to holding dopaminergic medications (22). The symptoms of NMS include hyperthermia, severe muscle rigidity, change in loss of consciousness (LOC) status, tachycardia, diaphoresis, incontinence, and elevation of creatine kinase levels (12). Patients should be aware that this is a risk, and the development of these and other related symptoms should be treated as a medical emergency.

Inter-Op Education

During the surgery, the patient will be an active participant in assessing the efficacy of the DBS technology. The patient will be sedated during the drilling of the burr holes, but will be awake during the targeting of the subthalamic nucleus (STN) and positioning of the lead wires. In the operating room the patient may have the opportunity to hear the neurons fire and may be asked to perform motor tasks to assess PD-symptom response to lead placement. The purpose of evaluating motor tasks during surgery is to ensure optimal benefit of the lead positioning. The patient will be under general anesthetic for tunneling the connection wire and neurostimulator placement. Preparing the patient for this unique surgery is essential, as the patient will be able to contribute as an observer and participant. Patients will report hearing and sometimes feel the drilling of the burr hole. Remembering that the patient is awake for much of this surgical procedure is important, as they will be able to recall conversations heard in the operating room.

Having the surgery team aware of the patient's medical and surgical history can ensure that medications are managed appropriately in the operating room and postoperatively. The patient will be assessed for comfort and considered for anti-anxiety medications in the operating room. Keeping blood pressure managed is imperative in stabilizing intracranial pressure (Chap. 9).

Post-Op Teaching

Wound Care

Care of surgical wounds and prevention of infection is reviewed with the patient for care at home. Incisions should be kept clean and dry for the first week following surgery. Sutures and staples are typically removed seven to 10 days post-op. Swelling and bruising around the eyes, behind the ear, and around the neurostimulator is expected.

Headache

Headaches post-op are normal for post-op days and can last a week. The headaches should respond to acetaminophen. If acetaminophen does not relieve the headache, the patient/ family should be instructed on how to contact the treatment team.

Pulmonary Embolism

With neurosurgery, there is a risk reported, up to 25%, of patients of post-op deep vein thrombosis potentially leading to a pulmonary embolism (13). In an article reviewing methods of prevention of DVTs, mechanical prophylaxis is the best method, as heparin has the risk of causing postoperative intracranial hemorrhage (14).

Post-Lesioning Effect

Educating the patient/family in the phenomenon of post-lesioning effect is important in the preoperative phase. The post-lesioning effect may dramatically improve functioning after surgery and is a good indication of overall surgical outcome. Patients should understand post-lesioning effect can last seven days or longer and the return of PD symptoms, in the immediate postoperative phase is not an indication of poor surgical outcome (2). Although one goal of DBS surgery is to reduce the need for anti-Parkinson medications, the patient should be educated in the combination role of pharmaconetics with DBS therapy. Medications will continue to be part of the treatment strategy after surgery. Optimization of the combination of the DBS device and PD medications may take three to six months post surgery. This involves adjusting the setting of the device and reducing medications as necessary (15).

Activities of Daily Living

The recovery period varies depending on patient's response. General guidelines are listed in Table 2.

Weight Gain

Symptoms, such as dyskinesias, tremor, and rigidity may improve post surgery, decreasing caloric expenditure (16). Informing the patient of this risk, and discussing an exercise plan and diet modifications is appropriate presurgery.

Table 2 Guideline for Recovery/Activity

Precaution	Guideline
Lifting precautions	Nothing heavier than a gallon of milk for one month
Sexual relations	As tolerated
Driving	No driving for one month—reassess at one month
Working/employment	As tolerated
Shower/bathing	Hand held shower head may be useful to shower, careful to keep incisions dry. No cream rinses
Sun exposure	Wear a loose hat or head covering in the sun
Bowel habits	Increase fiber in diet, stool softener, no straining with bowel movements

Length of hospital stay depends on the patient status and surgery complications. On average, patients can anticipate a two to five day admission (see chap. 10). Post-op patients are not permitted to drive home from the hospital and should arrange an alternative method of transportation.

Assessment of Gait

It is important for the patient to realize that freezing of gait problems and falling will not generally improve with DBS surgery. If the symptoms did not respond to dopaminergic medication presurgery, there is no expectation that gait disturbances will improve post surgery. Physical-therapy referral is encouraged after surgery to retrain muscles, to teach normal gait mechanics, and strengthen muscles (15).

LONG-TERM STIMULATION MANAGEMENT: PATIENT EXPECTATIONS

The following section focuses on preparing the patient/family for expectations of living with PD after DBS surgery. By discussing this information with the patient/family in the preoperative stage, they will gain additional knowledge to prepare them for living successfully with DBS technology.

Food and Drug Administration MRI Warning (Table 3)

The Food and Drug Administration (FDA) has issued a warning regarding MRI interfering with DBS systems. An MRI scan is performed after DBS surgery is

Table 3 FDA/MRI Warning

FDA	Medtronic
FDA public health notice recommends that physicians "explain to the patient what MRI procedures are and stress that they must consult with the monitoring physician before having any MRI exam to find out whether it can be performed safely."	MRI systems generate powerful electromagnetic fields that can produce a number of interactions with implanted components of the active neurostimulation system. Some of these interactions, especially heating are potentially hazardous and can lead to serious injury or death. Implantation of the active brain stimulation system is contraindicated for patients who will be exposed to MRI using full body transmit radio frequency coil a receive-only head coil or a head transmit coil that extends over the chest area.

Abbreviation: FDA, Food and Drug Administration.
Source: Courtesy of the FDA and Medtronics.

Table 4   Diathermy Warning

Diathermy definition	Contraindication
Diathermy is the use of high frequency electrical current to generate heat within some part of the body for therapeutic indications. Energy from diathermy can be transferred throughout your implanted system, can cause tissue damage and can result in severe injury or death.	Shortwave diathermy, microwave diathermy, or therapeutic ultrasound diathermy (referred to as diathermy) is contraindicated with an implanted neurostimulation system. Injury can occur during diathermy treatment whether the neurostimulator system is turned on/off.

completed to assess lead placement and to rule out complications of surgery. This MRI is completed with a head coil, 1.5 Teslar MRI unit and the neurostimulator turned off and voltage set to zero. This is the only type of MRI procedure permitted post implantation. Patients should carry an FDA warning card and an ID card from the vendor of the device, wear a medic alert bracelet and tell health care providers about MRI precautions, in order to ensure compliance (17).

Diathermy Warning (Table 4)

Diathermy (the use of heat therapy) is contraindicated after surgery. Commonly, diathermy is used in dentistry, but can be used for other therapies. There is a serious risk that the diathermy therapy can produce heat, traveling up the connection wire and into the brain, resulting in destruction of brain tissue and possible death (18).

Emergency Cardiac Care (Table 5)

Automatic defibrillation has the potential to interfere with a DBS system causing dysfunction of the system and serious damage to the patient. If a cardiac arrest occurs and if time permits, the patient should be defibrillated using posterior-anterior positioning of cardiac pads (19). The use of a medic alert bracelet should be used as a tool to alert other health care providers about the DBS system. Patients should follow-up with their neurologist regarding cardioversion to evaluate the function of the neurostimulator system (20).

Table 5   Emergency Cardiac Warning

Damage to pulse generators may be caused by external defibrillation. In the event of a cardiac event:
   Adjust the voltage to zero and turn the device off if possible
   Place defibrillator pads at least two inches away from device
   Use anterior-posterior positioning of cardiac pads

Initial Programming

The timing of the initial programming session varies with the practice of each treatment team. Interoperatively, the neurosurgical team may have tested for efficacy of electrode placement and determined the contacts to be used in initial programming. This information can be helpful to the programmer in configuration of the electrodes for symptom management. Some teams choose to program immediately postoperatively with low voltage and others choose to delay programming until the postoperative lesioning effect has resolved (15).

The patient/family should be familiar with the staff assigned to programming the neurostimulator and be assured that the treatment team will be working collaboratively to optimize symptom control, and utilizing both DBS technology and traditional pharmacotherapy. Providing the patient with written instruction for programming sessions is helpful in setting the stage for their role in the treatment team (Table 6 programming).

The commitment to the long-term management of DBS technology should be discussed. The patient/family should receive information on the need for a long-term relationship with a health professional, skilled at programming the neurostimulator. Appointments for programming may be frequent in the first six months for programming and medication changes. Later, appointments may be scheduled as routine office visits in the years to follow. Although, there is some debate about the effects of DBS on the progression of PD, it is important to remind the patient/family that there is no present evidence to suggest that DBS arrests the progression of PD. Stimulation parameters will be adjusted for disease progression, just as medications have been adjusted prior to surgery.

Life span of the Kinetra neurostimulator is two to five years. The timing of neurostimulator replacement is dependent on parameters set by the programmer. At each programming session, the patient should be advised on the status of the

---

Table 6 Patient Education for Programming Sessions

The patient is an important member of the treatment team. The following guidelines are designed to assist the patient in being prepared for programming sessions.

Write down questions ahead of time to ask your heath care provider at the programming session.

Bring a list of all medications. Please include prescription medications, over the counter medications, herbals, vitamins, and supplements. Include the dose and what time you take the medications.

Get a good nights rest and eat before coming to the programming session.

Make a list of your most troublesome symptoms.

Call your health care provider before the initial programming session to ask if you should be "on" or "off" medications.

Allocate sufficient time to be at the programming session. Ask your provider for length of visit.

---

neurostimulator battery and the projected life. Thus loss of efficacy can be avoided with a planned outpatient surgical procedure to replace the neurostimulator in a timely manner before it becomes depleted.

The advances in DBS technology have led to the development of hand-held devices to assist the patient/family in stimulation management. In preoperative teaching the patient/family will benefit from an understanding of the hand-held device, which will be issued postoperatively. The hand-held technology available to the patient will be determined by the choice of equipment implanted by the neurosurgeon. For example, the Kinetra neurostimulator, manufactured by Medtronic, has a companion hand-held device that gives the patient the opportunity to adjust neurostimulator parameters: voltage, pulse width, and frequency (Fig. 2). The device has a lighted coding system to perform a system check on the neurostimulator. The hand-held devices are a remarkable addition in managing Parkinson's symptoms in the community, thus reducing unnecessary office visits and promoting patient independence in self care. However, as with PD medications, the patient/family should execute adjustments following specific guidelines discussed with their health care provider. Each hand-held device is accompanied by an instruction booklet, for patients.

Patient/families frequently have questions regarding environmental interference with DBS equipment. The most beneficial source of information on this topic is the Medtronic web site. This web site provides the patient/family with current information on commonly asked questions regarding living with DBS technology. The web site includes a patient manual, which explains how the DBS system works, tips for caregivers, risks, benefits, troubleshooting, and electrical interference. A table is provided in the Medtronic patient manual, which identifies common equipment and procedures that may produce electrical interference with the neurostimulator (Table 7).

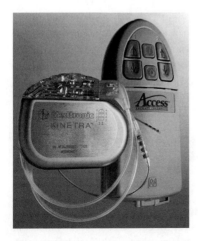

Figure 2 Neurostimulator and hand-held patient programmer. *Source*: Courtesy of Medtronic.

Table 7 Environmental Interference with Internal Pulse Generator Devices

The following is a sample of procedures and equipment identified as "likely" to produce
interference with the deep brain stimulation system
External defibrillation
Diathermy
Electric power generators
Lithotripsy
Ham radio antenna
Therapeutic magnets
Magnetic resonance imaging radiation therapy

Source: Courtesy of Medtronic.

Table 8 Educational Web Sites for Deep Brain Stimulation

Rewired for life, http://www.rewiredforlife.org
Medtronic, http://www.medtronic.com
Medic alert, http://www.medicalert.org

The most frequently asked questions from patients/families involve
routine medical procedures such as electrocardiogram (EKGs) and dental
work. Neurostimulators may cause electrical artifact with some portable
EKG monitors. The interference is greater in patients with bilateral neurostimulator implants. The procedure for decreasing the interference with the
EKG machine is to turn the neurostimulator off with the hand-held device.
The hand-held device should be used to turn the device on after the procedure is completed. Routine dental work can be performed with the use
of prophylactic antibiotics prior to dental procedures (21).

With rapidly changing technology, the World Wide Web has become a
valuable resource for patient education. The Medtronic Company maintains an
up-to-date website with information for patients and health professional.
Through the Medtronic portal, the patient can read the section on commonly
asked questions and locate health care professionals qualified to program neurostimulators. Rewired for Life is a nonprofit organization, which maintains a
website for patients/families who are interested in information on DBS.

REFERENCES

1. Levine C. Family caregivers: burdens and opportunities. In: Morrison RS, Meier DE,
   eds. Geriatric Palliative Care. New York: Oxford, 2003:376–385.
2. Sanghera MK, Desaloms JM, Stewart RM. High frequency stimulation of the
   subthalamic nucleus for the treatment of Parkinson's disease—a team perspective.
   J Neurosci Nurs 2004; 36(6):301–311.
3. Fahn S, Elton R, UPDRS Development Committee. Unified Parkinson's disease rating
   scale. In: Fahn S, Mardsen C, Calne D, Goldstein M, eds. Recent Developments in
   Parkinson's Disease. Flarham Park, New Jersey: Macmillan Healthcare Information,
   1987:153–163.

4. Goetz CG, Stebbins GT, Blasucci LM, Grobman MS. Efficacy of a patient-training videotape on motor fluctuations for on-off diaries in Parkinsons's disease. Mov Disord 1997; 12(6):1039–1041.
5. Reimer J, Grabowski M, Lindvall O, Hagell P. Use and interpretation of on/off diaries in Parkinson's disease. J Neurol Neurosurg Psychiat 2004; 75:396–400.
6. Defer GL, Widner H, Marie RM, Reny P, Levivier M, and the Conference Participants. Core assessment program for surgical interventional therapies in Parkinson's disease (CAPSIT-PD). Mov Disord 1999; 14:572–584.
7. Voon V, Saint-Cyr J, Lozano AM, Moro E, Poon YY, Lang AE. Psychiatric symptoms in patients with Parkinson's disease presenting for deep brain stimulation surgery. J Neurosurg 2005; 103(2):246–251.
8. Sage JI. Pain in Parkinson's disease. Current Treatment Option in Neurology 2004; 6:191–200.
9. Crane MK, Wittink M, Doukas DJ. Respecting end-of-life treatment preferences. Am Fam Physician 2005; 72:1263–1268, 1270.
10. Umemura A, Jaggi JL, Hurtig HI, Siderowf AD, Colcher A, Stern MB, Baltuch GH. Deep brain stimulation for movement disorders: morbidity and mortality in 109 patients. J Neurosurg 2003; 98:779–784.
11. Lyons KE, Wilkinson SB, Overman J, Pahwa R. Surgical and hardware complications of subthalamic stimulation. Neurology 2004; 63:612–616.
12. Nicholson D, Chiu W. Neuroleptic malignant syndrome. Geriatrics 2004; 59(8): 36, 38–40.
13. Browd SR, Ragel BT, Davis GE, Scott AM, Skalabrin EJ, Couldwell WT. Prophylaxis for deep venous thrombosis in neurosurgery: a review of the literature. Neurosurg Focus 2004; 17(4):E1.
14. Stewart RM, Desaloms JM, Sanghera MK. Stimulation of the subthalamic nucleus for the treatment of Parkinson's disease: postoperative management, programming, and rehabilitation. J Neurosci Nurs 2005; 27(2):108–114.
15. Danish SF, Burnett MG, Ong JG, Sonnad SS, Maloney-Wilensky E, Stein SC. Prophylaxis for deep venous thrombosis in craniotomy patients: a decision analysis. Neurosurgery 2005; 56(6):1286–1292.
16. Macia F, Perlemoine C, Coman I, Guehl D, Burbaud D, Cuny E, et al. Parkinson's disease patients with bilateral subthalamic deep brain stimulation gain weight. Mov Disord 2004; 19(2):206–212.
17. Medtronic Deep Brain Stimulation 3387, 3389 Implant Manual. Minneapolis: Medtronic, 2005.
18. Henderson JM, Tkach J, Phillips M, Baker K, Shellock FG, Rezai AR. Permanent neurological deficit related to magnetic resonance imaging in a patient with implanted deep brain stimulation electrodes for Parkinson's disease: a case report. Neurosurgery 2005; 57(5):E1063.
19. Heath S. The Emergency Care of the Patient with Deep Brain Implants. Unpublished procedure. Department of Veterans Affairs, San Francisco VA Medical Center PADRECC: San Francisco, California, 2001.
20. Yamamoto T, Katayama Y, Fukaya C, Kurihara J, Oshima H, Kasai M. Thalamotomy caused by cardioversion in a patient treated with deep brain stimulation. Sterotactic Func Neurosurg 2000; 74:73–82.
21. Medtronic Patient Manual: Your Activa Therapy. Minneapolis: Medtronic, 2003.
22. Ward, C. Neuroleptic malignant syndrome in a patients with Parkinson's disease: a case study. J Neurosci Nurs 2005; 37(3):160–162.

5

Surgical Technique for Leksell Frame Based Deep Brain Stimulation of the Subthalamic Nucleus

Uzma Samadani

*Department of Neurosurgery, Hospital of the University of Pennsylvania,
Philadelphia, Pennsylvania, U.S.A.*

Shabbar F. Danish

*Department of Neurosurgery, Hospital of the University of Pennsylvania, and
Department of Bioengineering, University of Pennsylvania,
Philadelphia, Pennsylvania, U.S.A.*

**Jurg L. Jaggi, Santiagio Figuereo, and
Gordon H. Baltuch**

*Department of Neurosurgery, Hospital of the University of Pennsylvania,
Philadelphia, Pennsylvania, U.S.A.*

INTRODUCTION

With 3000 deep brain stimulation procedures performed annually in the United States alone, technique for the procedure will clearly have some variability. In this chapter, we will describe our technique using the Leksell frame and Medtronics Stealth Station image guidance systems for implantation of unilateral or bilateral subthalamic deep brain stimulator leads. We will also describe how we perform placement and connection of the internal pulse generator. This protocol can be adapted for use with other frames and systems.

PREOPERATIVE PREPARATION

Patients are instructed not to take aspirin, plavix, coumadin, or other hemolytic agents for an appropriate interval prior to the surgery in order to ensure normal coagulation during the perioperative period. Parkinsonian medications are discontinued either the night prior or the morning of surgery depending on the

71

severity and quality of the patient's symptoms. Other medications, and in particular those for blood pressure, are administered the morning of the surgery.

Due to the risk of thrombo-embolic event in the perioperative period (1,2),
we administer 5000 units of subcutaneous heparin and place TED hose (Tyco
Healthcare, Mansfried, Massachusetts, U.S.A.) upon admission to the hospital
on the day of surgery, which is approximately one hour prior to frame placement.
Intravenous lines are placed and perioperative antibiotics are administered prior
to entering the operating room.

LEKSELL FRAME FIXATION

In the operating room, viscous lidocaine saturated cotton is used to anesthetize the
ear canal, while telemetry, pulse oximetry, and cuff blood pressure monitoring
devices are placed. The preassembled Leksell G-frame (Elekta Instruments, Atlanta,
Georgia, U.S.A.) is then temporarily held with ear bars to the patient's head under
conscious sedation using propofol with the patient in the sitting position propped
with pillows. The tilt of the Leksell frame is parallel to the lateral canthal-meatal
line, which is itself parallel to the anterior commissure-posterior commissure
(AC-PC) line. The scalp areas for the four pin sites are cleansed with topical
alcohol and infiltrated with lidocaine/marcaine. The frame is then fixed via four
sharp pins at these sites and the temporary ear bars are removed. Ideal frame placement centered at the midline and parallel to the canthal-meatal line will result in no
pitch (up/down), roll (tilt), or yaw (turning right or left) displacement. The magnetic
resonance imaging (MRI) localizer is attached to the frame and the patient is taken
for MRI with telemetry monitoring after placement of a Foley catheter.

MAGNETIC RESONANCE IMAGING

Imaging for targeting is performed using a 1.5 Tesla MRI unit (Signa, General
Electric) (3). The optimal modes for visualization of target anatomy are the
fast spin echo inversion recovery and the standard T2 weighted sequences. If
the surgeon additionally wishes to make a three-dimensional model of the
cortex showing surface vessels, as seen in Figure 1, for planning of the coronal
burr hole entry point, then gadolinium-enhanced images should also be obtained.

Sagittal images are obtained first, to identify the AC-PC line. The scan
angle is then set such that axial images are obtained parallel to the AC-PC
line, and coronal images are obtained orthogonal to it. Details of the scanning
parameters are given in Table 1.

TARGETING VIA INDIRECT LOCALIZATION ACCORDING
TO THE SCHALTENBRAND ATLAS

First, the anterior commissure and posterior commissure are identified and the
distance between the two points is measured. This intercommisural length
should approximate 24 to 30 mm.

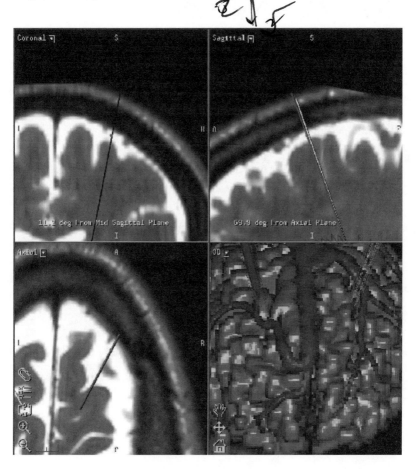

Figure 1   In the *lower right* quadrant, a gadolinum-enhanced reconstruction of the cortex is shown. Appropriate thresholding allows visualization of the superficial veins, aiding proper placement of the burr hole. (*See color insert.*)

Next, we determine the frame coordinates of the anterior and posterior commissure. Beginning with an axial section parallel to the AC-PC line superior to the level of the subthalalmic nucleus (STN), straight crosshairs are drawn from the corners of the Leksell frame to establish the midpoint of the frame, as seen in Figure 2. In an ideal scenario, the frame is perfectly centered on the head, but more often small allowances have to be made. By convention, the center of the Leksell frame is designated with coordinates 100, 100, 100 in the X, Y, and Z planes. X increases in value to the left, Y increases in value moving anterior, and Z increases in value moving inferior. The anterior and posterior commissure can then be assigned values by measuring their distance from the center of the frame. For example, if the frame is off center by two millimeters to the left, which means the AC-PC line is 2 mm to the right, then the resulting X for

Table 1 Magnetic Resonance Imaging Parameters for Preoperative Localization of the Subthalamic Nucleus

Sequence	Scan timing	Scanning range	Acquisition timing
Sagittal T1	TE = 23	FOV = 27	Freq = 256
	TR = 34	Sl-Th = 4	Phase = 192
	ETL = 2		NEX = 2
	RBW = 15.63		
Oblique inversion recovery	TE = 30	FOV = 27	Freq = 256
	TR = 4000	Sl-Th = 2.0	Phase = 192
	TI = 180		NEX = 2
	ETL = 18		
	RBW = 15.63		
Axial T2	TE = 90	FOV = 27	Freq = 256
	TR = 3000	Sl-Th = 2.5	Phase = 224
	ETL = 7		NEX = 2
	RBW = 15.63		
Coronal T2	TE = 130	FOV = 27	Freq = 256
	TR = 2500	Sl-Th = 2.5	Phase = 224
	ETL = 14		NEX = 3
	RBW = 15.63		
Post gadolinium T1	TE = 23	FOV = 27	Freq = 256
	Flip = 10	Sl-Th = 1.3	Phase = 256
	RBW = 31.25		NEX = 2

Abbreviations: ETL, echo train length; FOV, field of view; Freq, frequency; NEX, number of excitations; RBW, receiver band width; Sl-Th, slice thickness (in mm); TE, echo time; TR, time to repetition.

both AC and PC will be 102 (Fig. 2). The difference between the Y values from AC to PC by definition must equal the intercommissural length. For example, if the intercommissural length is 28 mm, and AC is at a Y of 116, PC should be measured at a Y of 88. The Z distance is obtained by adding 40 mm to the average of the height of the section measured at the frame on each side (Fig. 2).

The midcommissural point is the point at the center of the AC-PC line. The STN should be located 12 mm lateral, 2 mm posterior, and 5 mm inferior to this point. As an example, if the X for AC and PC is 99, the target STN X on the left would be 111 and for the right STN X would be 87. Occasionally, in a smaller or more scaphocephalic head we will adjust the lateral distance to 11 mm, and in a larger head we will adjust to 13 mm laterally. Target STN Y can be obtained either by averaging the AC and PC Y values then subtracting 2, or by adding half the intercommissural distance minus 2 to the PC Y value. For example, if AC Y is 116 and PC Y is 88, then STN target Y is 100. The STN Z value is obtained by adding 5 to an average of the AC and PC Z values. If for example,

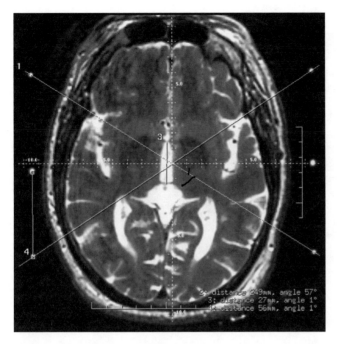

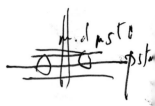

Figure 2 AC and PC coordinates are obtained via manual targeting at the magnetic resonance imaging console. The intersection of the cross hairs indicates the center location of the frame. Lateral, anterior–posterior and superior–inferior offsets are measured as outlined in the text.

the AC and PC Z values are both 92 (and hence the midcommissural point has a Z of 92), then the target Z value will be 97 mm.

TARGETING VIA DIRECT LOCALIZATION ON THE MRI SCAN

The principle behind direct targeting is that a straight line drawn through the anterior margin of the red nucleus will bisect the STN as shown in Figure 3. Also, a line drawn through the middle of the red nucleus will lie at the posterior edge of the STN.

Direct targeting is not used to calculate the target STN X value, since this is calculated to be 12 mm from the midline. Direct localization to calculate the target STN Y and Z values can be performed on both the axial and coronal MRI. Crosshairs are drawn to identify the center of the frame. A straight line is then drawn through the anterior margin of the red nucleus and the distance from the center of the frame to the straight line is measured to obtain the target Y value. The Z value is obtained by measuring the height at the sides of the frame, and averaging these two values and adding 340 mm to obtain the height in the center.

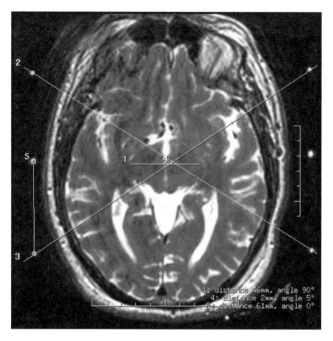

Figure 3 A tangent drawn at the anterior border of the red nuclei intersects subthalamic nucleus (STN) and permits an independent assessment of the anterior–posterior as well as superior–inferior coordinates of STN.

TARGETING WITH THE STEALTH

The coordinates for the STN target can also be obtained with FrameLink Software for the Medtronic (Minneapolis, Minnesota, U.S.A.) Stealth-Navigation System. The MRI is uploaded into the Stealth Station computer and the coordinates of the stereotactic frame, anterior commissure, and posterior commissure are registered. The computer then calculates the coordinates of the bilateral STN targets in the X, Y, and Z planes.

We generally use a point on the coronal suture at the mid-pupillary line as our entry point. This provisional entry point is marked on the MRI image so that a simulated trajectory can be visualized going through the cortex on the MRI scan. We use a three-dimensional reconstruction of the cortex and its overlying veins to avoid placing our entry point directly on top of a large vein (Fig. 1). The azimuth (medial–lateral) and declimation (anterior–posterior) angles for the entry point to the target are then calculated by the computer and manually adjusted as needed. In an ideal simulated trajectory, the electrode traverses gyri rather than sulci en route to the target to minimize the risk of local hemorrhage. In patients with large ventricles, the simulated trajectory will almost invariably traverse the ventricle. We attempt to minimize the loss of cerebrospinal fluid (CSF) during the operation to prevent ventricular collapse and brain shift via placement of gelfoam over the entry point. We do not generally move the burr hole laterally to avoid the ventricle.

The Stealth system software can also superimpose a digitized Schaltenbrand and Wahren Atlas image on the MRI scan from the patient, as shown in Figure 4. This superimposed image can be used as a framework to assess the accuracy of the Stealth coordinates.

The coordinates obtained through indirect, direct, and Stealth guided methods are then compared. Some evidence suggests that targeting based on the red nucleus is most reliable for STN localization (4,5), so we tend to weigh the direct localization data most heavily in determining the optimal target coordinates.

PLACEMENT OF THE GUIDING CANNULA

Upon return from MRI to the operating room the patient is positioned supine with the head slightly flexed and fixed with a frame adapter in the Mayfield head-holder. Mild propofol sedation may be administered for patient comfort and

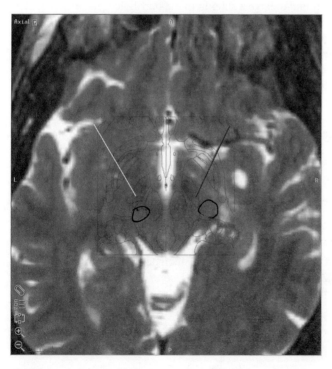

Figure 4 A typical overlay of the Schaltenbrandt and Wahren atlas on a T2 weighted axial magnetic resonance imaging scan on Framelink. Subthalamic and the red nuclei are clearly visible allowing for direct targeting parameters.

oxygen is given by nasal cannula. Additional lidocaine/marcaine is injected into each of the four pin sites to prevent pain during the duration of the operation. We do not generally shave any hair at the incision sites as this has not been demonstrated to decrease infection rates (6,7). Surgical lubricant and combs are used to create hair partings at the suture lines prior to sterile preparation and draping. The stereotactic arc is set according to the X, Y, and Z coordinates and attached to the Leksell frame. Round target markers (cross hairs) for fluoroscopic visualization are attached to the arc and the fluoroscope is draped and checked for optimal positioning to obtain a true lateral head image with the center of the target at the STN target.

Sagittal linear skin incisions are made extending approximately 3 to 4 cm anterior and 1 to 2 cm posterior to the coronal suture after infiltration with lidocaine. A 14 mm diameter burr hole is made with a perforating drill, just anterior to the coronal suture at the site recommended by Stealth planning. The silastic burr hole ring from the Medtronic lead kit (DBS lead 3389) that will ultimately be used for immobilizing the lead is applied to the burr hole to ensure secure fit, and then removed. If the ring does not fit, as is occasionally the case for patients with very thin skulls, a small cutting burr on a drill is used to expand the inner table until the ring is found to have a snug fit in the burr hole. The dura is cauterized and opened sharply and the underlying pia is also cauterized. The needle guide is brought into alignment with the pial opening and the actual azimuth and declimation angles of approach are obtained from the arc and entered on the Stealth Station computer. The simulated trajectory is then obtained from the Stealth Station and again confirmed to avoid traversing sulcal vessels.

When the procedure is to be performed bilaterally, we make both incisions and burr holes, prior to opening to the dura on the first side, to avoid loss of CSF.

The guiding cannula with its stylet is then inserted into the brain slowly and gently until 15 mm above the target as confirmed with fluoroscopy. The stylet is removed and the recording microelectrode is inserted and attached to its drive.

After the burr holes are completed, all propofol sedation is stopped and the patient is slowly wakes up. By the time microelectrode recordings are initiated, the patient will be able to speak clearly and follow basic instructions throughout recording and intraoperative macrostimulation. During the microelectrode recording period all electronic equipment that can interfere with the recording signal is turned off or is unplugged. These include the operating and room lights, Bovie, bipolar machines, the sequential compression devices, and even the operating room table itself. The suction is also shut off to minimize noise contamination of the acoustic recording signal.

MICROELECTRODE RECORDING

Anatomical localization based on the MRI scan pinpoints the STN target within a few millimeters, and microelectrode recording further increases the accuracy to enable placement of the DBS lead at the center of the STN. The microelectrodes we utilize have a tungsten tip diameter of approximately 10 microns and impedance of 1 MΩ at 1000 Hz (FHC Inc. Bowdoinham, ME.) At 15 mm above the STN target we begin recording. As the microelectrode is advanced in 0.1 mm increments, filtered action potentials generate a signal displayed on a screen, which is also fed to an audio amplifier for sound monitoring. Fluoroscopic confirmation of the target approach is obtained at 5 mm intervals, 2 mm before target, and target. Structures traversed during microelectrode recording en route to the STN include the zona reticulata and zona incerta. The STN is identifiable by increased neuronal firing of large asymmetrical spikes and lower rate biphasic spikes. We further advance the electrode through the STN to the substantia nigra pars reticulata (SNr) in order to estimate the length of STN traversed by each trajectory. Additional confirmation of the target is obtained by sensorimotor stimulation of the contralateral limbs, which increases neuronal firing at the STN. Generally, the target point is moved slightly, if necessary, according to the functional mapping of the first trajectory. A separate chapter of this text is devoted to microelectrode recording for STN DBS.

INTRAOPERATIVE MACROSTIMULATION

Following anatomic localization and microelectrode recording to physiologically confirm the target, the electrode is removed and the burr hole ring is applied. The DBS lead is placed through the cannula and slowly advanced to the target from 10 mm above, under direct fluoroscopic guidance. The DBS lead has four contacts (0–3), and generally the most distal of these (0) is placed at or just slightly beyond the target point. The Medtronic Model 3387 and 3389 DBS leads both have four contacts measuring 1.5 mm in length. The 3387 leads are spaced 1.5 mm apart and the 3389 leads are 0.5 mm apart to enable more contact within the STN. One case report suggests greater success stimulating pre-STN to suppress levodopa-induced dyskinesias with the 3389 (8). We generally use the Model 3389 DBS for our patients with PD.

Once the DBS lead has been placed at target, it is connected to a hand-held pulse generator for macrostimulation. The stimulation voltage is slowly increased while the patient is being assessed for PD symptom relief. The patient is asked to recite speech and report any parasthesias. The stimulation voltage is further increased to find the threshold value for side effects. To guard against signal spread into the internal capsule, low frequency stimulation (5 Hz) is also performed which should not elicit any tonic contraction. If there are no adverse effects of stimulation, then the lead is carefully held in place while the cannula and stylet are removed. Under direct fluoroscopic visualization to prevent movement, the lead is secured to the burr hole ring and the cover is applied to fix its position.

In cases where bilateral lead placement is to be performed, attention is then shifted to the other side of the brain, where the second lead is placed with similar technique. After both leads have been placed, the anesthesiologists are informed that they may liberalize sedation to make the patient comfortable.

If the procedure is performed bilaterally, one lead is carefully tunneled so that its connector is brought out into the contralateral incision. The residual lead length from the tunneled lead is coiled around its ipsilateral burr hole cover to avoid having too much lead under the incision. The incision on the tunneled side is then copiously irrigated with half-strength Betadine® mixed with saline and closed with interrupted vicryl sutures on galea and staples on skin, with meticulous attention to avoid catching the traversing lead with a stitch. The second incision, with a short length of the contralateral lead and the ipsilateral lead coiled around its own burr hole cover, is also irrigated with Betadine®, and temporarily closed with a single vicryl stitch through the galea at the center of the incision and staples for the skin. The Leksell head frame is removed in preparation for implantation of the internal pulse generator (IPG).

IMPLANTATION OF THE PROGRAMMABLE INTERNAL PULSE GENERATOR

General endotracheal anesthesia is administered for the implantation phase of the procedure. A small retroauricular area is shaved on the side where the IPG is to be implanted and the head, neck, and infraclavicular regions are prepared and draped. The scalp incision with both leads is reopened. The leads are carefully disentangled so that tunneling may be performed without dislodging them. A 4 cm separate incision is made 5 to 6 cm inferior and parallel to the clavicle after infiltration with local anesthetic. A tunneler is passed first from the cranial parasagittal incision to a separate retroauricular stab incision and subsequently from the retroauricular to the infraclavicular incision. An extension lead is tunneled through from chest to burr hole and then attached to the DBS lead with a silicon boot to cover the connection. The internal pulse generator is connected to the extension wires and placed in the infraclavicular pocket. Copious irrigation with Betadine®/saline is performed and the incisions are closed in two layers. We use staples on the head and running subcuticular biosyn for the infraclavicular pocket. Anesthesia is reversed and the patient is taken to the recovery room after extubation.

POSTOPERATIVE CARE

After recovery from anesthesia the patient is taken for MRI to confirm appropriate placement of DBS leads and absence of any bleed. Patients are monitored in the intensive care unit overnight, restarted on all parkinsonian medications, and transferred to the neurosurgical floor on the first postoperative day. Antibiotics are administered intravenously for two days following the surgery and subcutaneous heparin injection is performed twice daily. Patients are discharged from the hospital on postoperative day two, or referred for rehabilitation as desired. The stimulators are turned on at suture removal approximately 10 days after implantation. Patients are subsequently re-evaluated several times after surgery for reprogramming of the stimulator to optimize symptomatology. After adequate symptom relief is attained, the patient is followed at 6 to 12 months intervals.

REFERENCES

1. Thobois S, Mertens P, Guenot M, et al. Subthalamic nucleus stimulation in Parkinson's disease: clinical evaluation of 18 patients. J Neurol 2002; 249(5):529–534.
2. Umemura A, Jaggi JL, Hurtig HI, et al. Deep brain stimulation for movement disorders: morbidity and mortality in 109 patients. J Neurosurg 2003; 98(4):779–784.
3. Simon SL, Douglas P, Baltuch GH, Jaggi JL. Error analysis of MRI and Leksell stereotactic frame target localization in deep brain stimulation surgery. Stereotact Funct Neurosurg 2005; 83(1):1–5.
4. Andrade-Souza YM, Schwalb JM, Hamani C, et al. Comparison of three methods of targeting the subthalamic nucleus for chronic stimulation in Parkinson's disease. Neurosurgery 2005; 56(suppl 2):360–368, discussion 360–368.
5. Pollo C, Meuli R, Maeder P, Vingerhoets F, Ghika J, Villemure JG. Subthalamic nucleus deep brain stimulation for Parkinson's disease: magnetic resonance imaging targeting using visible anatomical landmarks. Stereotact Funct Neurosurg 2003; 80(1-4):76–81.
6. Sheinberg MA, Ross DA. Cranial procedures without hair removal. Neurosurgery 1999; 44(6):1263–1265, discussion 1265–1266.
7. Winston KR. Hair and neurosurgery. Neurosurgery 1992; 31(2):320–329.
8. Alterman RL, Shils JL, Gudesblatt M, Tagliati M. Immediate and sustained relief of levodopa-induced dyskinesias after dorsal relocation of a deep brain stimulation lead. Case report. Neurosurg Focus 2004; 17(1):E6.

6

Frameless Stereotaxy for Placement of Deep Brain Stimulators

Gregory G. Heuer, Jurg L. Jaggi, Gordon H. Baltuch, and John Y. K. Lee

Department of Neurosurgery, Hospital of the University of Pennsylvania, Philadelphia, Pennsylvania, U.S.A.

Over the past decade computer-based neuronavigation systems have found a greater role in the neurosurgery operating room (OR). Particularly in neuro-oncologic surgery, frameless systems have become increasingly used to guide and provide volumetric tumor resections (1–9). These systems provide the surgeon with the intraoperative ability to correlate the operative anatomy to the preoperative imaging. To utilize these systems, the patient undergoes specialized preoperative imaging. This imaging is then registered into a computer platform to generate a three-dimensional image that can be used in the operating room. These frameless neuronavigation systems have been shown to be particularly useful in defining normal anatomy and in tailoring resections, and have accuracy comparable to frame based systems (10). Additionally, systems have been modified to guide the placement of biopsy needles into target lesions (11–14). Studies on frameless image guided needle biopsies have demonstrated that such systems can be accurate to the millimeter scale (15). Because of the successful experience with needle-guided biopsies, these systems were thought to be potentially applicable to the placement of deep brain stimulator leads.

The current standard for target localization in placement of deep brain stimulator leads is frame-based, commonly utilizing a Cosman-Roberts-Wells or Leksell frames. During a typical frame based procedure the patient is brought into the operating room where a frame is rigidly attached to the patient's skull. Next, the patient is imaged by CT or magnetic resonance imaging (MRI), and the stereotaxic coordinates and target are defined. The target can be set in three ways: indirect localization of target based on the AC-PC line; direct localization of the visualized target; and a combination of the two. The target, entry point, and trajectory are set on the day of the surgery by the surgical team. The frame allows for great flexibility in the choice of these three variables.

Recent advances in computer-based systems may allow for replacement of frame-based lead placement. There are currently two types of frameless systems being used, a platform based system and a complete frameless system. Additionally, direct placement of leads using intraoperative imaging has been tested.

Platform Systems

When a platform system is used, a custom prosthesis is individually manufactured for each patient, in essence generating a miniature stereotaxic head frame for each patient. The prototypical platform system is the MicroTargeting Platform System with STarFix Guidance (FHC Inc, Bowdoinham, Maine, U.S.A.) (16).

The use of such a system involves multiple steps. Preoperatively, a number of mounting anchors (Acustar, Z-Kat, Inc., Hollywood, Florida, U.S.A.) are placed into the skull of the patient surrounding the presumptive burr hole location. The bone anchors must be placed in an outpatient setting and can be placed one to two weeks prior to the definitive surgery.

Next, locator pins are placed into the bone anchors and a CT scan is performed to register the anchors. Most frameless systems utilize bone fudicials to register the patient's head and brain into stereotaxic space. Unlike the skin, applied-fudicial markers often used for neuro-oncologic procedures, these fudicials are rigidly attached to the skull. Preoperative MRI and CT scans are obtained and a CT-MR fusion is performed on the workstation in order to define the stereotaxic target. On the workstation, a virtual platform is generated based on the location of the bone fudicials and the intended target (Fig. 1). This data file is then downloaded and sent to the manufacturer. The manufacturer (FHC Inc, Bowdoinham, ME) creates a custom platform that is then shipped to the neurosurgeon in one to three days for sterilization and use.

The day of the surgery, the patient is brought into the operating room and the custom platform is attached to the skull of the patient via the mounting anchors (Fig. 2A). The micro-electrode recording instruments and micro-drive are then attached to the platform and the standard placement of the electrode and leads are performed.

In a clinical study of this type of design, 21 patients had electrodes implanted (9 unilateral and 12 bilateral), of which 20 implanted electrodes could be studied, the remainder of the implanted electrodes could not be studied due to technical

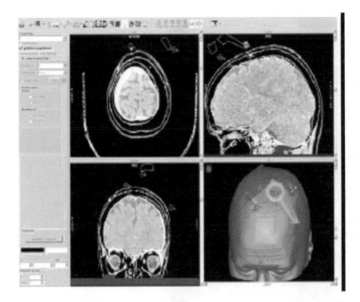

Figure 1 Workstation generation of virtual platform. (*See color insert.*)

errors with the postoperative scans. The authors found that the mean absolute electrode placement error is below 2.7 mm, which the authors found comparable to similar studies preformed for the Leksell frame (17).

Complete Frameless Stereotaxic Systems

A second design for frameless stereotaxic is the use of a skull mounted guide. Unlike the previously described platform system that utilizes a miniature frame, these systems more closely resemble those systems utilized for volumetric resection of brain tumors or stereotaxic biopsies. In oncologic procedures, fudicials, which can be visualized on preoperative imaging, are placed on the patient. Next, when the patient is secured in the operating room, the location of the fudicials are registered with optical laser or magnetic field, and in doing so the location of the skull and brain is also registered.

A prototypical frameless system is the NeXframe (Image Guided Neurologics, Inc., Melbourne, Florida, U.S.A.). Similar to the platform system, patients have bone-mounted fudicials (Stryker-Leibinger, Kalamazoo, MI, U.S.A.) placed in the outpatient setting, although the fudicials can be placed the same day as the surgery. Small skin incisions are made in five locations on the head of the patient and a screw is placed into the skull of the patient. These screws can be seen on CT scans and therefore serve as fudicials on the preoperative scans. Rigid bone fudicial markers are used as it is felt that they provide greater accuracy compared to the rather mobile skin fudicials. The patient

(A)

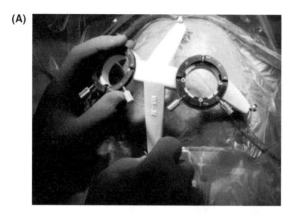

(B)

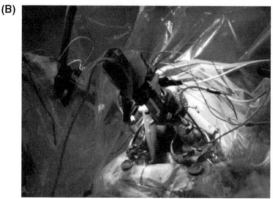

Figure 2 Intraoperative use of platform system: (**A**) attachment of platform to bone anchors and (**B**) attachment of micro-drive and recording equipment to the platform. (*See color insert.*)

undergoes preoperative CT and MRI scans. Unlike the platform-based system, no custom prosthesis needs to be manufactured, therefore the scans can be pre-formed either days before or on the same day as the surgical procedure. As with the platform system, an MRI and CT-MR fusion are performed on the work-station in order to define the stereotaxic target.

The patient is then brought into the operation room where a skull-mounted trajectory guide is placed over the burr hole (Fig. 3A). The bone-mounted fudi-cials are then registered into an image-guided workstation using an optical laser system (Fig. 3B) (ex. Stealth Station, Medtronic Inc., Minneapolis, Minnesota, U.S.A.). The target is localized directly and the trajectory to this target is then determined on the workstation platform (Fig. 4).

When tested in a laboratory setting in a plastic skull phantom model, this type of system has been shown to be accurate, with a mean localization error of 1.25 mm. (18,19). In a clinical study using such a system 38 patients were

(A)

(B)

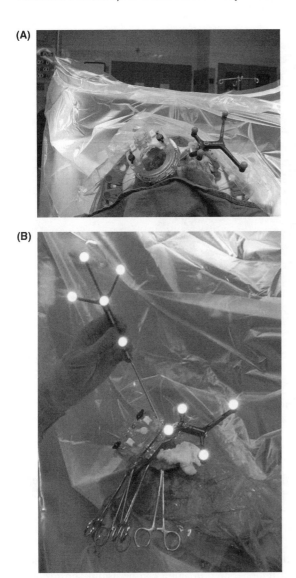

Figure 3   (**A**) Skull-mounted trajectory guide with attached optical image-guidance arc. (**B**) Registration of guide and skull mounted fudicials using an optical system. *Source*: From Ref. 20. (*See color insert.*)

implanted (47 electrodes total), of which 42 cases were analyzed postoperatively (20). The authors compared the placement of the electrodes using the Leksell frame and the frameless system and found no significant difference in the accuracy of the two groups. The error in the actual and expected lead locations was

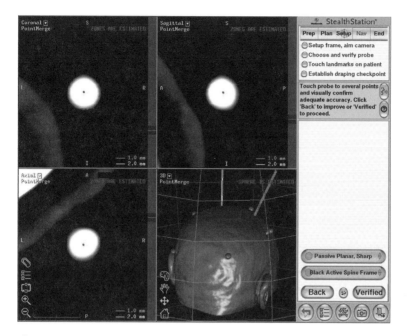

Figure 4   Image guidance platform for determination of trajectory. *Source*: From Ref. 20. (*See color insert.*)

found to be greatest in the Z-plane, 1.7 mm in the frame-based group and 2.0 mm in the frameless group.

INTRAOPERATIVE MAGNETIC RESONANCE GUIDANCE

Both frame based systems and the previously described systems rely on preoperative imaging for localization. Because of this reliance, these systems are unable to account for brain shift that may occur during surgery.

Intraoperative MRI has been used to guide and tailor resections of brain tumors (21,22) and in other types of functional surgery (23,24). The MRI for these procedures is performed during the surgical procedure. The results of these and other studies suggest that intraoperative imaging can be useful and result in more complete resection of intracranial pathology and less complications.

One study has been performed utilizing intraoperative MRI for placement of deep brain stimulators (25). In this study, the authors utilized a modified skull-mounted trajectory guide. A similar modified system has been used for intraoperative MRI guided brain biopsies (26). A fluid-filled stem is attached to the trajectory guide with a spherical tip that can be imaged and used to align the guide to the proper trajectory for the imaged target. Next, a titanium mandrel is passed down the trajectory and its location confirmed with imaging. Lastly, a peel away sheath is passed down the mandrel to serve as a conduit for the lead, and then the lead is passed and its location confirmed with imaging.

In skull phantoms, such a system had a maximum error of 2 mm. The system was then tested in five patients, in the placement of a total of eight electrodes. The lead was correctly placed in seven of the eight patients on the first pass; one lead required a second pass to placement. The mean error on the first pass was 1 mm with a range of 0.1 to 1.8 mm.

DISCUSSION

These frameless systems have not replaced frame-based systems at most centers. The frame-based systems have flexibility in adjusting the entry point, trajectory, and the target by adjusting the coordinates on the frame, intraoperatively. The frameless systems do not yet have as much freedom in adjustment. Also, unlike frameless systems, the final target can be easily confirmed with fluoroscopy when a frame is used.

Frameless systems have some advantages over traditional frame-based systems. Patient comfort may be higher with these systems because there is not a large frame attached to the patient during the entire procedure. Also, the total OR time may be reduced with these systems as the imaging and some of the operative planning can be and in some instances must be performed prior to bringing the patient to the OR. Lastly, these systems have a number of disposable units, reducing the concern for general wear on the equipment.

The application of frameless systems to placement of deep brain stimulators is still in the development stage. As these systems evolve, they have the possibility to increase accuracy, patient comfort, and possibly patient outcome.

REFERENCES

1. Gumprecht HK, Widenka DC, Lumenta CB. BrainLab VectorVision Neuronavigation system: technology and clinical experiences in 131 cases. Neurosurgery 1999; 44(1):97–104, discussion 5.
2. Linskey ME. The changing role of stereotaxis in surgical neuro-oncology. Journal of Neuro-Oncology 2004; 69(1–3):35–54.
3. Haberland N, Ebmeier K, Hliscs R, et al. Neuronavigation in surgery of intracranial and spinal tumors. J Cancer ResClin Oncol 2000; 126(9):529–541.
4. Lee JY, Lunsford LD, Subach BR, Jho HD, Bissonette DJ, Kondziolka D. Brain surgery with image guidance: current recommendations based on a 20-year assessment. Stereotact Funct Neurosurg 2000; 75(1):35–48.
5. Spetzger U, Laborde G, Gilsbach JM. Frameless neuronavigation in modern neurosurgery. Minim Invas Neurosurg 1995; 38(4):163–166.
6. Sipos EP, Tebo SA, Zinreich SJ, Long DM, Brem H. In vivo accuracy testing and clinical experience with the ISG viewing wand. Neurosurgery 1996; 39:194–203.
7. Golfinos JG, Fitzpatrick BC, Smith LR, Spetzler RF. Clinical use of a frameless stereotactic arm: results of 325 cases. J Neurosurg 1995; 83(2):197–205.
8. Barnett GH, Kormos DW, Steiner CP, Weisenberger J. Use of a frameless, armless stereotactic wand for brain tumor localization with two-dimensional and three-dimensional neuroimaging. Neurosurgery 1993; 33(4):674–678.

9. Reinhardt HF, Horstmann GA, Gratzl O. Sonic stereometry in microsurgical procedures for deep-seated brain tumors and vascular malformations. Neurosurgery 1993; 32(1):51–57.

10. Dorward NL, Alberti O, Palmer JD, Kitchen ND, Thomas DG. Accuracy of true frameless stereotaxy: in vivo measurement and laboratory phantom studies. Technical note. J Neurosurg 1999; 90(1):160–168.

11. Grunert P, Espinosa J, Busert C, et al. Stereotactic biopsies guided by an optical navigation system: technique and clinical experience. Minim Invas Neurosurg 2002; 45(1):11–15.

12. Frighetto L, De Salles AA, Behnke E, Smith ZA, Chute D. Image-guided frameless stereotactic biopsy sampling of parasellar lesions. Technical note. J Neurosurg 2003; 98(4):920–925.

13. Germano IM, Queenan JV. Clinical experience with intracranial brain needle biopsy using frameless surgical navigation. Comput Aided Surg 1998; 3(1):33–39.

14. Gralla J, Nimsky C, Buchfelder M, Fahlbusch R, Ganslandt O. Frameless stereotactic brain biopsy procedures using the Stealth Station: indications, accuracy and results. Zentralblatt fur Neurochirurgie 2003; 64(4):166–170.

15. Dorward NL, Paleologos TS, Alberti O, Thomas DG. The advantages of frameless stereotactic biopsy over frame-based biopsy [see comment]. Brit J Neurosurg 2002; 16(2):110–118.

16. Fitzpatrick JM, Konrad PE, Nickele C, Cetinkaya E, Kao C. Accuracy of customized miniature stereotactic platforms. StereotactFunct Neurosurg 2005; 83(1): 25–31.

17. Cuny E, Guehl D, Burbaud P, Gross C, Dousset V, Rougier A. Lack of agreement between direct magnetic resonance imaging and statistical determination of a subthalamic target: the role of electrophysiological guidance. J Neurosurg 2002; 97(3):591–597.

18. Henderson JM. Frameless localization for functional neurosurgical procedures: a preliminary accuracy study. Stereotact Funct Neurosurg 2004; 82(4):135–141.

19. Henderson JM, Holloway KL, Gaede SE, Rosenow JM. The application accuracy of a skull-mounted trajectory guide system for image-guided functional neurosurgery. Comput Aided Surg 2004; 9(4):155–160.

20. Holloway KL, Gaede SE, Starr PA, Rosenow JM, Ramakrishnan V, Henderson JM. Frameless stereotaxy using bone fiducial markers for deep brain stimulation. J Neurosurg 2005; 103(3):404–413.

21. Black PM, Moriarty T, Alexander E, III, et al. Development and implementation of intraoperative magnetic resonance imaging and its neurosurgical applications. Neurosurgery 1997; 41(4):831–842, discussion 42–45.

22. Black PM, Alexander E, III, Martin C, et al. Craniotomy for tumor treatment in an intraoperative magnetic resonance imaging unit [comment]. Neurosurgery 1999; 45(3):423–431, discussion 31–33.

23. Buchfelder M, Ganslandt O, Fahlbusch R, Nimsky C. Intraoperative magnetic resonance imaging in epilepsy surgery. J Magn Reson Imaging 2000; 12(4): 547–555.

24. Buchfelder M, Fahlbusch R, Ganslandt O, Stefan H, Nimsky C. Use of intraoperative magnetic resonance imaging in tailored temporal lobe surgeries for epilepsy. Epilepsia 2002; 43(8):864–873.

25. Martin AJ, Larson PS, Ostrem JL, et al. Placement of deep brain stimulator electrodes using real-time high-field interventional magnetic resonance imaging. Magn Reson Med 2005; 54(5):1107–1114.
26. Truwit CL, Liu H. Prospective stereotaxy: a novel method of trajectory alignment using real-time image guidance. J Magn Reson Imaging 2001; 13(3):452–457.

7

Neurophysiology of the Microelectrode Track During Subthalamic Nucleus and Globus Pallidus Internus Targeting

Shabbar F. Danish

Department of Neurosurgery, Hospital of the University of Pennsylvania, and Department of Bioengineering, University of Pennsylvania, Philadelphia, Pennsylvania, U.S.A.

Jason T. Moyer

Department of Bioengineering, University of Pennsylvania, Philadelphia, Pennsylvania, U.S.A.

Jurg L. Jaggi

Department of Neurosurgery, Hospital of the University of Pennsylvania, Philadelphia, Pennsylvania, U.S.A.

INTRODUCTION

The debate over the need for microelectrode recordings (MERs) during movement disorder deep brain stimulation (DBS) surgery is still unsettled (1). There are proponents who unequivocally state that MERs are an absolute necessity for successful DBS surgery. Others point to the fact that clinical outcome is not improved with MERs, and no well-designed studies exist to prove that they are essential and lead to improved placement of the stimulating electrodes. Although there might be some agreement that for ablative procedures MERs are a requirement, the "reversibility" of DBS surgery weakens that argument and leaves room for discussion. The answer to this fundamental question hinges on the ability of accurate targeting. As better imaging techniques and targeting software platforms are evolving, the accuracy of the electrode placement is improving and the need for MERs is diminishing. However, since direct visualization of subthalamic nucleus (STN) and globus pallidus internus is difficult at best, most neurosurgeons rely on complimentary tools, such as MER or intra-operative stimulation, to ascertain proper placement of DBS leads. Clearly, there is no better way than physiological target confirmation to assure an optimal outcome of the surgical procedure.

RECORDING OF ELECTRICAL POTENTIALS

It has been known for some time that electrical potentials are the basics of information transfer and processing of cellular function. Fundamental experiments and developments of electrical models helped in the understanding of action potentials and led to a great wealth of information. Although highly developed glass electrodes are generally utilized to explore the intracellular milieu on mainly isolated cells in research environments, intra-operative MERs are of extracellular nature mainly due to the physical electrode properties and the requirement of identifying neuronal characteristics during surgical procedures.

Extracellular spikes are recorded as the potential difference between an active electrode with a relatively small electrode tip near a neuronal structure and a much bigger reference electrode somewhere in the interstitial space. During neuronal inactivity, a generally small steady-state potential exists and its polarity is depending on the difference of the positivity between active and reference electrodes. Brief biphasic spikes as are recorded when a depolarization wave traverses the neuron and transient potential gradients are formed as seen in Figure 1. The neuronal surface

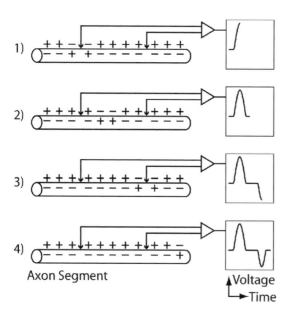

Figure 1 In principle, the generation of a biphasic potential recorded from a neuronal structure is depicted.

potential changes from a positive resting level to a brief negative state, and after repolarization, back to the positive value. Given an electrode arrangement described above, a biphasic spike is recorded. Many factors affect the spike formation but the physical location of the electrode in relation to the neuronal structure is assumed to be an important one.

RECORDING SYSTEMS

MER systems are complex in design and are nowadays often integrated into the surgical targeting platform. Despite their complexity, they all consist of the same basic components and include preamplifier, amplifier, low- and high-pass filters, speaker(s) for acoustic analysis, and a display system which is generally computer based and allows for on-line analysis as well as archival of the data. Although during the pioneering phase of MERs, home-built recording systems were the norm, commercially available systems with extensive data analysis capabilities are dominating nowadays. Over time, instrumentation has been miniaturized to the point to make simultaneous recordings of up to five parallel tracks feasible even in the constraint space of a cramped operating room.

Many different electrodes are available, although insulated tungsten wires tapered to narrow tip with a 10 to 50 μm exposure are commonly used and are suitable single-unit recordings. The corresponding impedances range from 0.5 to 1.5 MΩ. Lower values yield generally lower noise levels and are preferable. From the electrode, the signal is amplified and band-pass filtered with separate low- and high-pass filters. Commonly used high-pass filter settings range from 10 to 500 Hz and low-pass filter settings from 1 to 50 kHz. Notch filters (60 Hz) and/or high-pass filters settings above 100 Hz are helpful in eliminating 60 Hz noise from the main power supply. For visual inspection of the recordings, a running display of 5 to 10 seconds is adequate and allows assessing and comparing signal frequencies. For waveform analysis of individual spikes, however, shorter sweep times are needed (1 to 5 m sec) and well as trigger capabilities to freeze a single trace.

NEUROPHYIOLOGY OF THE SUBTHALAMIC NUCLEUS MICROELECTRODE TRACK

Given a typical stereotactic setup, a microelectrode track typically begins 15 mm above the target and, depending on the angles of approach, four major anatomical structures are normally traversed (Fig. 2). These are the anterior thalamus or reticular formation, zona incerta (ZI), STN, and substantia nigra pars reticulata (SNr). Thalamic neurons are usually encountered within the first several millimeters of recording, followed by a relatively silent ZI. The clearest indicator that the electrode has breached STN is the dramatic increase in signal background level followed by intense, irregular neuronal activity. Frequently, a brief pause in STN activity is observed as the electrode further passes through the lamina between dorsal and ventral part of STN. On exiting STN, a sudden drop in background activity is observed and is followed by a period of silence before the electrode enters the SN. Typical recordings for these main structures are given in Figure 2B.

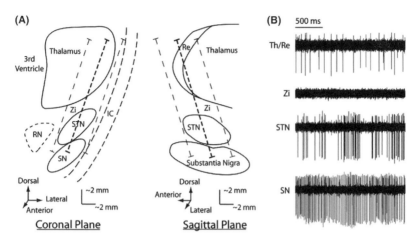

Figure 2   Coronal and sagittal sections of the STN with several microelectrode recording tracks as described in the text are shown. *Abbreviations*: IC, internal capsule; Re, reticulum; RN, red nucleus; SN, substantia nigra; STN, subthalamic nucleus; Th, thalamus; ZI, zona incerta.

Thalamus

Thalamic activity usually consists of large amplitude discharges without significant background spiking from more distant cells. Single units may either spike tonically or burst-like. Neurons in the reticular thalamic formation tend to fire quite regularly at lower frequency than anterior thalamic neurons, with frequent pauses. Bursting cells are almost always anterior thalamic cells. Both reticular and anterior thalamic cells may respond to sensorimotor stimulation, especially active movements.

Zona Incerta

The ZI is a flat thin layer of gray matter located dorsal of the subthalamus. It is a very quiet territory, although occasionally there is some isolated neural activity, somatic or axonal, characterized by rare and sharp discharges of equidistant nature. The length of the ZI is variable and depends on the angles of the trajectory.

Subthalamic Nucleus

Typically, it is the loudest structure encountered on an average track. Entry into the nucleus is most easily recognized by the rapid increase in the background activity. The increase in activity owes to the high density of neurons within STN. Even in the absence of single-unit discharges, the obvious change in the background intensity is a reliable marker of STN entry. The change in background signal has been quantified as a change in spectral density and is used to assist in localizing the STN along the microelectrode track (2,3). Often, the STN exhibits a very characteristic, audible oscillation at very low frequency

(<2 Hz; visible in STN trace). The underlying cause of this is unknown, although it may reflect correlated bursting activity between cells in the STN.

Three different types of neuronal activity have been described in the STN: irregular, tonic, and bursting. It has been estimated that 55% to 65% of the STN neurons fire irregularly, whereas 15% to 25% fire tonically and 15% to 50% present bursting activity (4). Many STN cells exhibit periodic discharge behavior and have been classified as either tremor cells (2–6 Hz) or high (>10 Hz) frequency periodic cells. Some cells exhibit both types of behavior. The mean firing rate of single STN cells has been reported as 37 ± 17 Hz (5). Higher rates are often observed and are most likely the result of multiunit recordings. Spike analysis algorithms which is usually done off-line allow for proper separation into individual units.

In single STN units, a sensory motor response can often be elicited by passive movements of the contralateral arm and leg as well as sensory stimulation of the contralateral face. Optimally, passive movements of the limb with the worst symptoms, usually arm or leg, gives a strong phasic response with generally increased spiking. The presence of a sensorimotor response provides confirmation of a satisfactory trajectory. In general, STN neurons that respond to movement are either irregular or tonic and are found in the dorsolateral STN. Bursting neurons do not usually respond to movement and are most often located in the ventral STN (6).

A brief (<1.5 mm) pause in activity of the electrode indicates passage from dorsal to ventral STN. Dorsal STN is usually more active than ventral STN. A potential explanation for this observation might be the increased amount of sensorimotor-related neurons in the dorsal STN, although it might also be the result of stimulation of fibers of passage coursing near the dorsal STN border (7–9).

Substantia Nigra

On exiting from the STN, the electrode is descended further along the track until SN is encountered. Although located beyond the target structure, SN serves as a "cornerstone" and is essential for physiological localization of the target. There is a noticeable drop in background activity between STN and SN. Single SN cells fire spikes at frequencies slightly higher than STN, for instance, 71 ± 23 Hz (5). Their discharge pattern is much more regular than in STN and consists of much less bursting activity. Acoustically, SN sounds more like a continuous buzz and is higher pitched compared to the irregular and spiky sound of STN. It is good practice to locate at least some SN neurons to confirm that indeed the entire STN has been traversed. Only under rare conditions as outlined below is the electrode advanced beyond STN without encountering SN activity within a few millimeters of STN.

IDENTIFYING THE OPTIMAL SUBTHALAMIC NUCLEUS TRAJECTORY

At least two different MER strategies are commonly used to identify the optimal target location. A complete mapping of the nucleus with at least four or more (simultaneous) tracks allows one to identify the outline of the STN and hence the exact location of the desired target area. However, the price for this complete physiological information is a significantly elevated surgical risk. Alternatively, the risk of complication is minimized if only the absolute minimal number of tracks is performed. In the best case, only one is needed and additional ones are performed only if the previous recordings indicate a poor location. In either case, a set of criteria is needed to help to decide whether either the completed track is adequate and no additional ones are required or which one of the multiple tracks is to be used for lead implantation. Clearly, the length of the STN as measured along the trajectory is a crucial indicator. Accounting for differences in the approach angles as well as across subject differences, a length of at least 4 to 5 mm indicates a passage of the trajectory very near the center of the nucleus and is satisfactory. Dense and "crisp" discharge patterns recorded in the STN indicate a viable and functional nucleus and will most likely yield a good DBS response. An identifiable region of sensorimotor activation will confirm the target location but is often elusive. Despite the reported inconsistencies of the STN somatopy in Parkinson's disease, a receptive field that overlaps with the locus of the most severe symptom is additional corroborating evidence of a good target location. Finally, stimulation of the target area with the microelectrode is another potential tool assisting in the decision process. Given its small size, microelectrodes allow fine localization of the somatopy. But as a result of the high electrode impedance, relatively high voltages are required to produce sufficient current, which in turn, tend to erode the electrode tip and significantly degrade or invalidate future recordings.

If a trajectory is found to be suboptimal based on the criteria outlined above, a new tract is initiated with a target location slightly distant from the previous one. The change in direction is based on the MER findings from one or more prior tracks. With each additional track, the topology is better described and the corrections tend to be more accurate. Fortunately, there are some unique features of the surrounding structures that help in deciding the direction of change. When the trajectory is too anterior, we will often encounter thalamic reticular cells at the top of the trajectory followed by a long length of silence or very sparsely firing neurons. The SN is encountered at the bottom of the track, essentially "skipping" the STN (Fig. 2A, right). There are times when there is complete silence at the top of the track and the only recorded neurons are those of the SN. In a trajectory which is too posterior, the thalamus is often more dense, followed by a length of silence, and then SN (Fig. 2A, right). Essentially, the main difference between a track that is too anterior versus too posterior is the density and length of the thalamus encountered. It is important to note that the STN may be encountered in both these situations, but that the length of STN along the track will be suboptimal, that is, less than 4 mm.

Medial and lateral displacements from the optimal trajectory tend to be needed less frequently. If a trajectory is positioned too lateral, it is common to not encounter any neural activity. The trajectory will not encounter any thalamic cells, subthalamic cells, or any part of the SN, basically following the internal capsule. Furthermore, the patient may complain of some "pulling" of the contralateral limbs as a result of internal capsule fiber interruption (Fig. 1, left). Medial tracks are characterized by increased density of thalamic firing, followed by a lack of SN firing at the bottom of the microelectrode track. It is possible that the red nucleus is traversed at the end of the track, but this is somewhat uncommon given the distance from the target. (Fig. 1A, left). Although these generalizations are helpful, many technical factors, individual idiosyncrasies, and the disease state influence the exact relationships between the gray and white matter structures along the microelectrode track.

NEUROPHYSIOLOGY OF GLOBUS PALLIDUS INTERNUS MICROELECTRODE TRACK

The globus pallidus is comprised of the external (GPe or lateral) and internal (GPi or medial) segments and forms part of the basal ganglia that includes the striatum lying dorsal and lateral to it. The internal capsule divides these two structures in the coronal planes that contain GPe and GPi. Although both segments receive major input from the striatum, their anatomical connections and functional roles differ (10). The classical model of basal ganglia function in PD predicts that the tonic ongoing firing rates of GPe neurons should be decreased and that of GPi should be increased compared with the normal condition (11). As a result, interruption of the GPi neurons should correct the clinical manifestations of hypoactive movement disorders.

The intended target for DBS is the lateral posteroventral segment of GPi, which is consistent with the functional heterogeneity within the globus pallidus (12–14). The target is usually located 2 to 3 mm anterior to the midcommissural point, 18 to 21 mm lateral to the midline, and 3 to 6 mm below the intercommissural line. When the guide cannula is placed, 15 to 20 mm above target, the encountered structures include the internal capsule, GPe, the lamina between the two segments, GPi, and the optic tract below. Each has its own distinct neural signature, which can be utilized for trajectory optimization (Fig. 3).

Two major types of neurons have been described in GPe. The first demonstrates slow-frequency discharges with firing rates of 40 to 60 Hz and pauses from 300 to 500 msec. The second type of GPe neuron is characterized by low-frequency discharges with bursts and a firing rate of 20 Hz, with grouped discharges occurring at irregular intervals and with intraburst firing frequencies at 300 to 500 Hz (15–17). GPe cells exhibit short bursts compared to those found in GPi. The border cells in the periphery of the GPe and GPi are characterized by low-frequency discharges (18,19).

In the GPi, neurons fire with discharge rates in the range of 70 to 120 Hz, with a mean firing rate of 91 $\pm$ 52 Hz, have fewer pauses and fire with an irregular pattern. The mean firing frequency of GPi cells has been shown to be significantly higher than for those in GPe (20,21). Although the classic papers

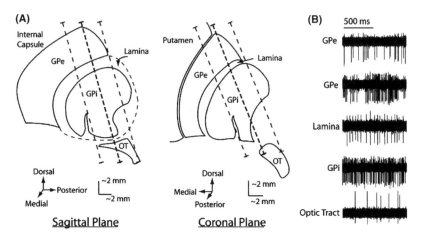

Figure 3 Coronal and sagittal sections of the pallidum with several microelectrode recording tracks as described in the text are shown. *Abbreviations*: GPe, globus pallidus, internal segment; GPi, globus pallidus, external segment; OT, optic tract.

describing pallidal physiology did not divide the GPi into dorsal and venral aspects, differences in firing rates of neurons in these regions have been described (4,8,15). GPi neurons demonstrate a continuous, high-frequency discharge that is distinct from the heterogeneous firing patterns among GPe cells (18). Cells in both GPe and GPi have been characterized according to burst and pause indices, as well as pause ratios, but these have generally shown overlapping ranges. Although mean firing rates do not completely characterize neuronal discharges, they remain an important differentiating factor between GPe and GPi (22). In addition, the differences in electrophysiological signatures cannot be determined by recording individual cells and only become apparent by examining several cells (23).

Tremor cells, cells with periodic oscillations in their firing rate that occur at the same frequency as the subject's tremor, have been identified in both GPe and GPi. The average firing rate of tremor cells is higher at 85 Hz than that of other GPi neurons (65 Hz) (19,24,25). Neurons that change their firing rate in response to passive movement (kinesthetic cells) are found in similar proportions in both GPe and GPi. These cells respond to several combinations of movement, including upper and lower limb movements and combined contralateral and ipsilateral limb movements (22).

IDENTIFYING THE OPTIMAL GLOBUS PALLIDUS INTERNUS TRACK

In determining the optimal track for lead placement, four basic physiological elements should be carefully examined. These are: general neuronal activity, tremor synchronous cells, the presence of kinesthetic responses, and increased firing rates to visual stimulation near the optic tract. Generally, the pallidum is traversed and after identifying the inferior boundary, the microelectrode is further advanced to explore the proximity of the optic tract by visual stimulation with a small flashlight, similar to a pupilar response test. After completion of the initial track, the recorded physiological properties are evaluated and a decision is made if further tracks are needed or if the current one is congruent with the anatomical structures as planned. If a trajectory is found to be suboptimal, a new tract is initiated with a target location slightly distant from the previous one. The guiding principles are as follows. A completely quiet track indicates either a rather medial or posterior location since little or no neuronal activity is encountered while the electrode is traversing the internal capsule. Whereas one encounters GPe and GPi in the absence of a visual response the trajectory may be too lateral. Moves in the anterior direction that are based on a best fit of the physiological data onto the Schaltenbrand atlas are much more likely to be incorrect compared to those in the posterior direction (23). The decision for placement within any given microelectrode track is usually based on the combined presence or absence of the physiological elements as depicted in Figure 3. As in the case of STN, passive limb movements might help in identifying the location of the trajectory. Kinesthetic responses are mostly found in the anterior part of the pallidum.

REFERENCES

1. Priori A, Egidi M, Pesenti A, et al. Do intraoperative microrecordings improve subthalamic nucleus targeting in stereotactic neurosurgery for Parkinson's disease? J Neurosurg Sci 2003; 47(1):56–60.
2. Liu X, Rowe J, Nandi D, et al. Localisation of the subthalamic nucleus using Radionics Image Fusion and Stereoplan combined with field potential recording. A technical note. Stereotact Funct Neurosurg 2001; 76(2):63–73.
3. Pesenti A, Rohr M, Egidi M, et al. The subthalamic nucleus in Parkinson's disease: power spectral density analysis of neural intraoperative signals. Neurol Sci 2004; 24(6):367–374.
4. Wichmann T, Bergman H, DeLong MR. The primate subthalamic nucleus. I. Functional properties in intact animals. J Neurophysiol 1994; 72(2):494–506.
5. Hutchison WD, Allan RJ, Opitz H, et al. Neurophysiological identification of the subthalamic nucleus in surgery for Parkinson's disease. Ann Neurol 1998; 44(4): 622–628.
6. Rodriguez-Oroz MC, Rodriguez M, Guridi J, et al. The subthalamic nucleus in Parkinson's disease: somatotopic organization and physiological characteristics. Brain 2001; 124:1777–1790.
7. Andrade-Souza Y SJ, Hamani C, Eltahawy H, Hoque T, Saint-Cyr J, Lozano A. Comparison of three methods of targeting the subthalamic nucleus for chronic stimulation in Parkinson's disease. Neurosurgery 2005; 56:360–368.
8. Bergman H, Wichmann T, Karmon B, DeLong MR. The primate subthalamic nucleus. II. Neuronal activity in the MPTP model of parkinsonism. J Neurophysiol 1994; 72(2):507–520.

9. Hamani C, Saint-Cyr J, Fraser J, Kaplitt M, Lozano A. The subthalamic nucleus in the context of movement disorders. Brain 2004; 127:4–20.
10. Parent A, Hazrati L-N. Functional anatomy of the basal ganglia: II. The place of the subthalamic nucleus and external pallidum in basal ganglia circuitry. Brain Res 1995; 20:128–154.
11. Albin R, Young A, Penney J. The functional anatomy of basal ganglia disorders. Trends in Neurosci. 1989; 12(10):366–375.
12. Gross RE, Lombardi WJ, Hutchison WD, et al. Variability in lesion location after microelectrode-guided pallidotomy for Parkinson's disease: anatomical, physiological, and technical factors that determine lesion distribution. J Neurosurg 1999; 90(3):468–477.
13. Gross RE, Lombardi WJ, Lang AE, et al. Relationship of lesion location to clinical outcome following microelectrode-guided pallidotomy for Parkinson's disease. Brain 1999; 122 (Pt 3):405–416.
14. Lang AE, Duff J, Saint-Cyr JA, et al. Posteroventral medial pallidotomy in Parkinson's disease. J Neurol 1999; 246(suppl 2):II28–41.
15. Hutchison WD, Levy R, Dostrovsky JO, Lozano A, Lang AE. Effects of apomorphine on globus pallidus neurons in parkinsonian patients. Ann Neurol 1997; 42:767–775.
16. Nini A, Feingold A, Slovin H, Bergman H. Neurons in the globus pallidus do not show correlated activity in the normal monkey, but phase-locked oscillations appear in the MPTP model of parkinsonism. J Neurophysiol 1995; 74:1800–1805.
17. Raz A, Feingold A, Zelanskaya V, Vaadia E, Bergman H. Neuronal synchronization of tonically active neurons in the striatum of normal and parkinsonian patients. J Neurophysiol 1996; 76:2083–2088.
18. Hayase N, Miyashita N, Endo K, Narabayashi H. Neuronal activity in GP and Vim of parkinsonian patients and clinical changes of tremor through surgical interventions. Stereotact Funct Neurosurg 1998; 71(1):20–28.
19. Hutchison WD, Lozano AM, Tasker RR, Lang AE, Dostrovsky JO. Identification and characterization of neurons with tremor-frequency activity in human globus pallidus. Exp Brain Res 1997; 113(3):557–563.
20. Magnin M, Morel A, Jeanmonod D. Single-unit analysis of the pallidum, thalamus and subthalamic nucleus in parkinsonian patients. Neuroscience 2000; 96(3):549–564.
21. Sterio D, Beric A, Dogali M, Fazzini E, Alfaro G, Devinsky O. Neurophysiological properties of pallidal neurons in Parkinson's disease. Ann Neurol 1994; 35(5): 586–591.
22. Favre J, Taha JM, Baumann T, Burchiel KJ. Computer analysis of the tonic, phasic, and kinesthetic activity of pallidal discharges in Parkinson patients. Surg Neurol 1999; 51(6):665–672, discussion 72–73.
23. Kirschman D, Milligan B, Wilkinson S, et al. Pallidotomy microelectrode targeting: Neurophysiology-based target refinement. Neurosurgery 2000; 46(3):613–624.
24. Lemstra AW, Verhagen Metman L, Lee JI, Dougherty PM, Lenz FA. Tremor-frequency (3–6 Hz) activity in the sensorimotor arm representation of the internal segment of the globus pallidus in patients with Parkinson's disease. Neurosci Lett 1999; 267(2):129–132.
25. Lozano A, Hutchison W, Kiss Z, Tasker R, Davis K, Dostrovsky J. Methods for microelectrode-guided posteroventral pallidotomy. J Neurosurg 1996; 84(2):194–202.

8

Complications and Avoidance

Atsushi Umemura

Department of Neurosurgery, Nagoya City University Medical School, Nagoya, Japan

INTRODUCTION

Deep brain stimulation (DBS) has been performed in the last decade for medically refractory Parkinson's disease (PD) as an alternative to ablative stereotactic neurosurgical procedures (1–7). DBS of the subthalamic nucleus (STN) and the globus pallidus internas has essentially replaced pallidotomy and thalamotomy as the procedure of choice for PD. In contrast to ablative stereotactic procedures, DBS does not require destructive brain lesions and, therefore, lessens the risk of permanent postoperative neurological deficits. Pathological studies have demonstrated that DBS does not cause damage to the adjacent tissue, except for mild gliosis around the implanted electrode track (8).

Although DBS is considered to be less morbid than ablative procedures, a significant incidence of adverse effects associated with the DBS procedure has been reported (9–13). This chapter reviews the DBS-related complications and discusses their avoidance.

MORBIDITY AND MORTALITY OF DEEP BRAIN STIMULATION FOR PARKINSON'S DISEASE

There is a significant incidence of adverse effects associated with the DBS procedure. Most of them are mild and transient, but some serious morbidity is also reported. Table 1 shows reported complications of DBS for PD. There are

Table 1 Complications of Deep Brain Stimulation for Parkinson's Disease

Surgery-related complications
   Intracerebral hemorrhage
   Subdural hematoma
   Venous infarction
   Seizure
   CSF leak
   Sterile seroma
   Pulmonary embolism
   Pneumonia
   Perioperative confusion
   Improper lead placement
Device-related complications
   Infection
   Skin erosion
   Electrode or wire break
   Lead migration
   IPG malfunction
Stimulation-related complications
   Dyskinesia
   Hemiballismus
   Dysarthria
   Paresthesia
   Diplopia
   ALO
   Weight gain
   Mania
   Depression
   Psychosis

Abbreviations: ALO, Apraxia of eyelid opening; CSF, cerebrospinal fluid; IPG, internal pulse generator.

three types of complications related to DBS, namely those related to surgery, to the device, and to stimulation. According to a recent systematic review, the mortality rate is 0.4%. There is a 9% incidence of device-related complications (infections, lead, and pulse generator problems) and a 2.8% incidence of intracerebral hemorrhage, with 0.7% overall incidence of permanent neurological deficits (7).

SURGERY-RELATED COMPLICATIONS

Intracerebral hemorrhage caused by insertion of the cannula or microelectrode into the brain is one of the typical and serious surgery-related complications that occur in stereotactic neurosurgery. The risk of intracerebral hemorrhage in stereotactic surgery is 1% to 8% (14). The incidence of hemorrhagic complications in the DBS procedure is lower than in radio frequency lesioning, a procedure that damages the vessel wall with heat. Reported rates of intracerebral hemorrhage in DBS surgery range from 0.3% to 3.6% per electrode track (15). However, the incidence of symptomatic hemorrhage or symptomatic hemorrhage with permanent neurological deficit seems to be less frequent. The use of microelectrode recording is controversial (16,17). In a report from the DBS for PD study group, the number of microelectrode passes used to determine target location correlated with the risk of hemorrhage (2.9 passes in patients without hemorrhage vs. 4.1 passes in patients with hemorrhage) (2). Gorgulho et al. (18) emphasizes that the combination of microelectrode recording and hypertension will increase the incidence of bleeding. Although microelectrode recordings are useful for improving the accuracy of target localization, it may increase the risk of intracerebral hemorrhage. Additionally, intracerebral hemorrhage may occur several hours after surgery (Fig. 1) (9). Careful control of perioperative blood pressure is important and may prevent this complication. Intraoperative systolic blood pressure should be maintained less than 140 mmHg. It is also important to screen patients for coagulopathy or recent use of antiplatelet agent before surgery.

To prevent hemorrhagic complication, the choice of entry point is very important. We pay close attention to superficial veins and sulci near the entry point. The recent availability of a computer guided surgery system has allowed

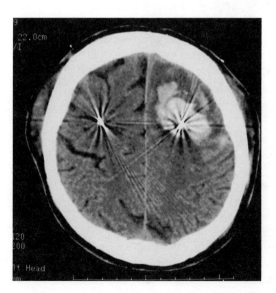

Figure 1 A computed tomography scan obtained six hours after surgery revealing subcortical hemorrhage at the site of deep brain stimulation implantation. This hematoma did not require evacuation but caused mild permanent hemiparesis.

us to simulate the electrode's trajectory and hence avoid penetrating deep vessels. Surgical planning with gadolinium-enhanced magnetic resonance (MR) image clearly identifies cortical veins (Fig. 2). This method is quite useful for avoiding the cortical vein at the entry point and for preventing hemorrhagic complications and venous infarction.

There is some evidence indicating intraoperative hemorrhage: bleeding from the cannula, unexpected electrical silence on microelectrode recording, displacement of the DBS electrode as seen on fluoroscopy, and so on. In such cases, we should control the patient's blood pressure at a lower level and watch the patient carefully. If deterioration of consciousness or a focal neurological deficit is found, the procedure should be interrupted and emergency computed tomography should be performed. On that occasion, leaving the stereotactic frame in place will be helpful for subsequent emergent stereotactic aspiration of hematoma when the patient's airway is secured (15).

Venous infarction is caused by coagulating a large draining vein that enters the dura at the site of the burr hole (Fig. 3). In addition to detailed surgical planning with gadolinium-enhanced MR image, we recommend placing the burr hole anterior to the coronal suture. In the case of a venous infarct, it will be more likely to be asymptomatic from this position.

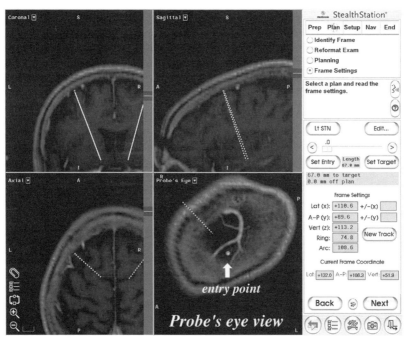

Figure 2 An example of deep brain stimulation surgical planning with gadolinium-enhanced T1-weighted magnetic resonance image. Cortical veins near the entry point are clearly shown, particularly in the probe's eye view.

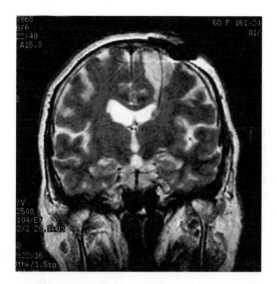

Figure 3 Coronal T2-weighted magnetic resonance image demonstrating a broad, high-intensity lesion that is consistent with venous infarction at the site of deep brain stimulation implantation.

The reported incidence of *postoperative seizures* related to the DBS procedure is 3.1% (7). However, prophylactic use of anticonvulsant agents in DBS surgery may increase the risk of medication-related complications and drug interaction in this mostly elderly population and may not be necessary. When seizure occurs postoperatively, antiepileptic medication should be administered for a certain period.

Cerebrospinal fluid leak, which causes subcutaneous fluid collection, may require surgical repair. On the other hand, *sterile seroma* at the site of the internal pulse generator (IPG) is easily drained by needle puncture.

Pulmonary embolism is a prominent source of mortality and morbidity in neurosurgical patients. The reported incidence of postoperative pulmonary embolism ranges from 0.4% to 4.9%; in those cases, the mortality rate ranges from 8.6% to 59.4% (19). Despite standard prophylaxis with pneumatic compression boots, fatal deep vein thrombosis can still occur. Patients at high risk include those with heart disease, obesity, polycythemia, paralysis of the lower extremities, and forced immobilization. Patients with PD may have increased risk of pulmonary embolism because of medication withdrawal during the day of surgery and resulting immobility. Hence, early rehabilitation is important, especially for patients with PD. Some studies showed effectiveness of low molecular weight heparin combined with compression stockings for the prevention of postoperative venous thromboembolism without causing excessive bleeding in neurosurgery (20–22).

Perioperative aspiration *pneumonia* is also a fatal complication. Patients with advanced PD sometimes have swallowing difficulties. These patients may be at risk for perioperative aspiration. Indication of surgery for such patients should be carefully reviewed.

Perioperative confusion is a common adverse effect after STN DBS surgery, especially in older patients (7,9). Perioperative confusion is usually transient and several factors may contribute to its pathogenesis, including penetration of the bilateral frontal lobe, long duration of brain surgery, and the withdrawal of dopaminergic medication.

Improper lead placement is a fundamental issue in the surgical procedure. In addition to proper surgical technique, fluoroscopy is useful for confirming the lead position during surgery. The physiology cannulas need to be maintained very well. Small bends may induce misplacement of the lead. We usually verify anatomical localization of the lead with MR image immediately after surgery.

DEVICE-RELATED COMPLICATIONS

Infection is one of the most probable device-related complications in DBS (7,9,11–13). Since the DBS procedure involves the implantation of a foreign body, the risk of infection is high. The reported incidence of infection in the DBS procedure is 3% to 10%. In general, infected DBS systems should be removed, as treatment with antibiotics without device removal is unlikely to be effective, and leaving an infected lead in place can potentially result in an intracranial infection (subdural empyema or brain abcess). Aseptic operative technique, intraoperative antibiotics, careful irrigation with antibiotic solution, and shorter surgical times are the best way to avoid infection. As a practical suggestion, administration of one dose of cefazolin sodium prior to surgery and two doses after surgery is recommended to reduce the chance of infection (12). It is controversial whether the patient's hair ought to be shaved to avoid infection. Miyagi et al. (23) showed that leaving the hair intact was not associated with any statistically significant lower infection rate. Industry may consider in the future coating DBS leads with antibiotics as in ventricular shunt catheters.

Skin erosion with or without infection sometimes occurs at the connector site as a late complication (beyond 12 months). The bulky lead connector used in the early days of the procedure might have contributed to this. The recently developed low-profile connector combined with proper placement under the scalp, and meticulous galea closure, should decrease the risk of skin erosion (9,12). Kinetra dual IPG used recently is large and may cause increased risk of skin erosion. Placing it in the flank may obviate this problem. A thin patient may be better off with two Soletra IPGs.

Electrode or wire break occurs, especially when the connector between extension cable and electrode is located below the mastoid (13,24,25). This fact suggests that to-and-fro movement of the DBS electrode with repeated head turning increases stress at the connector site and causes eventual disruption.

It is recommended that the connector between the extension cable and electrode is placed in the parietal subgalea. Electrode break will result in complete revision requiring intracranial procedure under stereotactic guidance.

Lead migration seems to occur when fixation of the lead to the skull is insufficient (12,13). If the lead does not remain correctly positioned, it will result in clinical failure. Downward dislocation of the connector, extension cable, or IPG is responsible for upward migration of the lead. Favre et al. (26) recommend the use of a titanium microplate to anchor the DBS lead to prevent lead migration. However, care is necessary in this technique to avoid crushing the electrode under the microplate. We use a Medtronic burr hole ring and cap to fix the lead and have not experienced any cases of lead migration.

Regarding *IPG malfunction*, shocking sensation or intermittent stimulation have been reported (12). Most of these complications occurred in patients with the previous Itrel II model IPG, not the recent Soletra IPG. Replacement of the IPG will be required in such cases. Acute battery failure may cause a parkinsonian crisis (27). Therefore, replacement of the IPG should be considered before complete depletion of the battery.

STIMULATION-RELATED ADVERSE EVENT

Stimulation-related adverse events are common in DBS. Stimulation of the STN may immediately induce *dyskinesia, hemiballismus, dysarthria, paresthesia,* and *diplopia* (7,9,28). However, these effects are usually reversible and can be avoided by adjusting the stimulation parameters.

Stimulation-induced dyskinesia in stimulation of the STN seems to indicate correct electrode placement. Therefore, a favorable outcome can be expected by careful adjustment of stimulation parameters and reduction of dopaminergic medication. Other stimulation-induced adverse effects seem to be caused by excessive stimulation of the corticobulbospinal tract located laterally, the medial lemniscus located posteriorly, or the oculomotor nerve fiber located medially to the STN (29). Stimulation parameters should be programmed to maximize symptom suppression and to minimize side effects. Postoperative MR imaging demonstrates anatomical localization of the electrode and is useful in selecting active contacts.

Apraxia of eyelid opening (ALO) is an infrequent side effect of STN DBS. Its incidence is approximately 5% (7). ALO is more frequently seen in patients who obtain a good anti-PD effect of STN DBS (30). The mechanism of ALO is not well understood. Originally, this symptom was observed in idiopathic PD and other degenerative diseases involving the basal ganglia (31). Most patients are successfully treated by injection of botulinum toxin (1,30). From our experience, postoperative modification of dopaminergic medication may be a cause of ALO.

Weight gain is one of the most common adverse effects after STN DBS (7,32,33). This weight gain occurs in the first three months and continues to increase slowly beyond one year. It is conceivable that weight gain after DBS is caused by the reduction of energy expenditure related to the control of dyskinesia, rigidity, and tremor. Additionally, changes in dopaminergic medication after STN DBS may modulate motivation for food intake (33). Therefore, candidates for STN DBS should be given nutritional counseling to prevent rapid and excessive weight gain (32).

Psychiatric problems including *mania*, *depression*, and other *psychosis* are also among the most common adverse effects in patients treated with STN DBS (3,5,7,34–36). These problems are frequently encountered in advanced PD patients treated with drugs alone. Hence, pre-existing psychiatric illness may be related to these complications. Further, the spread of stimulation to the limbic circuit seems to be a cause of altered mood states. Mania is usually transient in the immediate postoperative period. Depression occurring several months after surgery often coincides with a significant reduction of dopaminergic medication and is generally alleviated by increasing the dose of the dopaminergic treatment. Severe depression after successful DBS has been reported even leading to suicide, therefore, great care should be taken with regard to the patient's emotional state (37). We consider that STN stimulation does not affect cognitive function, but this issue is still controversial (3,5,35).

CONCLUSION

In general, DBS seems to be a relatively safe procedure. Serious complications with permanent sequelae are rare, but there are nonetheless significant incidences of adverse effects in DBS procedure. Surgery-related and device-related complications can be reduced with increased surgical experience and the introduction of new surgical equipment and techniques, such as the use of computer-based surgical planning.

REFERENCES

1. Limousin P, Krack P, Pollak P, et al. Electrical stimulation of the subthalamic nucleus in advanced Parkinson's disease. N Engl J Med 1998; 339:1105–1111.
2. The Deep-brain Stimulation for Parkinson's Disease Study Group. Deep-brain stimulation of the subthalamic nucleus or the pars interna of the globus pallidus in Parkinson's disease. N Engl J Med 2001; 345:956–963.
3. Krack P, Batir A, Blercom NV, et al. Five-year follow-up of bilateral stimulation of the subthalamic nucleus in advanced Parkinson's disease. N Engl J Med 2003; 349:1925–1934.
4. Jaggi JL, Umemura A, Hurtig HI, et al. Bilateral stimulation of the subthalamic nucleus in Parkinson's disease: surgical efficacy and prediction of outcome. Stereotact Funct Neurosurg 2004; 82:104–114.
5. Rodoriguez-Oroz MC, Obeso JA, Lang AE, et al. Bilateral deep brain stimulation in Parkinson's disease: a multicentre study with 4 years follow-up. Brain 2005; 128:2240–2249.

6. Schüpbach WMM, Chastan N, Welter ML, et al. Stimulation of the subthalamic nucleus in Parkinson's disease: a 5 year follow up. J Neurol Neurosurg Psychiatry 2005; 76:1640–1644.

7. Hamani C, Richter E, Schwalb JM, et al. Bilateral subthalamic nucleus stimulation for Parkinson's disease: a systematic review of the clinical literature. Neurosurgery 2005; 56:1313–1324.

8. Haberler C, Alesch F, Mazal PR, et al. No tissue damage by chronic deep brain stimulation in Parkinson's disease. Ann Neurol 2000; 48:372–376.

9. Umemura A, Jaggi JL, Hurtig H, et al. Deep brain stimulation for movement disorders: morbidity and mortality in 109 patients. J Neurosurg 2003; 98:779–784.

10. Beric A, Kelly PJ, Rezai A, et al. Complications of deep brain stimulation surgery. Stereotact Funct Neurosurg 2001; 77:73–78.

11. Oh MY, Abosch A, Kim SH, et al. Long-term hardware-related complications of deep brain stimulation. Neurosurgery 2002; 50:1268–1276.

12. Lyons KE, Wilkinson SB, Overman J, et al. Surgical and hardware complications of subthalamic stimulation. A series of 160 procedures. Neurology 2004; 63: 612–616.

13. Blomstedt P, Hariz MI. Hardware-related complications of deep brain stimulation: a ten year experience. Acta Neurochir 2005; 147:1061–1064.

14. Binder DK, Rau GM, Starr PA. Risk factors for hemorrhage during microelectrode-guided deep brain stimulator implantation for movement disorders. Neurosurgery 2005; 56:722–732.

15. Rosenow JM, Rezai AR. Surgical technique and complication avoidance. In: Baltuch GH, Stern MB, eds. Surgical Management of Movement Disorders. Boca Raton: Taylor & Francis, 2005:45–62.

16. Hariz MI, Fodstad H. Do microelectrode techniques increase accuracy or decrease risks in pallidotomy and deep brain stimulation? A critical review of the literature. Stereotact Funct Neurosurg 1999; 72:57–169.

17. Palur RS, Berk C, Schulzer M, et al. A metaanalysis comparing the results of pallidotomy performed using microelectrode recording or macroelectrode stimulation. J Neurosurg 2002; 96:1058–1062.

18. Gorgulho A, DeSalles AAF, Frighetto L, et al. Incidence of hemorrhage associated with electrophysiological studies performed using macroelectrodes and microelectrodes in functional neurosurgery. J Neurosurg 2005; 102:888–896.

19. Inci S, Erbengi A, Berker M. Pulmonary embolism in neurosurgical patients. Surg Neurol 1995; 43:123–129.

20. Cerrato D, Ariano C, Fiacchino F. Deep vein thrombosis and low-dose heparin prophylaxis in neurosurgical patients. J Neurosurg 1978; 49:378–381.

21. Nurmohamed MT, van Riel AM, Henkens CMA, et al. Low molecular weight heparin and compression stockings in the prevention of venous thromboembolism in neurosurgery. Thromb Haemost 1996; 75:233–238.

22. Agnelli G, Piovella F, Buoncristiani P, et al. Enoxaparin plus compression stockings compared with compression stockings alone in the prevention of venous thromboembolism after elective neurosurgery. N Engl J Med 1998; 339:80–85.

23. Miyagi Y, Shima F, Ishido K. Implantation of deep brain stimulation electrodes in unshaved patients. J Neurosurg 2002; 97:1476–1478.

24. Schwalb JM, Riina HA, Skolnick B, et al. Revision of deep brain stimulator for tremor. J Neurosurg 2001; 94:1010–1012.

25. Mohit AA, Samii A, Slimp JC, et al. Mechanical failure of the electrode wire in deep brain stimulation. Parkinsonism Relat Disord 2004; 10:153–156.
26. Favre J, Taha JM, Steel T, et al. Anchoring of deep brain stimulation electrodes using a microplate. J Neurosurg 1996; 85:1181–1183.
27. Chou KL, Siderowf AD, Jaggi JL, et al. Unilateral battery depletion in Parkinson's disease patients treated with bilateral subthalamic nucleus deep brain stimulation may require urgent surgical replacement. Stereotact Funct Neurosurg 2004; 82:153–155.
28. Hariz MI. Complications of deep brain stimulation surgery. Mov Disord 2002; 17(suppl 3):S162–S166.
29. Pollak P, Krack P, Fraix V, et al. Intraoperative micro- and macrostimulation of the subthalamic nucleus in Parkinson's disease. Mov Disord 2002; 17(suppl 3): S155–S161.
30. Krack P, Fraix V, Mendes A, et al. Postoperative management of subthalamic nucleus stimulation for Parkinson's disease. Mov Disord 2002; 17(suppl 3):S188–S197.
31. Boghen D. Apraxia of lid opening: a review. Neurology 1997; 48:1491–1503.
32. Barichella M, Marczewska AM, Mariani C, et al. Body weight gain rate in patients with Parkinson's disease and deep brain stimulation. Mov Disord 2003; 18:1337–1340.
33. Macia F, Perlemoine C, Coman I, et al. Parkinson's disease patients with bilateral subthalamic deep brain stimulation gain weight. Mov Disord 2004; 19:206–212.
34. Takeshita S, Kurisu K, Trop L, et al. Effect of subthalamic stimulation on mood state in Parkinson's disease: evaluation of previous facts and problems. Neurosurg Rev 2005; 28:179–186.
35. Funkiewiez A, Ardouin C, Caputo E, et al. Long term effects of bilateral subthalamic nucleus stimulation on cognitive function, mood, and behaviour in Parkinson's disease. J Neurol Neurosurg Psychiatry 2004; 75:834–839.
36. Piasecki SD, Jefferson JW. Psychiatric complications of deep brain stimulation for Parkinson's disease. J Clin Psychiatry 2004; 65:845–849.
37. Burkhard PR, Vingerhoets FJ, Berney A, et al. Suicide after successful deep brain stimulation for movement disorders. Neurology 2004; 63:2170–2172.

9

Programming Deep Brain Stimulation

Jurg L. Jaggi

Department of Neurosurgery, Hospital of the University of Pennsylvania, Philadelphia, Pennsylvania, U.S.A.

INTRODUCTION

Deep brain stimulation (DBS) is a complex medical treatment. The success of this intervention depends on a variety of components including proper patient selection, accurate surgical placement of the electrode, effective programming of the stimulator and adequate follow-up medication management. While the former two are one-time events, the latter two are reoccurring interventions over the lifespan of the therapy. As the strength of a chain is determined by its weakest link, the overall success of DBS is determined by its weakest component as well. In general, stimulator programming represents the weakest link and does not infrequently break the chain, diminishing or eliminating potential benefits of DBS. Fortunately, programming is a reoccurring event and allows for correction or reprogramming, and hopefully improved outcome. While individual components of this therapy are performed by highly trained neurosurgeons and neurologists, programming is often relegated to health care professionals with inadequate training and experience. As a result, the full potential benefit of this therapy is not always attained and the efficacy of DBS is potentially diminished.

Like any medical intervention, the proper definition of a successful outcome is essential so that all contributing factors can be evaluated in terms of their relative importance. Although each patient rates the severity of the many symptoms differently, the main objective is a reduction or cessation of the most disabling ones. In general, stricter inclusion criteria lead to better outcomes (1) and patient satisfaction. For ethical and possibly legal reasons, however, inclusion criteria are often relaxed and the symptom control resulting from DBS is less than optimal. These facts should be discussed with patients prior to surgery so that their expectations are realistic. Today's patients are mostly computer literate and Internet savvy and have researched the scientific literature as well as pertinent Parkinson's disease (PD) websites. As a result, expectations are often inflated from the many excerpts of success stories. The optimally attainable result from DBS surgery is comparable to the best presurgical response to dopaminergic medication (2). In other words, patients rarely do better after surgery than during their best on-time prior to surgery (3). The big benefit, however, is the lack of motor fluctuations and/or disabling dyskinesia following the procedure.

CONSIDERATIONS PRIOR TO PROGRAMMING

DBS is used as a therapy in an increasing number of diseases with different target locations (4). Although subthalamic nucleus (STN) (5) is the evolving target location for PD, globus pallidus (GPi) (6) and ventral intermediate nucleus of the thalamus (VIM) (7) are other valid locations used for specific symptom control. VIM targets are often found in tremor predominant PD patients who had their surgery prior to the FDA approval of STN-DBS in early 2002. Hence, it is important to ascertain the target location prior to the initial (as well as follow-up) programming, especially if the surgical procedure was performed elsewhere. In addition, it is very helpful if post-op imaging data is available and exact electrode positions can be determined. This can be done by simple visual inspection of the scans (Fig. 1) or with imaging software that permits one to measure the electrode position in relation to anatomical landmarks (8). If the preop targeting scans are available, merging of pre- and post-op scans allows determination of the exact electrode position in terms of frame coordinates and assessing the severity of postoperative shifts in the brain anatomy. Based on a thorough review of the imaging data, an optimal electrode contact is identified for the initial programming as outlined subsequently.

Following DBS surgery, most patients experience a temporary improvement in the symptoms as a result of the lesion effect. Surgical placement of micro- and macroelectrodes disrupts the local circuitry sufficiently to reduce the overactivity of the target nucleus (9). As a result, less inhibitory signal reaches the motor cortex, which in turn reduces bradykinesia and rigidity (10). As the brain heals, the temporarily improved PD symptoms slowly return to preoperative levels usually within a day or two. If not properly informed, patients invariably come to the conclusion that this is an indication of a surgical failure and become distressed and even depressed about it. Preoperative counseling and extensive discussion of the lesion effect prevents this from occurring. Since this transient phenomenon makes an accurate motor assessment difficult, it is best to wait until it has subsided. As an acceptable compromise, we generally wait a week and begin programming when patients return for suture removal.

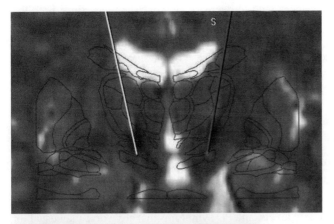

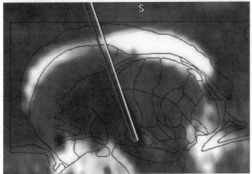

Figure 1 Interpolated coronal (*top*) and sagittal (*bottom*) magnetic resonance imaging (MRI) sections showing planned and actual trajectory of deep brain stimulation (DBS), electrodes. The trajectory is angled approximately 10° lateral from the vertical axis in the coronal section and approximately 30° anterior from the vertical in the sagittal section.

REVIEW OF ELECTRICAL PROPERTIES

The currently available DBS electrodes consist of four cylindrical platinum-iridium contacts of 1.27 mm in diameter and 1.5 mm in lengths. They are spaced either 0.5 (Medtronic, 3389) or 1.5 mm (Medtronic, 3387) from each other resulting in a total length of 7.5 and 10.5 mm, respectively. While each of the contacts can be programmed to be cathodic (−), anodic (+), or switched off, the case of the stimulator can only be cathodic or off. If the stimulator case is used as the cathode, the stimulation mode is said to be monopolar, else bipolar. The main parameters to be programmed are voltage, pulse width, and frequency. Although other modes are possible, generally a continuous stimulation mode is utilized for PD. For a given voltage, pulse width and frequency, the resulting current is dependent on the impedance, which is mainly affected by the electrode-tissue interface. After implantation, the impedances tend to decrease slowly over time. Since both the Soletra (Medtronic 7426) and Kinetra (Medtronic 7428) are voltage-controlled stimulators, that is, a constant voltage is maintained, the stimulation current slowly increases concurrently with the decrease of the impedance. This results in an increase of stimulation over time without any change in the programmed stimulation parameters. The only way to assess this "silent" increase is by performing a "therapy measurement" during each programming session and documenting changes in current and/or impedance.

INITIAL PROGRAMMING

Patients arrive at the clinic for the initial programming session with high expectations and most of the time, as instructed, in an off-medication state. This generally leads to high anxiety levels, and PD symptoms that are worse than usual. In addition, recuperation from surgery is generally far from complete which further limits the time window of a cooperative patient and a practical neurological steady state. Given these limitations, extended initial programming sessions are somewhat less productive and hence should be limited to no more than one hour. Prior to any programming a complete motor assessment of the patient is required to serve as a baseline exam. Nonmotor functions such as speech, vision, and mood should also be documented as they may be affected by DBS. Although different programming strategies can be employed, a standard approach has evolved over the years (11,12).

Starting with the more symptomatic side, the contralateral electrode is placed in monopolar mode with the optimal electrode contact, as identified from intraoperative stimulation and postoperative imaging data, selected as negative pole (cathode) and the stimulator case as positive pole (anode). A pulse width of 60 to 90 μS and a frequency of 130 Hz are selected (13). If the patient is tremor predominant, a higher frequency, that is, 185 Hz, might be considered (14). After turning the stimulator on, the voltage is slowly increased to 1 V while carefully observing the patient. At that point a therapy measurement can be performed to assess the functionality of the DBS system. Any change in the patient's symptoms should be documented. As the voltage is gradually increased in 0.1 V increments while again carefully observing the patient, repeat assessments with documentation should be done at least at every 0.5 V intervals. Usually, rigidity is improved with little delay for STN or GPi stimulation, although the full magnitude of change might take a day to develop. Tremors should be evaluated at rest as well as under action positions. Postural tremors often are different between flexed or extended upper limb conditions, and both should be evaluated. Tremors respond quickly to STN, GPi, and VIM stimulation, although sometimes a brief initial worsening is seen prior to the elimination of tremor.

As the voltage is further escalated, side effects may arise in addition to effective symptom relief. Significant side effects will eventually prevent any further escalation of the voltage. At this point, a "window of opportunity" is

Table 1 Programming Information for Case Study 1: Bilateral Globus Pallidus with Kinetra

Right												Date	Left											
0	1	2	3	C	V	PW	F	Cur	Imp	Bat	Comments		0	1	2	3	C	V	PW	F	Cur	Imp	Bat	Comments
−				+	2.0	90	130				Screen, 1 wk	3/17/2004	−				+	2.0	90	130				Screen
−				+	2.4	90	130	26	918	3.32	ACed to 2.1	4/14/2004	−				+	2.4	90	130	26	918	3.32	Same
−				+	2.7	90	130					6/9/2004	−				+	2.7	90	130				
−				+	2.8	90	130				ACed to 2.8	9/15/2004	−				+	3.0	90	130				ACed to 2.8
−				+	2.8	90	130			3.25	n/c	11/10/2004	−				+	3.2	90	130			3.25	
−				+	3.0	90	130	26	1230	3.18		3/21/2005	−				+	3.2	90	130	52	700	3.18	
−				+	3.1	90	130	26	1275	3.12		9/28/2005	−				+	3.4	90	130	52	700	3.12	
−				+	3.1	90	130					3/21/2006	−				+	3.4	90	130				

Note: 0, 1, 2, and 3 refer to the electrode contacts.

Abbreviations: ACed, patient used the Access Controller to change settings inbetween visits; C, stimulator case; Cur, current in microamps; F, frequency in Hertz; Imp, impedance in Ohm; Bat, battery voltage in Volts; PW, pulse width in microseconds; V, voltage in Volts.

Table 2 Programming Information for Case Study 2: Bilateral Subthalamic Nucleus with Soletras

Right													Left											
0	1	2	3	C	V	PW	F	Cur	Imp	Bat	Comments	Date	0	1	2	3	C	V	PW	F	Cur	Imp	Bat	Comments
												12/20/2001												Screening
												1/16/2002	—			+		2.5	90	130				Stim was off
—			+		1.1	90	185				Inpatient	4/9/2002	—			+		2.5	90	130				n/c
—			+		1.3	90	185	23	1244	3.7		4/17/2002	—			+		2.5	90	130				
—			+		1.7	90	185	35	1252	3.7		5/8/2002	—	+				5.0	90	130	98	1419	3.7	n/c
—		+			4.5	90	185	135	1019	3.7		6/12/2002	—	+				5.0	90	130	96	1318	3.7	
—		+			4.7	90	185	149	1050	3.7		3/19/2003	—	+				5.0	90	130	98	1272	3.7	
											Dead battery	8/11/2004	—	+				5.0	90	130	86	1450	3.67	n/c
—		+			3.6	90	185				New battery	8/24/2004	—	+				3.6	90	185				
—		+			4.2	90	185				Doing well	10/20/2004	—	+				4.4	90	185				New battery

Note: 0, 1, 2, and 3 refer to the electrode contacts.

Abbreviations: Bat, battery voltage in Volts; C, stimulator case; Cur, current in microamps; F, frequency in Hertz; Imp, impedance in Ohm; PW, pulse width in microseconds; V, voltage in Volts.

Table 3 Programming Information for Case Study 3: Bilateral Subthalamic Nucleus with Soletras

				Right								Date					Left						
0	1	2	3	C	V	PW	F	Cur	Imp	Bat	Comments		0	1	2	3	C	V	PW	F	Cur	Imp	Bat	Comments
+	−				2.3	90	130					10/29/2003	−	+				2.3	90	130				
+	−				2.9	90	130	18	2000	3.7		11/19/2003	−	+				2.6	90	130	19	2000	3.7	
+	−				2.2	90	130	25	1784	3.7		12/17/2003	−	+				2.6	90	130	20	2000	3.7	n/c
	−	+			2.8	90	130	30	1133			1/14/2004	−	+				2.6	90	130	20	2000	3.7	
	−	+			2.5	90	130	37	1051	3.7		1/16/2004	−	+				2.6	90	130	20	2000	3.7	n/c
	−	+			2.5	90	130	31	1200	3.7		2/25/2004	−	+				2.8	90	130	21	2000	3.7	
	−	+	+		3.2	90	130	29	1260	3.74		7/21/2004	−	+				2.8	90	130	26	2000	3.74	n/c
	−	+	+		3.5	90	130	25	1964	3.74		12/15/2004	−	+				3.1	90	130	25	1057	3.74	
	−	+	+		3.5	90	185	27	1943	3.74		1/19/2005	−	+				3.1	90	170	41	1027	3.72	
			+			90	185	75	818	3.74		7/20/2005	−	+				3.1	90	170	54	972	3.72	
+	−				3.1	90	185	64	842	3.74		10/11/2005												Dead battery
+	−				2.9	90	185				New battery	10/13/2005	−	+				2.8	90	170	44	1073	3.69	New battery
+	−				2.8	90	185	59	874	3.69		10/19/2005	−	+				2.8	90	170	45	1067	3.71	
	−	+	+		3.0	90	185	59	874	3.69	Was 2.9	11/2/2005	−	+				2.9	90	170	50	1054	3.71	
	−	+	+		3.0	90	130	73	839	3.71	No dyskinesia	11/7/2005	−	+				2.6	90	130	50	1054	3.71	
	−	+	+		3.0	90	130	45	863	3.71		11/16/2005	−	+				2.6	90	130	34	1081	3.71	
	−	+	+		3.0	90	130	37	881	3.71		12/14/2005	−	+				2.8	90	130				n/c

Note: 0, 1, 2, and 3 refer to the electrode contacts.

Abbreviations: Bat, battery voltage in Volts; C, stimulator case; Cur, current in microamps; F, frequency in Hertz; Imp, impedance in Ohm; PW, pulse width in microseconds; V, voltage in Volts.

defined as the range from lowest voltage where symptom relief was achieved to that voltage value where significant side effects limit any further increase. A wider range allows for better therapy options and is more desirable. DBS induced changes in symptoms and evolving side effects take time to develop, ranging from seconds to hours and even days. Therefore, during a relatively short programming session mostly incomplete changes are observed.

Upon completion of the screening of the first electrode contact, the stimulator is turned off and sufficient time is allowed for the symptoms to reach base line level before proceeding with the next electrode contact. In reality, however, base line levels often seem to worsen because this time-consuming programming procedure is taxing the patient considerably. This must be considered when establishing the "therapeutic window;" otherwise, an objective comparison of the efficacy of the four electrode contacts is not possible. In frail patients, the screening of bilateral leads might require two separate programming sessions. A thorough screening procedure should clearly identify which of the four contacts of the DBS lead yields the most beneficial symptom relief which subsequently is selected and cautiously activated at a low voltage of 0.5 to 1.0 V. Often this voltage is below the window of opportunity and no immediate effect is noticed. However, since the latencies of some clinical benefits and side effects are considerable, it may take a day for the full effect to develop. It is prudent to initially set the stimulator conservatively for multiple reasons: many patients live quite a distance from the clinical center and an unscheduled visit for corrective programming action often represents hardship. Also, slow but constant progress is a more positive experience for the patients than temporary, anxiety provoking setbacks. Finally, these settings are usually not dyskinesia inducing when the patients resume their medication regimen, and no immediate change is required. Many patients who undergo bilateral procedures have the dual channel Kinetra stimulator implanted. This device allows patients to make adjustments to one of the stimulation parameters, usually the voltage, with the aid of the Access controller within a predetermined range of values. Our patients are instructed to increase the stimulation voltage by 0.2 V or two clicks bilaterally after the first and the second week of the initial programming, and to call the office if they experience any adverse events. The stimulator is programmed to limit patient adjustments to maximal ± 0.4 V or four clicks. Most calls are a result of stimulator-induced dyskinesias and are easily corrected by the neurologist reducing dopaminergic medication. One month after surgery, patients return for the final surgical visit as well as follow-up programming.

FOLLOW-UP PROGRAMMING

A thorough physical exam and a complete inventory of patient findings are performed first, which allows a comparison with the preprogramming exam and an objective review of benefit and potential side effects attained from DBS. At this point, patients are almost recovered from the surgical interaction and are accustomed to DBS. Anxiety levels are greatly reduced. Often habituation or adaptation to stimulation is observed after the initial programming and PD symptoms are more pronounced again. An increase in the stimulation parameters counteracts this reduction in response effectively. Generally, after several adjustments the stimulation effects remain effective and constant, and no more waning is observed over shorter periods of time. The stimulation parameters are usually not sufficiently incremented to be in the therapeutic range to deliver optimal symptom relief at this point. Hence, a more copious increase in stimulation is indicated. Before proceeding, however, it is advisable to discuss with the patient's neurologist a strategy on dopaminergic medication reduction, as patients most likely will show signs of induced dyskinesias following a significant increase in stimulation.

As stimulation is increased, the potential for inducing adverse reactions is also increased. Again, a thorough discussion with the patient on what the various signs are and how to reduce them is helpful in alleviating apprehension and stress as well as emergent phone calls. Patients with a Kinetra stimulator can reduce the settings and often ease side effects to the point that they are tolerable until they are addressed at the next scheduled programming visit.

After successful adjustments when patients experience great symptomatic relief from DBS, side effects may develop that are bothersome or afflictive to the point that they are not tolerable on a long-term basis. Current spread from the electrode reaches adjacent structures to the target and interferes with neurologic function. As the electrode trajectory is usually angled slightly lateral to medial and anterior to posterior from burr hole to target location (Fig. 1), changing the active electrode to its nearest neighbor might alleviate the undesirable effect. For example, if persistent parasthesias are intolerable, which usually indicates a too posterior stimulation location, a superior electrode contact might relieve them, as the new stimulation focus is now more anterior in addition to slightly more superior and lateral. Figure 2 shows the effects of DBS to sub-optimal electrode positions and what effects might be expected. If switching to an adjacent electrode contact does not prove successful in alleviating undesired effects, restricting the current spread by using bipolar mode might help. Instead of the stimulator case, an adjacent contract is used as the positive pole or anode. Often times, only by trial and error are the optimal + and − contacts found. Generally speaking, when switching to bipolar mode, more stimulation, at least 0.5 V, is needed to provide similar symptom relief. On rare occasions, double negative and positive bipolar mode is needed if a singular configuration is not sufficient. Whenever the active negative electrode is changed to another contact during a reprogramming session, adaptation occurs again and it might take several programming session to reach a stable setting. After the initial programming phase, which can take several months, the adjustments tend to get smaller as only fine-tuning is needed. Generally speaking, GPi stimulation seems to require fewer adjustments as compared to STN. Often patients are under the impression that any ailment can be corrected with stimulator

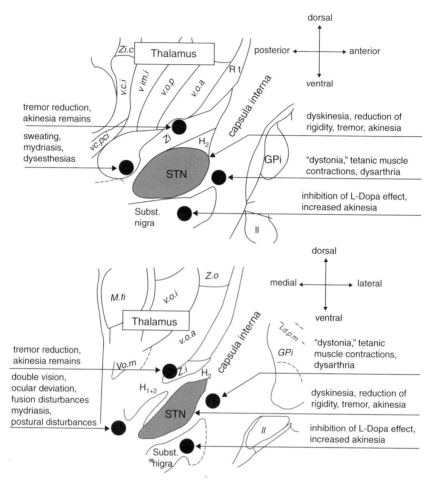

Figure 2 Stimulation-induced effects and adverse effects with high-frequency stimulation of the STN and its adjacent structures. Sagittal section 12 m lateral to the anterior commissure-posterior commissure line (*top*) and frontal section 1.5 mm behind the midcommissural point (*bottom*). *Abbreviations*: GP; globus pallidus; STN, subthalamic nucleus. *Source*: From Ref. 11.

adjustments. It should be emphasized that once the optimal setting is reached, going beyond that does not increase the benefit from stimulation. On the contrary, overstimulation can acutely worsen the condition as current spread reaches beyond the target nucleus and negatively affect other neuronal activity.

DBS requires energy and is supplied by a battery built into the stimulator. The life span of a battery depends on the stimulation parameters and typically extends over several years. A typical setting (amplitude 3.0 V, pulse width 60 μS, frequency 130 Hz, simple bipolar mode, continuous mode, and a given impedance of 1000 Ω) yields a life span of 81 months or $6\frac{3}{4}$ years for the Soletra (15) and approximately 84 months or seven years for the Kinetra (16) powering two leads. Practical experience teaches us, however, that the actual longevity is usually shorter than the numbers calculated. A low battery status is indicated by a blinking green light on the patient's Access Review (Medtronic 7438) or Access (Medtronic 7436) controller, respectively. As these blinking light thresholds are set rather low, immediate remediation is required if stimulation is not to be interrupted due to battery failure. In patients with advanced stages of PD, crisis situations can develop quickly with disabling adverse effects when battery depletions are encountered (17). A better way to avoid these potentially dangerous situations is by carefully monitoring battery status during every programming visit. With sufficient data points, the end-of-life date can be predicted and battery replacements can be scheduled in a more timely fashion. Hence, it is advisable to schedule follow-up appointments in shorter intervals, for example, three months, rather than the more customary 6 to 12 months when approaching the predicted battery depletion date.

APPROACH TO CHALLENGING PATIENTS

Occasionally, despite extensive programming efforts, only marginal symptom relief is attained. In this case, a thorough review by the neurologist is indicated to assure that no latent or active comorbid conditions are interfering with the DBS therapy. The medication regimen should also be reassessed as the response might be altered following DBS surgery. Also, if not performed as a postoperative procedure, follow-up magnetic resonance imaging (MRI) scans might be indicated and reviewed with the neurosurgeon to confirm proper location of the leads and absence of any pathology. If no cause for the lack or diminished response can be identified, an extended programming session might prove beneficial in finding the elusive setting with more satisfactory results. The session should start with a complete electrical assessment of the hardware to rule out any technical problems. The "electrode impedance" function on the n'Vision programmer is used for that purpose. It is often necessary to increase the test voltage to 3 V or more volts with preset pulse width (210 μS) and frequency (30 Hz), patient permitting, to achieve sufficient measurement accuracy and avoiding threshold values as indicated by either a " $<$ " or " $>$ " sign in the readout. It is important that adequate time is allocated and a well-prepared strategy is followed to increase the chance of success. Often, as a last resort, nonstandard or creative electrode contact selections such as double negative bipolar might prove effective if monopolar configuration is not tolerable.

Occasionally, a patient returns to the clinic with a complaint of loss or significant reduction of stimulation benefit. A careful review of the history will provide some insight about the rate of regression, and the condition can often be classified as either a rapid or a slow decline. The former condition is often related to hardware failures or the onset of a significant clinical event such as pneumonia. Proper remediation generally restores the previously potent benefit. In the case of the slowly declining patients, medication compliance issues are often found to be the cause as patients often reduce their dopaminergic medications on their own. The disease also might have worsened, progressing at a more accelerated pace. In this case, a follow-up visit with the neurologist is strongly recommended.

PROGRAMMING EXAMPLES

Case Study 1

A 54-year-old man who was diagnosed with PD in 1998 was operated in early 2004. His major symptoms included bradykinesia, gait freezing, and motor fluctuations with peak dose dyskinesias. He was a participant in the NIH/VA Cooperative Study Program 468 at our institution, randomized to GPi as his target location. The operative procedure included MRI based targeting and microelectrode recordings and was uneventful. One week after surgery he returned for a surgical follow-up visit and his DBS devices were first programmed. After a careful screening procedure, both electrodes were placed in monopolar mode as shown in Table 1. His medications remained unchanged from preoperative levels and included Mirapex, Stalevo, and Sinemet. Gradually his symptoms improved as stimulation voltages were increased during subsequent visits. Approximately six months after surgery, he reported a cessation of dyskinesias and very rare occasions of gait freezing. A further increase in the stimulation voltages only minimally decreased the occasional hesitation freezing episodes. An increase of his dopaminergic medication did not further reduce these infrequent episodes.

Conclusions

Despite the relatively high initial levels of stimulation, minimal benefits were observed at first. Only after six months and some further increases in stimulation voltages were gait-freezing episodes finally reduced to very few and dyskinesias were completely eliminated. Further increases in stimulation did not yield significant additional gains. Stimulator derived benefit are slow to evolve for GPi targets and sufficient time has to be given for symptom control to develop. Only then should further therapy escalating measures been taken.

A closer inspection of the Table 1 reveals that the right DBS current did not increase beyond 26 μA as the voltage is changed from 2.4 to 3.1 V. As the electrode impedance increased during the same time interval from 918 to 1275 Ω, it negated any gains in current and hence stimulation. More frequently, however, a decrease of the impedance is observed over time, which, in turn, enhances the stimulation effect. This is clearly seen on the left electrode data in Table 1. The current doubled as a result of an increase in stimulation voltage and a concurrent decrease in the electrode impedance.

Case Study 2

A 59-year-old women with a 13-year history of PD was operated on in late 2001 for a left DBS placement. Her symptom was a moderate right upper extremity tremor primarily on the right with some rigidity and bradykinesia, all of which became increasingly medication resistant. The surgical procedure was uneventful and MRI targeting and microelectrode recordings (MER) assisted localization resulted in effective placement of the leads in the STN . Nine days after surgery her electrode was screened and programmed. Table 2 summarizes her programming sessions. The patient did not tolerate monopolar stimulation as she felt lightheaded. A "wide" bipolar setting was used and provided effective tremor relief. She was quite pleased with the result and did not return for programming for about a year when suddenly her left hand tremor reappeared. The Soletra stimulator was found to be off. Restarting the device controlled the tremor again and the patient was advised to regularly check the status of the device. Over time the patient's left hand started to tremor to a point that made daily house work difficult. She was scheduled for a right DBS placement and several months later underwent a successful procedure. The new electrode was screened and programmed in monopolar mode during her hospital stay. The settings were increased in subsequent programming sessions.

Two months later during the 6/12/02 visit, the patient complained about the persisting left upper extremity tremor. An increase in the monopolar setting from 1.7 to 2 V arrested the tremor but produced lightheadedness. So she was switched to bipolar mode at 1−2+ then to 2−3+ as only approximately 90% tremor suppression was achieved on the former setting. At 4.5 V complete suppression was noted with no concurrent adverse events. On 3/19/2003, a small adjustment was needed to retain full tremor suppression. The patient was quite happy with the symptom control and did not return to the clinic until a year and a half later when suddenly her left hand was shaking worse than ever before. The battery for the left DBS device must have expired since no readings could be obtained with the n'Vision programmer (Medtronic 8840). She was scheduled as an outpatient for bilateral stimulator replacements, and following surgery both devices were reprogrammed before she left the hospital. An attempt was made to utilize more battery efficient parameters as seen in Table 2. Although full tremor control was achieved initially, several weeks later the settings had to be increased due to recurring tremors.

Conclusions

It is not always possible to limit the stimulation voltage to 3.6 V or less in order to optimize battery longevity. However, before voltages are increased beyond that threshold, it is advantageous to explore if a gradual increase in the frequency to 185 Hz, and possibly in the pulse width to 120 μS, would not yield additional symptomatic benefit.

If the patient is followed by an outside neurologist, as in this case, it is important that he or she is instructed to return for periodic programming visits so that electrical properties and battery status can be monitored. Although a 6 to 12 month interval is adequate initially, it must be shortened as the anticipated battery depletion date approaches. Sudden battery failure and concurrent worsening of the symptoms might put the patient at significant risk, which is avoidable with proper planning as discussed before.

Case Study 3

A 48-year-old man received his bilateral DBS implants in late 2003. He was first diagnosed with PD in 1998. Prior to surgery he was on Sinemet and his main problem was wearing off abruptly with subsequent severe freezing. Again, MRI based targeting with microelectrode recordings were utilized to implant bilateral, narrow-spaced leads in the STN. The Soletra stimulators were placed during the same session. After a brief and uneventful hospital stay he returned one week later for initial programming. After a careful screening, bipolar settings were activated as outlined in Table 3. While symptoms on his right extremities were controlled rather quickly, the left side required more programming sessions to achieve a satisfactory result. An attempt was made again to use a monopolar mode on the right, but after some period of time, the setting was returned to bipolar mode. Late in 2005, he was exhibiting slight dyskinetic movements at times but they were not interfering with his daily activities. In October 2005, after experiencing significant off time for several days, he came to the clinic for evaluation. His left Soletra stimulator was found unresponsive to the n'Vision as well as the older-programmer model (Medtronic 7432) and he was scheduled for surgical replacement of both devices. Since an exhausted battery is rather unlikely given his programming history, a technical defect was suspected and the device was returned to Medtronic for evaluation. The new stimulators were programmed slightly lower, by 0.2 and 0.3 V, with the plan to increase it if needed during the follow-up visit, one week later.

Instead, a further decrease in the stimulator settings was needed as the patient experienced significantly increased dyskinesia in the form of body rolling motion shortly after the outpatient DBS replacement procedure. It took several sessions and a close interaction with his neurologist to limit these dyskinetic movements and avoid significant freezing episodes that usually followed.

Conclusions

No cause for the suddenly increased sensitivity for dyskinesia could be identified with a neurologic exam and MRI scanning. After two months of systematic medication and programming adjustments, a satisfactory balance was found which eliminated the alternating dyskinesia and freezing episodes and allowed the patient to resume his work full-time again. A careful inspection of the impedance might indicate changing conditions at the electrode-tissue interface. A decrease in the impedance led to an increase in current despite lower voltage settings and might have contributed to this transient dyskinetic phase.

KEY TO SUCCESSFUL DEEP BRAIN STIMULATION PROGRAMMING

During each programming session, careful documentation of all symptoms with complete concurrent stimulation parameters settings is most important. This is imperative if the patient has been followed for some time and the chart has grown in size to the point that reconstructing the past history becomes challenging. Without a complete overview of past settings, the quest for improved stimulation parameters may easily return a patient to a previously used and apparently inadequate setting. This adds to the patient's as well as programmer's frustration and wastes valuable clinic time and resources. Not making the same mistake twice should be the guiding principle, which will invariably lead to success in DBS programming.

REFERENCES

1. Welter ML, Houeto JL, Tezenas du MS, et al. Clinical predictive factors of subthalamic stimulation in Parkinson's disease. Brain 2002; 125(Pt 3):575–583.
2. Jaggi JL, Umemura A, Hurtig HI, et al. Bilateral stimulation of the subthalamic nucleus in Parkinson's disease: surgical efficacy and prediction of outcome. Stereotact Funct Neurosurg 2004; 82(2–3):104–114.
3. Limousin P, Krack P, Pollak P, et al. Electrical stimulation of the subthalamic nucleus in advanced Parkinson's disease. N Engl J Med 1998; 339(16):1105–1111.
4. Volkmann J. Deep-brain stimulation for the treatment of Parkinson's disease. J Clin Neurophysiol January 2004; 21(1):6–17.
5. Weaver F, Follett K, Hur K, Ippolito D, Stern M. Deep brain stimulation in Parkinson disease: a metaanalysis of patient outcomes. J Neurosurg 2005; 103(6):956–967.
6. Follett KA. Comparison of pallidal and subthalamic deep brain stimulation for the treatment of levodopa-induced dyskinesias. Neurosurg Focus 2004; 17(1):E3.
7. Lee JY, Kondziolka D. Thalamic deep brain stimulation for management of essential tremor. J Neurosurg 2005; 103(3):400–403.
8. Danish SF, Jaggi JL, Moyer JT, Finkel L, Baltuch GH. Conventional MRI is inadequate to delineate the relationship between the red nucleus and subthalamic nucleus in Parkinson's disease. Stereotact Funct Neurosurg 2006; 84(1):12–18.
9. Benazzouz A, Piallat B, Pollak P, Benabid AL. Responses of substantia nigra pars reticulata and globus pallidus complex to high frequency stimulation of the subthalamic nucleus in rats: electrophysiological data. Neurosci Lett 1995; 189(2):77–80.
10. Dostrovsky JO, Lozano AM. Mechanisms of deep brain stimulation. Mov Disord 2002; 17(suppl 3):S63–S68.
11. Volkmann J, Fogel W, Krack P. Postoperative Patient Management. Stimulation of the subthalamic nucleus for Parkinson's disease. Medtronic, Minneapolis, Minnesota, U.S.A., 2001.
12. Fraix V, Pollak P. Postoperative Patient Management. Stimulation of the internal globus pallidus and the subthalamic nucleus for Parkinson's disease. Medtronic, Minneapolis, Minnesota, U.S.A., 2001.
13. Volkmann J, Herzog J, Kopper F, Deuschl G. Introduction to the programming of deep brain stimulators. Mov Disord 2002; 17(suppl 3):S181–S187.

14. Plaha P, Patel NK, Gill SS. Stimulation of the subthalamic region for essential tremor. J Neurosurg 2004; 101(1):48–54.
15. Soletra Neurostimulator for Deep Brain Stimulation. 2002. Medtronic, Minneapolis, Minnesota, U.S.A.
16. Kinetra Dual Neurostimulator for Deep Brain Stimulation. 2002. Medtronic, Minneapolis, Minnesota, U.S.A.
17. Chou KL, Siderowf AD, Jaggi JL, Liang GS, Baltuch GH. Unilateral battery depletion in Parkinson's disease patients treated with bilateral subthalamic nucleus deep brain stimulation may require urgent surgical replacement. Stereotact Funct Neurosurg 2004; 82(4):153–155.

10

Medication Adjustment After Deep Brain Stimulation Surgery of the Subthalamic Nucleus

Grace S. Lin Liang

The Parkinson's Institute, Sunnyvale, California, U.S.A.

INTRODUCTION

Over the past decade, deep brain stimulation (DBS) surgery has emerged as a powerful treatment modality for advanced Parkinson's disease (PD). DBS of the subthalamic nucleus (STN) has been shown to provide both immediate and long-term benefit in ameliorating the cardinal motor features of bradykinesia, rigidity, tremor, and gait impairment (1–8). For many patients, the impetus for undergoing surgery arises from the limitations of pharmacotherapy, which may include erratic fluctuations in medication duration and effect, as well as adverse effects of increasing doses of medications, such as levodopa-induced dyskinesias and neuropsychological effects.

Given that many patients are on complex medication regimens with multiple drugs and frequent dosing prior to DBS, the careful adjustment of medications following DBS surgery, in conjunction with managing stimulation parameters, is essential in providing the best possible outcome of the procedure. Okun et al. (9) evaluated a series of 41 patients who were referred to two movement disorder centers because of suboptimal outcomes following DBS surgery. Of these 41 DBS "failures," 30 (73%) were found to require changes in their parkinsonian medications. Three of the patients improved markedly with medication adjustment alone, and 17 others improved after adjustment of the medications and DBS programming. These findings emphasize the critical need for a thorough understanding of both of these modalities of treatment, and continual assessment and adjustment based on the unique needs of the individual patient, both in the immediate postoperative period and after years of chronic DBS therapy.

Dopaminergic Medications

In moderate-to-advanced PD, pharmacological therapy still centers around the dopaminergic agents, namely the levodopa preparations and dopamine agonists. The levodopa formulations are a combination of levodopa and a dopa-decarboxylase inhibitor, either carbidopa or benserazide, and are available in both immediate- and controlled-release forms. The catechol-*O*-methyl-transferase inhibitors, entacapone and tolcapone, may be used as adjuncts to levodopa to inhibit its metabolism, and thus extend its half-life and concentration area under the curve (10–12). Selegiline and rasagiline are inhibitors of monoamine oxidase-B, the other enzyme also responsible for degradation of dopamine in the brain. Levodopa is still the most potent pharmacological agent available for the relief of parkinsonian symptoms. The dopamine agonists are effective and may be used as monotherapy for relief of PD symptoms, but in moderate to severe stages of the disease, are more frequently used in conjunction with levodopa. The dopamine agonists that are currently available in the United States include bromocriptine, pergolide, cabergoline (which is not FDA-approved for treatment of PD), pramipexole, and ropinirole. Lisuride and piribedil are dopamine agonists available in Europe and other countries. Apomorphine is a water-soluble highly potent dopamine agonist with a rapid onset and short half-life. It is available in injectable form, used as "rescue" therapy for "off" periods.

After DBS surgery, overall dopaminergic medication dose requirements have been reduced significantly in multiple studies evaluating outcomes of the procedure, ranging from 19% to 100% average reductions in dose (1,2, 4–7,13). Several patients have been able to be maintained on DBS therapy and off of dopaminergic medications entirely, even up to five years after surgery (7,14–16). The rationale for reduction of medications is several-fold. With DBS there is improvement in patients' motor function and reduction in duration of "off" time, and thus lower or less frequent doses of the medications may be able to provide the same level of overall motor function (8). Furthermore, the procedure itself or STN stimulation may induce increased dyskinesias postoperatively, possibly because of a functional subthalamotomy effect (1,17,18). Tapering of the dopaminergic medications in this situation may lessen the likelihood of dyskinesias. In addition, the dose-dependent side effects of the medications, both short-term and long-term, may warrant a reduction in dose as DBS stimulation is increased to supplement or replace the effect of medications for alleviating parkinsonian symptoms.

Anticholinergic Medications

Drugs in the class of anticholinergic medications used to treat PD include benz-tropine, trihexyphenidyl, biperiden, and ethopropazine (not available in the United States), which are central muscarinic receptor antagonists. With the many medications currently available for PD treatment, the primary utility of the anticholinergic drugs now is for treatment of tremor. They are also sometimes used as an adjunctive medication for treating dystonia that can occur in PD, usually as an "off" phenomenon (19). However, they do not appear to provide as much benefit in treating the akinesia and rigidity of PD when compared with dopaminergic drugs (20). With reduction of tremor after DBS, the anticho-linergic medications can be tapered lower or eliminated from the regimen as tolerated. Reduction of anticholinergic medications can be beneficial because of both central and peripheral side effects, which can be bothersome, especially in patients who are elderly or have some cognitive impairment. Central side effects include sedation, confusion, memory impairment, and psychosis. Autonomic effects such as dry mouth, orthostatic hypotension, constipation, and urinary retention are also common with the anticholinergics and can be particularly problematic in PD patients who have underlying autonomic dysfunc-tion. Many of these central and peripheral adverse effects are reversible with reduction or discontinuation of the medications.

Amantadine

Amantadine may have several pharmacological mechanisms of action that mediate its effects on PD symptoms. Some studies suggest that amantadine may increase dopamine release and synthesis (21,22), and inhibit dopamine reuptake (22). It also has anticholinergic effects, perhaps, also mediated by N-methyl-aspartate (NMDA) receptors (23). Amantadine is often used in moder-ate to advanced PD as an adjunctive medication to the dopaminergic agents, usually at doses between 100 and 500 mg/day. It has mild anti-parkinsonian effects for relieving tremor, bradykinesia, and rigidity, and has been shown to reduce motor fluctuations and the duration of "off" time (24). In patients who are candidates for DBS, dyskinesias are another complication of chronic levodopa therapy, which become increasingly severe with increasing doses and duration of levodopa use. Amantadine has been shown to be effective in reducing dyskinesias (25–27). Its antidyskinetic effects may be related to its mild antagonism of glutamate NMDA receptors, which have been implicated as possibly involved in the development of levodopa-induced dyskinesias (28).

One of the benefits of DBS that has been described is reduction in levodopa-induced dyskinesias with chronic stimulation (18,29). The reduction in dyskinesia severity has been reported to range from 30% to 92% in various outcomes studies (1–3,7,16,30). Russmann et al. (31) evaluated dyskinesia sever-ity with levodopa challenge in 12 patients who had undergone chronic DBS. Six of the patients did not require medications to treat parkinsonian symptoms after DBS, and the reduction in average dyskinesia severity in this group was 96%, with only one out of six patients experiencing dyskinesia. The other six patients, whose dopaminergic medication doses were reduced 62% from baseline, had only 47% reduction in dyskinesia severity. The results suggested that the reduction of dyskinesias in STN DBS patients was partially dependent on the degree of dopaminergic medication reduction and may indicate some reversibility of sensitivity to levodopa-induced dyskinesias. However, in another study, Wenzelburger et al. (32) found that even in some patients with no reduction in dopaminergic medication, dyskinesia severity was still reduced after STN stimulation, which indicates that DBS may also have an intrinsic antidyskinetic effect independent of medication reduction. Thus, with improvement in the duration and severity of dyskinesias after surgery, the need for amantadine may be lessened and a gradual taper of the medication can be done. This would be particularly useful in patients who may have side effects from amantadine. These include cognitive impairment and confusion, dry mouth, and constipation, which may be from the anticholinergic effects of the drug. Amantadine may also cause peripheral edema and livedo reticularis, which is often reversible with reduction of the dose. However, the taper should be gradual, for example, by 100 mg/day every one to two weeks, because of the possibility of acute worsening of symptoms with sudden discontinuation of the medication (33,34). In some patients, some nonmotor symptoms may also have benefit from amantadine, and thus the response to dose reduction should be undertaken with careful monitoring of symptoms.

Considerations for the Timing and Progression of Medication Adjustment

There have been few assessments and no systematic controlled trials of the optimal protocol for medication reduction following STN DBS surgery. Most studies report outcomes in terms of change in overall dopaminergic medication daily dose, and do not differentiate between dopamine agonists and levodopa. Other PD medications such as the catechol-O-methyl transferase (COMT) inhibitors, selegiline, amantadine, and anticholinergics are usually not included in the conversion to levodopa equivalents. In an earlier series, medications were reduced by 60% within the first month, and maintained at about 65% below baseline for at least 12 months (17). Another study followed a protocol of initially reducing dopaminergic medications 30% immediately postsurgery, then adjusting further according to amount of improvement with stimulation; dopaminergic medication reduction was 51% at 12 months (35). Thobois et al. (36) assessed the timing of medication adjustments in a series of 18 consecutive patients who underwent STN DBS. Perioperatively, the nondopaminergic medications were first reduced or eliminated, which included the anticholinergic medications, selegiline, entacapone, apomorphine, and amantadine. To reduce the risk of postoperative confusion, the anticholinergics, and in some cases the dopamine agonists, were reduced preoperatively. After STN stimulation was initiated, the only medications still in use after the first month were levodopa, ropinirole, and bromocriptine. They reduced levodopa first preferentially because of the shorter half-life and simpler titration, and 45% of patients were able to discontinue levodopa. At the 12-month follow-up, one-third of patients were not on medication, 28% of the patients were either on monotherapy with levodopa or a dopamine agonist, and 39% on a combination of the two. The majority of medication reduction occurred during the first month, and the doses of the medications were approximately reduced to half in 12 months. Often, reducing both the individual doses of medications and the frequency of administration can be achieved because of the reduction in severity of fluctuations with STN DBS.

Vingerhoets et al. (16) performed a study in which anti-parkinsonian medications were held prior to surgery. In the first postoperative week, the stimulator was turned on and adjusted frequently, on an average twice daily in the first week, and every one to two weeks thereafter during the first two months, to optimize patient motor scores primarily with the stimulator. The anti-parkinsonian medications were only gradually and progressively reinstated if the DBS did not bring motor function to the same level as the preoperative medication "on" state, with a goal of using the least amount of medication necessary. Of the 20 patients they studied, 10 patients were maintained off medications and on stimulation alone for up to two years. Overall, medications were reduced by 79% at last follow-up. However, others have argued that medications should not be reduced rapidly or aggressively postoperatively. One reason is that there can be variability in clinical function during the initial recovery period of several months, which may partially be due to a microlesioning effect from the surgery, as well as stabilization of stimulation parameters and effect (37,38). Furthermore, patients may also have nonmotor symptoms that are responsive to the medications, and rapid tapering of the medications may cause intolerable exacerbations of these symptoms even while the motor symptoms are sufficiently reduced by the DBS. Uncovering restless legs symptom has been described following STN DBS (39). Changes in mood and cognition including apathy, depression, and even suicide, have also been seen after STN DBS, possibly related to decreases in dopaminergic medications following surgery (7,38,40).

Case Study

The patient noted gradual loss of dexterity at age 62 and was diagnosed with PD. He was started on carbidopa/levodopa and had an excellent response. He began to develop levodopa-induced dyskinesias around age 69. By age 75, he was having increasing motor fluctuations with delayed onset of medication effect and wearing off sometimes after one to two hours, with occasional dose failures. However, during his medication "on" time, he was able to walk without difficulty, and had minimal tremor and rigidity. The peak-dose dyskinesias were moderate-to-severe in intensity and occurred about 30% to 50% of the day. At the time of surgery, he was taking 1.5 to 2 tablets of carbidopa/levodopa 25/100 every three hours during the daytime (1000 mg levodopa), controlled release carbidopa/levodopa 50/200 at night, entacapone 100 to 200 mg five times daily, ropinirole 3 mg four times daily, and amantadine 100 mg twice daily. He underwent implantation of STN DBS electrodes bilaterally without complication at age 76. Shortly after the surgeries, the wearing off and dyskinesias were significantly decreased, and his total levodopa requirements were 800 mg/day, with entacapone 200 mg five times daily and ropinirole 3 mg three times daily. Amantadine was tapered-off two months later, but the patient continued to have some mild dyskinesias. Therefore, the dose of entacapone was then decreased to 100 mg five times daily. However, he continued to have wearing-off after about three hours, manifested primarily by gait-freezing and slurred speech. With further increases in stimulation amplitude over the following months, his gait improved, and the dose of levodopa was reduced to 400 mg daily. Because of complaints about short-term memory impairment, a plan to gradually taper ropinirole in conjunction with further monitoring and stimulator adjustment was made.

This case illustrates several considerations common to the patients who undergo STN DBS therapy. Through extensive preoperative testing of overall mobility and motor function, responsiveness to levodopa and neuropsychological status, he was determined to be a good DBS candidate. Preoperatively, he was taking levodopa in combination with a COMT inhibitor, dopamine agonist, and amantadine, for severe, frequent fluctuations and dyskinesias. Following surgery, the addition of DBS provided improvement in bradykinesia, rigidity, and gait, but also a mild increase in dyskinesias that necessitated reductions in dopaminergic medications. Because of his age and cognitive status, a primary goal of the management of his therapy is to find a balance between maximizing mobility and motor function with minimal fluctuations, and minimizing cognitive or other side effects of the medications.

SUMMARY

Although substantial or even complete reduction of anti-parkinsonian medications can often be achieved after DBS, it should not be a primary goal of postoperative medication adjustment. Medication reductions may provide the benefit of potentially lessening adverse or toxic effects of the drugs, but may also unmask nonmotor features of PD that are still responsive to dopaminergic therapy. Therefore, medication regimens need to be assessed frequently both in the immediate postoperative period of recovery from the procedure, and with each DBS adjustment thereafter, tailored to the individual symptoms and goals of the patient.

REFERENCES

1. Limousin P, Krack P, Pollak P, et al. Electrical stimulation of the subthalamic nucleus in advanced Parkinson's disease. N Engl J Med 1998; 339:1105–1111.

2. The Deep Brain Stimulation for Parkinson's Disease Study Group. Deep-brain stimulation of the subthalamic nucleus or the pars interna of the globus pallidus in Parkinson's disease. N Engl J Med 2001; 345:956–963.

3. Simuni T, Jaggi JL, Mulholland H, et al. Bilateral stimulation of the subthalamic nucleus in patients with Parkinson disease: a study of efficacy and safety. J Neurosurg 2002; 96:666–672.

4. Romito LM, Scerrati M, Contarino MF, Bentivoglio AR, Tonali P, Albanese A. Long-term follow up of subthalamic nucleus stimulation in Parkinson's disease. Neurology 2002; 58:1546–1550.

5. Pahwa R, Wilkinson SB, Overman J, Lyons KE. Bilateral subthalamic stimulation in patients with Parkinson disease: long-term follow up. J Neurosurg 2003; 99:71–77.

6. Kleiner-Fisman G, Fisman DN, Sime E, Saint-Cyr JA, Lozano AM, Lang AE. Long-term follow up of bilateral deep brain stimulation of the subthalamic nucleus in patients with advanced Parkinson disease. J Neurosurg 2003; 99:489–495.

7. Krack P, Batir A, Van Blercom N, et al. Five-year follow-up of bilateral stimulation of the subthalamic nucleus in advanced Parkinson's disease. N Engl J Med 2003; 349:1925–1934.

8. Rodriguez-Oroz MC, Obeso JA, Lang AE, et al. Bilateral deep brain stimulation in Parkinson's disease: a multicentre study with 4 years follow-up. Brain 2005; 128:2240–2249.

9. Okun MS, Tagliati M, Pourfar M, et al. Management of referred deep brain stimulation failures: a retrospective analysis from 2 movement disorders centers. Arch Neurol 2005; 62:1250–1255.

10. Bonifati V, Meco G. New, selective catechol-*O*-methyltransferase inhibitors as therapeutic agents in Parkinson's disease. Pharmacol Ther 1999; 81:1–36.

11. Nutt JG. Effect of COMT inhibition on the pharmacokinetics and pharmacodynamics of levodopa in parkinsonian patients. Neurology 2000; 55:S33–S37; discussion S38–S41.

12. Heikkinen H, Saraheimo M, Antila S, Ottoila P, Pentikainen PJ. Pharmacokinetics of entacapone, a peripherally acting catechol-*O*-methyltransferase inhibitor, in man. A study using a stable isotope techique. Eur J Clin Pharmacol 2001; 56:821–826.

13. Ostergaard K, Sunde N, Dupont E. Effects of bilateral stimulation of the subthalamic nucleus in patients with severe Parkinson's disease and motor fluctuations. Mov Disord 2002; 17:693–700.

14. Molinuevo JL, Valldeoriola F, Tolosa E, et al. Levodopa withdrawal after bilateral subthalamic nucleus stimulation in advanced Parkinson disease. Arch Neurol 2000; 57:983–988.

15. Valldeoriola F, Pilleri M, Tolosa E, Molinuevo JL, Rumia J, Ferrer E. Bilateral subthalamic stimulation monotherapy in advanced Parkinson's disease: long-term follow-up of patients. Mov Disord 2002; 17:125–132.

16. Vingerhoets FJ, Villemure JG, Temperli P, Pollo C, Pralong E, Ghika J. Subthalamic DBS replaces levodopa in Parkinson's disease: two-year follow-up. Neurology 2002; 58:396–401.

17. Moro E, Scerrati M, Romito LM, Roselli R, Tonali P, Albanese A. Chronic subthalamic nucleus stimulation reduces medication requirements in Parkinson's disease. Neurology 1999; 53:85–90.

18. Krack P, Pollak P, Limousin P, Benazzouz A, Deuschl G, Benabid AL. From off-period dystonia to peak-dose chorea. The clinical spectrum of varying subthalamic nucleus activity. Brain 1999; 122(Pt 6):1133–1146.

19. Poewe WH, Lees AJ, Stern GM. Dystonia in Parkinson's disease: clinical and pharmacological features. Ann Neurol 1988; 23:73–78.
20. Schrag A, Schelosky L, Scholz U, Poewe W. Reduction of Parkinsonian signs in patients with Parkinson's disease by dopaminergic versus anticholinergic single-dose challenges. Mov Disord 1999; 14:252–255.
21. Scatton B, Cheramy A, Besson MJ, Glowinski J. Increased synthesis and release of dopamine in the striatum of the rat after amantadine treatment. Eur J Pharmacol 1970; 13:131–133.
22. Von Voigtlander PF, Moore KE. Dopamine: release from the brain in vivo by amantadine. Science 1971; 174:408–410.
23. Stoof JC, Booij J, Drukarch B, Wolters EC. The anti-parkinsonian drug amantadine inhibits the *N*-methyl-D-aspartic acid-evoked release of acetylcholine from rat neostriatum in a non-competitive way. Eur J Pharmacol 1992; 213:439–443.
24. Shannon KM, Goetz CG, Carroll VS, Tanner CM, Klawans HL. Amantadine and motor fluctuations in chronic Parkinson's disease. Clin Neuropharmacol 1987; 10:522–526.
25. Metman LV, Del Dotto P, LePoole K, Konitsiotis S, Fang J, Chase TN. Amantadine for levodopa-induced dyskinesias: a 1-year follow-up study. Arch Neurol 1999; 56:1383–1386.
26. Verhagen Metman L, Del Dotto P, van den Munckhof P, Fang J, Mouradian MM, Chase TN. Amantadine as treatment for dyskinesias and motor fluctuations in Parkinson's disease. Neurology 1998; 50:1323–1326.
27. Adler CH, Stern MB, Vernon G, Hurtig HI. Amantadine in advanced Parkinson's disease: good use of an old drug. J Neurol 1997; 244:336–337.
28. Chase TN, Oh JD. Striatal mechanisms and pathogenesis of parkinsonian signs and motor complications. Ann Neurol 2000; 47:S122–S129, discussion S129–S130.
29. Krack P, Limousin P, Benabid AL, Pollak P. Chronic stimulation of subthalamic nucleus improves levodopa-induced dyskinesias in Parkinson's disease. Lancet 1997; 350:1676.
30. Volkmann J. Deep brain stimulation for the treatment of Parkinson's disease. J Clin Neurophysiol 2004; 21:6–17.
31. Russmann H, Ghika J, Combrement P, et al. L-dopa-induced dyskinesia improvement after STN-DBS depends upon medication reduction. Neurology 2004; 63:153–155.
32. Wenzelburger R, Zhang BR, Poepping M, et al. Dyskinesias and grip control in Parkinson's disease are normalized by chronic stimulation of the subthalamic nucleus. Ann Neurol 2002; 52:240–243.
33. Wilson JA, Farquhar DL, Primrose WR, Smith RG. Long term amantadine treatment. The danger of withdrawal. Scott Med J 1987; 32:135.
34. Factor SA, Molho ES, Brown DL. Acute delirium after withdrawal of amantadine in Parkinson's disease. Neurology 1998; 50:1456–1458.
35. Jaggi JL, Umemura A, Hurtig HI, et al. Bilateral stimulation of the subthalamic nucleus in Parkinson's disease: surgical efficacy and prediction of outcome. Stereotact Funct Neurosurg 2004; 82:104–114.
36. Thobois S, Corvaisier S, Mertens P, et al. The timing of antiparkinsonian treatment reduction after subthalamic nucleus stimulation. Eur Neurol 2003; 49:59–63.
37. Kleiner-Fisman G, Saint-Cyr JA, Miyasaki J, Lozano A, Lang AE. Subthalamic DBS replaces levodopa in Parkinson's disease. Neurology 2002; 59:1293–1294.

38. Krack P, Fraix V, Mendes A, Benabid AL, Pollak P. Postoperative management of subthalamic nucleus stimulation for Parkinson's disease. Mov Disord 2002; 17(suppl 3):S188–S197.
39. Kedia S, Moro E, Tagliati M, Lang AE, Kumar R. Emergence of restless legs syndrome during subthalamic stimulation for Parkinson disease. Neurology 2004; 63:2410–2412.
40. Funkiewiez A, Ardouin C, Krack P, et al. Acute psychotropic effects of bilateral subthalamic nucleus stimulation and levodopa in Parkinson's disease. Mov Disord 2003; 18:524–530.

11

Rehabilitation After Deep Brain Stimulation

Keith M. Robinson and L. Sue Traweek

Department of Physical Medicine and Rehabilitation, University of Pennsylvania, Philadelphia, Pennsylvania, U.S.A.

INTRODUCTION

High frequency deep brain stimulation (DBS) procedures have become more common to treat medically refractory Parkinson's disease (PD) in those who are experiencing "tolerance" to dopaminergic agents as manifested by dyskinesias and rapid motor fluctuations. Their efficacy has been optimal for suppressing the isolated clinical signs that usually are responsive to dopaminergic agents (tremor, rigidity, and bradykinesia), but not necessarily efficacious when considering gait and postural disturbances, speech impairments, motor blocks, cognitive/behavioral difficulties, dysautonomia, and other motoric and nonmotoric signs that are either usually not responsive to dopaminergic agents or are manifestations of later stage disease. Functional status and quality of life have been generally reported as improved after DBS procedures (1–5).

High-frequency stimulation of three subcortical structures that are encompassed among the neural networks that control movement have been studied: the ventralis intermedius nucleus (Vim) of the thalamus, the internal segment of the globus pallidus (GPi) of the basal ganglia, and the subthalamic nucleus (STN) of the basal ganglia. High-frequency stimulation or physiological ablation of these structures has been viewed as comparable to surgical or anatomic ablation (thalamotomy and pallidotomy), however reversible (2,3). Historically, thalamic stimulation has been the preferred procedure to treat tremor-predominant PD. However, it has been less effective for controlling other parkinsonian signs. Thalamic stimulation, thus, has largely been replaced by STN stimulation, which has been comparable to thalamic stimulation for control of tremor, and more effective for controlling other parkinsonian signs. STN and GPi stimulation have been viewed as relatively comparable for controlling parkinsonian signs, particularly when "off" dopaminergic medications, primarily contributing to improved regulation of motor fluctuations. STN stimulation has been reported to be less effective to control on-medication dyskinesias than GPi stimulation. Yet, STN stimulation more often has allowed for significant reductions in doses of dopaminergic medications, with associated decreased dyskinesias. STN-DBS has been observed to sustain its therapeutic effects beyond one year, whereas GPi-DBS anecdotally has led to "treatment failure" in a small number of patients after one year. GPi-DBS has required higher stimulation "dosing" than STN-DBS, but STN-DBS has required more intensive postsurgical observation associated with its relatively higher prevalence of adverse events, particularly neuropsychiatric. STN stimulation has evolved to become the preferred procedure over GPi. Only one randomized controlled trial that compares these stimulation procedures has been completed, however other such studies are in process (6–9).

The neurophysiologic mechanisms that underpin the reported efficacy of high-frequency DBS are not completely understood. During dopamine depletion within the substantia nigra compacta of the basal ganglia that occurs in PD, hyperactivity of the STN concurrently has been observed and is considered a hallmark of the disease. STN hyperactivity provides "over-excitation" of the GPi. "Overexcitation" of the GPi provides "over-inhibition" of the Vim of the thalamus. This inhibition provides "overexcitation" of the supplementary motor and dorsolateral prefrontal cortices that, in turn, results in parkinsonian motor signs. Physiological ablation using high-frequency DBS inhibits or re-balances this component of the neural network with the aim of dampening the classic levodopa-responsive parkinsonian clinical signs (2,3,6,10).

The expanding evidence-based outcome data are still considered insufficient to provide universal support for recommending DBS to treat medically refractory PD (7,11). The possibility of neuroprotective effects after DBS has not been firmly established but continues to be explored by neuroscientists. Thus, the current view of DBS procedures to treat PD is that they are essentially palliative; they provide support to stabilize the levodopa-responsive manifestations of the neurodegenerative process, but they do not retard the disease process (2–5,7).

When considering the rehabilitation needs of those individuals with PD who have DBS procedures, there have been no reported investigations of focused rehabilitation interventions. However, a substantial amount of investigation has been accomplished that can guide the rehabilitation process for this patient population to serve the purposes of defining realistic presurgical expectations and postsurgical outcomes, as well as for defining the rehabilitation service needs and practices to be provided immediately after surgery, during the initial year after surgery, and thereafter.

DEFINING REALISTIC PRESURGICAL EXPECTATIONS

Referral for DBS procedures by rehabilitation specialists to neurologists and neurosurgeons of appropriate individuals with PD, and rehabilitating those who are selected as candidates after these procedures, require knowledge of which patients are considered the best candidates for DBS and what patients should expect during their acute hospital stay, and inpatient rehabilitation stay if indicated.

Patient Selection

DBS has been considered most appropriate for those having a younger age of disease onset, and before the associated limitations in everyday life activities have progressed to threaten autonomous self-care, safe mobility, meaningful communication, and social and occupational role participation. Poor outcome after DBS is more likely in older individuals ($>$70) because they may have more manifestations of later-stage disease that are considered levodopa-resistant (2,7,12,13). Moreover, older patients are more likely to have more advanced comorbid medical conditions that increase surgical risks of adverse events and have associated disability independent from that associated with PD. With the exception of dyskinesias, motor signs that persist during the best "on-medication" state after receiving a suprathreshold dose of short-acting levodopa are unlikely to respond to DBS (4). Thus, a levodopa-challenge test has been recommended by some neurologists and neurosurgeons to assist with predicting surgical outcome (13). However, limiting the assessment for selecting appropriate individuals for DBS to the level of disease impairment, that is, in controlling the cardinal clinical signs of PD, is not enough. For each individual, these clinical signs must be explicitly linked to the level of disability and/or interference with participation in essential daily activities that contribute to quality of life in the areas of self-care, mobility, communication, and social role performance (7).

Several studies have articulated predictive factors influencing patient selection for DBS (14–16). Such factors include: lower age; better control of motor signs presurgically as clinically observed between the off-medication and the on-medication conditions as an indicator of levodopa responsiveness; and longer disease duration. Additionally, two specific levodopa-responsive clinical factors have emerged as positively predictive of outcome during the first postsurgical year: relatively more decrease in rigidity and relatively more improvement in postural stability, as observed presurgically between the off- and on-medication conditions.

Immediate Postsurgical Management

Except for patients who have tremor-predominant PD, the stimulators usually are not turned on until at least one week after the procedure. Thus, most patients who have DBS are restarted on their usual dopaminergic medications no later than the evening of the day of surgery, and they are expected to get out of bed and re-establish self-care and mobility no later than the first postsurgical day. Physiatry, physical therapy, and social work referrals are highly recommended in order to assess mobility and balance, and to determine whether there is an increase in the burden of care on informal caregivers (spouses, adult children/grandchildren, and friends) with whom the individuals with PD share their households. Moreover, occupational therapy and speech therapy assessments can be useful immediately postsurgically to define if there are difficulties in self-care abilities, swallowing, and communication that require further treatment.

For those patients who live alone, defining informal caregivers who can provide household supervision, physical assistance and transportation, and perform personal care and household chores is essential. If multidisciplinary assessments indicate a decline in the functional abilities of the individual in comparison to the presurgical functional baseline, or point to a lack of availability of informal caregivers, particularly for those who live alone, then continued rehabilitation services should be offered, either inpatient or at home. In the best of circumstances, that is, when there are no immediate postsurgical complications, when the informal caregivers are available, and when the patient quickly re-establishes baseline mobility, self-care, swallowing, and communication, the patient should be offered home nursing and physical therapy for wound and mobility "check-outs." Otherwise, more comprehensive rehabilitation services should be offered. The decision to choose inpatient or home rehabilitation services is influenced by several psychosocial factors including the "disability tolerance" of the informal caregivers, the geographical accessibility of informal caregivers to inpatient rehabilitation programs, and the "consuming power" that the patient has to purchase rehabilitation services as dictated by his/her health insurance plan. For example, if the patient develops a postsurgical delirium or other complications, and has not quickly re-established his/her baseline functional status, or if the caregiver has health problems with associated disability, and/or if the caregiver works and cannot be available during daytime hours, during the initial postsurgical week, then the "disability tolerance" of the patient–caregiver dyad may be compromised and an inpatient rehabilitation stay should be pursued. Or, if the patient and caregiver have traveled a great distance to a regional center to have DBS, the caregiver may be required to expend resources on travel, parking, and hotels. To reduce the necessity of daily long distance travel and parking/hotel expenses, many inpatient rehabilitation programs will offer the means for caregivers to "live in" by setting up a folding bed. The patient–caregiver dyad must be viewed as "client": thus, the caregiver should be encouraged to participate in as many therapy sessions as possible for educational purposes. Insurance plans, in general, have been convivial in their approval for inpatient rehabilitation after DBS given that the need for these expensive services has not been universal, and lengths of stay have been relatively short.

Our longitudinal study of 39 patients with PD who had STN-DBS revealed several findings that can provide a context for planning immediate postsurgical rehabilitation services:

1. The mean acute hospital length of stay for all patients was 3.5 days.
2. Forty-one percent of our study patients were admitted to inpatient rehabilitation; their mean inpatient rehabilitation length of stay was 7.3 days.
3. The need for inpatient rehabilitation was associated with the occurrence of nonlife threatening postsurgical complications, specifically, delirium (10.3%), worsening dysphagia without aspiration (10.3%), drug rash (5.1%), urinary retention (5.1%), urinary tract infection (2.6%), *Clostridium difficile* pseudomembraneous enterocolitis (2.6%), seizure (2.6%), atrial fibrillation (2.6%), chest pain (2.6%), and acute renal failure (2.6%). Among the 22 observed postsurgical complications, 17 of these were observed in patients who required inpatient rehabilitation.
4. Our subgroup of study patients who were admitted to inpatient rehabilitation after STN-DBS, when compared to the subgroup of patients who were immediately discharged home after STN-DBS, were significantly older; had significantly higher disease severity on the Modified Hoehn and Yahr Staging scale; scored significantly lower presurgically on the mobility subscale of the Functional Independence Measure; walked significantly slower presurgically on the Timed Get Up and Go test; and had significantly slower speed of cognitive processing during verbal fluency and verbal working memory tasks (17).

Knowledge of immediate postsurgical complications is essential for planning and providing postsurgical rehabilitation services after DBS. The occurrence of complications has been extremely low and usually transient. Postsurgical mortality and serious morbidity have been reported to be no more than 3%, and most often, these occurrences have been associated with intracerebral and subdural hemorrhagic events, cerebral venous infarctions, seizures, hardware infections, deep venous thromboses and pulmonary emboli (2,3,7). The reported undesirable transient effects after STN-DBS included delirium (24%), delayed wound healing/scalp cellulitis/skin erosion (8%), and cerebrospinal fluid leak (<2%) (18). Rare (<1%) neuropsychiatric postsurgical complications have included mania, delusions, hallucinations, and depression associated with suicidal attempts. These latter events were thought to be associated with the relatively abrupt decreases in dopaminergic agents sometimes necessary after STN-DBS. A hypothesized "therapeutic lesioning" effect has been observed; a reduction in parkinsonian motor signs before the initiation of stimulation has been thought to be associated with immediate postsurgical edema and micro-hemorrhages resulting from wire placement (5).

Postsurgical pain control after DBS has rarely been problematic. Pain usually was associated with the scalp wire entry and chest wall electrode sites. Short-acting nonopioid analgesia (acetaminophen) was usually effective, so consistent use of short-acting opioids was rarely necessary to reduce wound pain or headache associated with scalp, facial, and chest wall muscle spasm. Nonsteroidal anti-inflammatory agents were avoided because of their bleeding risk. Facial edema, particularly periorbital, was common and resolved relatively quickly over several days. The suture/staple sites on the scalp can be distracting to those patients who become disinhibited because of delirium after DBS procedures. Soft mitts have been reported to be useful for minimizing trauma and the risk of infection; a low dose of an atypical neuroleptic agent such as quetiapine, typically started at bedtime, can modulate such behavior. The subcutaneous wires that traverse between the scalp and chest wall typically have not induced limitations in head/neck range of motion (18).

SHORT-TERM AND LONG-TERM OUTCOMES

The study of DBS postsurgical motor functioning has primarily entailed short-term longitudinal observation of individuals during the initial year after the procedure. Increasingly, observations are extending beyond one year, or the long-term. Outcome measurement after DBS has encompassed a variety of tools to assess isolated and more integrative clinical signs (impairment-level), functional status (disability- or activity participation-level), and quality of life. Most of the measurement tools used to observe outcome after DBS were developed as PD-specific tools to serve the purpose of consistent observation across various clinical centers that care for individuals who have PD and related disorders. These have ubiquitously included the Uniform Parkinson's Disease Rating Scale (UPDRS), and the Schwab and England Activities of Daily Living (ADL) Scale (19).

The UPDRS is a 42-item tool that broadly assesses clinical signs of PD and associated functional status. It encompasses four subscales that measure: (*i*) mentation/behavior/mood; (*ii*) activities of daily living (ADL); (*iii*) motor performance; (*iv*) and complications of therapy (including dyskinesias and rapid motor fluctuations). These subscales methodologically are not pristine in that they combine impairment-based and disability/activity participation-based measures, more heavily weighted toward measurement at the impairment level. Few investigators have been rigorous in distinguishing impairment- and activity participation-based measurement when assessing postsurgical motor functioning in those who have PD by either adapting the UPDRS or by using alternative measurement tools (20,21). However, the methodological weaknesses of the

UPDRS have been counterbalanced by the strength of the provision of a universal measurement "language" among movement disorders specialists that has been applied over many years of use.

The Schwab and England ADL Scale is an ordinal scale that measures functional status or burden of care. It more explicitly measures activity participation across basic and instrumental ADL, articulated as the ability to perform "chores." Historically, the use of this scale has assured that impairment-based measurement, that is, the UPDRS, has been linked clinically to disability- or activity-based measurement when observing outcomes in the treatment of PD (22).

Lang and Widner (2002) (13) have promoted the application of the Core Assessment Program for Neurosurgical Interventions and Transplantation in Parkinson's Disease (CAPSIT-PD) as an additional strategy for observation of postsurgical outcomes after DBS procedures. This measurement scheme includes the UPDRS as its primary functional outcome measure along with a series of timed motor tasks that measure upper limb repetitive movements (pronation/supination, finger tapping, finger dexterity) and walking.

The observed outcomes after DBS presented below will be summarized briefly since they are discussed in more detail in other chapters of this book.

Outcomes After Vim-DBS

Short-term longitudinal studies of Vim-DBS have confirmed its efficacy for controlling tremor and handwriting ability, but not gait, in those with tremor-predominant PD. Several aspects of quality of life have been reported as significantly improved including ADL performance and affective/emotional state (20,23,24).

Several long-term longitudinal studies observed patients with tremor-predominant PD, and demonstrated significant improvements in tremor-specific and ADL scores that were sustained over means of 18 to 49 months; improvements in global scores of motor control were not sustained (25–27). Pinter et al. (28) cross-sectionally studied postural control and gait in seven patients who were assessed at an average of 19.6 months after Vim-DBS to treat tremor-predominant PD. On-stimulation conditions were associated with significant decreases in the latencies of gait initiation along with significant improvements in static postural sway, but not in postural stability in response to external provocations. Vim-DBS continues to be offered to treat essential tremor, action tremor associated with multiple sclerosis, and post-traumatic and poststroke tremors (29,30).

Outcomes After GPi-DBS

Several longitudinal studies have observed significantly improved motor and functional outcomes after GPi-DBS during the initial year after surgery, particularly during the off-medication/on-stimulation condition (31–33). This translates pragmatically into a decrease in rapid motor fluctuations associated with more consistent and sustained ability to participate in daytime functional activities; into increased safety for getting out of bed in the middle of the night for toileting when the effect of nighttime dosing of medications may be minimal; and into increased ability for getting out of bed in the morning to initiate self-care rituals before or as morning medications take effect. Moreover, significant decreases in on-medication dyskinesias during the initial postsurgical year were observed. This pragmatically translates into less interference of medication-induced dyskinesias on the performance of daytime functional activities.

Krystlowski et al. (34,35) observed several aspects of gait and postural control, cross-sectionally, during the initial year after GPi-STN; improvements in gait (increased stride length, decreased single and double support time) but not in postural control (preparatory postural adjustments) were observed. Quality of life has been reported as improved during the initial year after GPi-DBS (30).

Several long-term outcome studies, after GPi-DBS, have reported observations that have spanned means of between 24 and 60 months. The most robust observation has been decreases in on-medication dyskinesias that are thought to be a direct effect of stimulation. Rapid motor fluctuations recurred in many study patients at one year after GPi-DBS. Improvements in functional status were not consistently reported (36–41).

Short-Term Outcomes After STN-DBS

Postsurgical outcomes after STN-DBS have been the most extensively studied among DBS procedures. The findings of some of these studies that have observed outcomes during the initial year will be summarized.

Functional Status

Improvements in motor and functional outcomes during the initial year after STN-DBS have been reported during longitudinal studies (42–52). Moreover, decreases in on-medication dyskinesias have been reported and are thought to be associated with using lower dosing of dopaminergic agents. In contrast, decreases in rapid motor fluctuations are postulated to be a result of chronic stimulation with a "stabilizing effect" whether medications are on board or not. Qualitative observation during several of these studies revealed that no parallel improvements in motor and functional status over time were observed when considering walking abilities, and when stratifying the study patients into performance-based subgroups (42–44,48,51). Linazasoro (52) has offered some caution regarding the generally reported positive results after STN-DBS. Specifically, he has argued that the outcome studies are too focused on motor function, while other aspects of outcome such as the emotional status, cognition, and quality of life have been inadequately reported. Thus, an unrealistic impression of the impact of STN-DBS on everyday life has been communicated.

To support this argument, Linazasoro has presented an update of 18 patients from his program who also were involved in a multicenter trial: 6/18 could be considered to have a good clinical outcome when assessed comprehensively; 12/18 could be considered to have an unsatisfactory outcome because adverse events occurred that precluded a good clinical outcome despite the improvements in motor function described in many; 4/12 of those with unsatisfactory results were withdrawn from the study, and will likely not be reported in the multicenter trial, except as having serious adverse events—two intracranial hemorrhages, one cerebral infarction from venous thrombosis, and one hardware infection requiring hardware removal. When commenting on the larger sample size that is being studied in the multicenter trial, 25% of the study patients were considered as having an unsatisfactory result when being assessed comprehensively (52).

Gait

Cross-sectional and longitudinal studies using clinical and gait laboratory measures have consistently observed improvements in gait during the initial year after STN-DBS (3,53–56). Several studies (53–56) have presented findings that support that the effects of dopaminergic agents and stimulation may be additive in increasing gait velocity, but perhaps by different mechanisms. Levodopa had more impact on improving stride length while stimulation had more impact on improving cadence. The improvements in stride length had a greater impact on increasing gait velocity. This observed dissociation between levodopa and stimulation infers that different but overlapping neural networks are being used to influence gait. Such observations lend some support for the hypothesis promoted by Morris et al. (57) that stride length is directly mediated by the basal ganglia, while cadence is mediated by the midbrain or spinal locomotion centers and indirectly mediated by the basal ganglia. Moreover, another observation regarding freezing of gait was that when freezing was present presurgically off-medications, it was decreased postsurgically either by dopaminergic agents, stimulation, or both; when freezing was present presurgically on-medications, it was similarly resistant to dopaminergic medication and stimulation postsurgically (54,55).

Posture and Balance

As with gait, posture and balance have also been observed to improve in the initial year after STN-DBS, during both cross-sectional and longitudinal studies that have used both clinical and balance laboratory-based measures of static posture, postural stability, and balance (58–61). One cross-sectional study performed by Rocchi et al. (2002) (60) observed a "normalization" of static postural sway only during off-medication/on-stimulation conditions with a worsening during on-medication/off stimulation and on-medication/on-stimulation conditions, suggesting that stimulation may facilitate sensory feedback systems that control posture while dopaminergic agents may be detrimental.

Fine Motor Control

Fine motor control during the initial year after STN-DBS has been studied cross-sectionally, using an array of tasks including precision grip (62), repetitive alternating finger tapping (63), and tracing (64). The reported findings generally support the hypothesis that the influence of dopaminergic agents and stimulation are additive. Parallel functional improvements can only be inferred from these studies.

Speech

One case of "speech initiation hesitation" has been described after STN-DBS. It was conceptualized as an idiosyncratic manifestation of freezing, postsurgically (65). Other investigators (66,67) have observed oral motor functions that support speech during the initial year after STN-DBS. Improvements in oral motor force and dysarthria scores (66), but not in phonemic articulation, intelligibility, and spontaneous expression (67) were observed. Thus, improvements observed at an impairment level of assessment did not necessarily translate into improvements in functional communication in everyday life.

Sexual Well-Being

Men under the age of 60 who had STN-DBS more consistently reported improvements in their sexual lives (68). Corresponding data for women were not available.

Urinary Function

Finazzi-Agro et al. (69) urodynamically studied five postsurgical patients with PD and detrusor hyperreflexia presenting as urinary frequency, urgency, and incontinence. A significant increase in bladder capacity and threshold for detrusor contractions was observed during the on-stimulation conditions; however, no change in other urodynamic parameters such as bladder compliance and initial desire to void were observed. While these findings were consistent with a decrease in detrusor hyperreflexia, it remains unclear whether STN-DBS really normalizes urinary patterns during everyday life.

Sleep-Wake Patterns

In several small sample longitudinal studies, based on subjective reporting and polysomnography, preSTN-DBS sleep disturbances were commonly reported in individuals with PD. When observed during the initial year after STN-DBS, sleep patterns were reported as improved in these studies, with less sleep fragmentation and less daytime somnolence. The direct effects of chronic stimulation, decreases in dopaminergic agents, and improvements in affective state have been implicated to underpin improved sleep–wake patterns after STN-DBS (70–74).

Quality of Life

Quality of life has been reported as almost ubiquitously improved during the initial year after STN-DBS when PD-specific (e.g., Parkinson's Disease Quality of Life scale or PDQL) and generic (e.g., the Nottingham Health Profile or NHP) measurement tools were used. All dimensions of quality of life (e.g., emotional and social functioning) have been reported as significantly improved, and there were usually significant correlations reported among the quality of life measures and UPDRS ADL and motor examination subscales (30,75–77).

Complications and Side Effects

Complications and side effects observed during the initial year after DBS procedures are discussed in other chapters of this book. It is important to recognize them, particularly since they may occur during postsurgical rehabilitation programs. Since the stimulator is magnetically sensitive, it must be turned off for magnetic resonance imaging studies, if necessary for diagnostic reasons, under the direction of the neurosurgery/neurology/neuroradiology team. Many of the overstimulation effects of target or adjacent tissues are transient and managed with close titration of stimulation and dopaminergic medications. Weight gain is common, during the initial year after DBS, and multifactorial: increased efficiency during eating meals associated with lessening of bradykinesia and tremor; lowering of resting energy expenditure from reduction of involuntary movements including dyskinesias; and decreased depression (78–80).

Long-Term Outcomes After STN-DBS

Several investigator groups have observed patients longitudinally between means of 16.3 and 60 months (21,81–96), and these studies have observed: (*i*) improvements in motor and functional status during the off-mediation/on-stimulation condition were sustained beyond one year, and these improvements were associated with reductions in rapid motor fluctuations, (*ii*) sustained decreases in the dosing of dopaminergic agents were variable, and usually associated with decreases in on-medication dyskinesias, (*iii*) in some patients, elimination of dyskinesias and rapid motor fluctuations were associated with completely stopping dopaminergic medications when stimulation alone could enhance motor control, thus reinforcing the suggestion that STN-DBS and dopaminergic medications are "equipotent," (*iv*) in younger STN-DBS patients (≤ 50 years old) who had disease durations of less than ten years, a return to full employment occurred within the initial year and was sustained thereafter for up to several years, (*v*) overstimulation effects were usually modifiable with changes in stimulation, and device failures were easily reparable with replacement of hardware components, and (*vi*) hardware infections were rare and treatable with hardware removal, antibiotics, and later hardware replacement. These reported positive long-term outcomes after STN-DBS have been associated with improvements in quality of life for both the individuals who had the surgery and their caregivers (97).

Long-term motor and functional outcomes in individuals over 70 years of age, who had STN-DBS, have been reported as less promising when compared to younger counterparts; the level of impairment/disability usually worsened in the older individuals beyond one year, and stabilized in younger counterparts (98).

The long-term outcomes after STN-DBS when observing impairment specific issues have been reported to be variable and continue to require further study for developing consensus and for considering their concurrent influence on functional status. For example, impaired static posture and postural instability are reported to be therapeutically resistant to STN-DBS (99). These findings differed from the generally positive short-term outcomes regarding postural control that have been reported by other investigators.

Outcomes After Multiple Procedures

When parallel comparisons of STN-DBS and GPi-DBS were performed during the initial postsurgical year, STN-DBS has been generally viewed as having better outcomes than GPi-DBS; however, both procedures have reported significant improvements utilizing several impairment- and activity participation-based measures (100). The improvements in gait, after STN-DBS, were observed to be almost exclusively associated with increased stride length, while after GPi-DBS, improvements in gait were associated both with increased stride length and faster cadence (101). The relatively better improvements in postural sway after STN-DBS than GPi-DBS were postulated to be caused by the concurrent decreased dosing of dopaminergic agents more consistently after the former procedure (102). As mentioned, the antidyskinetic effect after GPi-DBS has been thought to be direct, while this effect after STN-DBS has been thought to be associated with postsurgical reductions in dopaminergic agents (103). No observed differences in fine motor control between STN- and GPi-DBS have been reported, yet both procedures appeared to induce improvements in hand grip force, hand/finger movement time, and coupling of grasping forces during a bimanual manipulation task (104). Several other studies observed oral-motor outcomes after DBS without making efforts for parallel comparisons of different stimulation sites (105–107), and the results have been conflicting.

In a published randomized controlled trial that directly compared GPi- and STN-DBS, Anderson et al. (8) reported their pilot data in which they randomized their study patients to be treated either with STN- or GPi-stimulation: the outcomes were relatively comparable when observing the motor examination of the UPDRS. Finally, Rodriguez-Oroz et al. (108) reported the long-term outcomes of 69 study subjects who had both STN- and GPi-DBS, and were observed longitudinally by eight investigator groups. Significantly, positive motor outcomes were demonstrated up to four years during the off-medication/on-stimulation condition. These findings were related to reported decreases in on-medication dyskinesias as well as in off-medication lessening of rapid motor fluctuations.

Cognitive/Behavioral Outcomes

When taking a broader view of the reported cognitive outcomes after DBS, what seemed most prevalent was the relative stability of intellectual functions across most domains during the initial postsurgical year, and particularly in those who were intact presurgically. These reported changes appeared to depend on which domain was being probed, what measurement tools were being used to probe them, and how much time had lapsed after the procedure. For example, improvements in executive functions as measured by tasks that probe visual organization and hypothesis generation, have been reported during the postsurgical year and up to three years thereafter (more so after STN- than GBi-DBS), although this finding of improvement did not generally hold true for tasks involving verbal fluency (2,109–118). Language skills such as word retrieval and verbal fluency were more consistently reported as worse, using several tasks during the initial year after STN-DBS (118–121). When more refined observations of language skills were observed, the decline was rationalized by slower cognitive processing. Factoring for slower processing speed, language skills were reported as improved based on more qualitative error analysis of verbal fluency tasks and spontaneous speech production (122–125). It is, thus, difficult to infer that new changes in cognition after DBS procedures will compromise learning during postsurgical rehabilitation.

Several investigator groups have observed the development of problematic behaviors after DBS procedures, more commonly reported after STN-DBS, and thought to be associated with too rapid lowering of dopaminergic agents, a practice that has been largely eliminated. Some investigators have speculated that these affective and behavioral changes may be directly related to STN-DBS stimulation (126). Those who have had mood and behavioral disorders presurgically have been considered to be more vulnerable for these to occur (127,128). Mood (anxiety and depression) appeared to be stable, and sometimes improved, during longitudinal observation during the initial year after GPi- and STN-DBS (111,117,118,122,129–132). When reported, mood disorders, usually transient, and extreme (suicide and mania), were rare after STN-DBS. Also, an array of disturbing "frontal lobe" syndromic behaviors have been rarely observed including, aggression, apathy, and hypersexuality. Psychotic behavior also was reported as rare (7,117,131,133–136).

Few investigators have observed mood and behavioral changes after DBS procedures in relation to the immediate interpersonal environment as defined by the patient–caregiver dyad. While early postsurgical affective and motoric improvements may result in more self-directive behaviors, such behaviors may not always be productive, and if so, may challenge longstanding patterns of interaction between "newly less dependent" patients and their caregivers.

Moreover, even when the patient–caregiver dyads adapt successfully to the "new" interpersonal homeostasis after DBS, the likelihood of future disease progression associated with recurrence of increased burden of care remains. It, thus, may be difficult for patient–caregiver dyads to reestablish presurgical interpersonal patterns over time (137).

REHABILITATION INTERVENTIONS IN PARKINSON'S DISEASE

Montgomery (138) has articulated empirically generated principles that underpin the feasibility of rehabilitation for those who have PD, in general, and after treatment with DBS, in particular:

1. Identification of environmental or contextual factors that enhance function: The best example of this is the use of external visual and auditory cueing strategies to enhance more fluid and goal directed movements, discussed later.

2. Selection of the most appropriate motor strategy from an array of possible strategies that can be used to complete a specific motor task: For example, balance training that teaches and reinforces the engagement of core and proximal leg (hip) muscle groups may be more effective than using distal muscle (ankle) groups to prevent falls in response to an external provocation.

3. Alteration of the individual's internal perception during functional activities: The best example of this is the application of Lee Silverman Voice Treatment to treat hypokinetic dysarthria, discussed later.

4. Implementation of procedural motor learning during rehabilitation treatments: These "learning how" systems underpin most motor learning/relearning during rehabilitation. Procedural motor learning is conceptualized as being "unconscious" or implicit, that is, not attentionally driven, and dependent on diffusely localized neural networks, rather than the frontal-hippocampal-thalamic neural networks that control conscious or explicit (attentionally-driven) learning. Several investigators (139,140) have hypothesized that procedural learning in those who have PD may be challenging because the neural networks that encompass the basal ganglia and control motor learning become impaired as an essential feature of the neurodegenerative process. The basal ganglia-cortical neural network is thought to support several components of motor learning including: early phase motor learning when novel information is being incorporated into established motor programs; translation of a newly learned motor task into automatic motor behavior using practice and rehearsal; "selection" of a specific motor program needed to execute a goal directed movement under specific sensory and environmental conditions; and

"switching" motor programs to facilitate sequential and rational motor behaviors.

Exercise interventions have been hypothesized to be neuroprotective in PD. Based on "forced exercise" studies in animals, the proposed mechanism that underpins neuroprotection is that exercise stimulates dopamine synthesis; this subsequently may support desired neurophysiological changes that facilitate improved movement (141,142). In parallel, when considering the relative stability of some of the therapeutic outcomes beyond one year in those with PD treated with DBS, it has been speculated that physiologic ablation may facilitate neural plasticity because the stimulation is continuous or repetitive and synchronized. Thus, it seems rational to apply rehabilitation treatments "to guide" plasticity that may underpin motor learning after these surgical interventions (138). This does not necessarily mean that DBS is reversing or preventing the progression of the neurodegenerative process in PD, but that it may be supporting the available-neural reserve that is available to allow learning/relearning to occur during rehabilitation treatments.

Several critical reviews of rehabilitation interventions directed toward those who have PD reported equivocally positive efficacy (143–145). However, several caveats from these reviews must be articulated: (*i*) less than half of the reviewed studies were randomized controlled trials, (*ii*) about one-third of the reviewed studies had sample sizes of less than 16 subjects, and (*iii*) more than half of the reviewed studies discontinued their observations at the completion of the intervention phases, and did not observe over time, whether the positive effects of various interventions were sustained. Dean et al. (145) asserted that a lack of evidence of efficacy does not necessarily suggest a lack of effect. Further investigation, particularly randomized controlled trials observing larger sample sizes of study patients, still need to be performed. An exploratory substrate of methodologically flawed studies have been completed and provide a basis for more refined hypotheses to be generated and explored during clinical trials that use more robust methodologies in the future.

Among the better performed multidisciplinary clinical trials, Sunvisson et al. (146) reported their observations of a model-driven treatment that combined nursing education and physical therapy. This intervention trial (twice weekly, two hour sessions, over five weeks) observed 43 study subjects with PD: significant improvements were reported at the end of the intervention phase and three months later in the ADL subscale of the UPDRS, and on performance based measures of mobility speed and integration of motor control, but not on the motor examination subscale of the UPDRS. Moreover, significant improvements three months after the end of the intervention phase were observed on the sickness impact profile (SIP); this delayed improvement in quality of life was explained by improved regulation of sleep–wake cycles. However, these positive outcomes were reported not to have much practical influence on improving the everyday lives of these study subjects based on the qualitative observations of these investigators.

Trend et al. (147) reported the results of their open trial of rehabilitation interventions provided to those with PD (N = 118) over six weeks, once weekly. This encompassed a structured therapeutic day of one-on-one and group sessions of physical, occupational, and speech therapies based at a day-hospital program: significant gains in gait, voice articulation, and quality of life were demonstrated. However, when these investigators (148) extended this line of investigation and observed another large sample (N = 71) of individuals with PD, and their caregivers, during a randomized controlled crossover trial that compared multidisciplinary treatment (similar to their open trial) and no treatment groups, the group comparisons at the crossover point (six months) demonstrated improvements that approached significance only in mobility speed during a stand-walk-sit test, and significant deterioration in the general health subscale, mental health subscale, and the mental health summary scores of the SF (Short Form)-36 health survey. Moreover, there was an increase in caregiver strain that approached significance. It is curious to observe that the methodologically more meticulously performed clinical trial of these investigators' treatment intervention was essentially a negative trial. These findings observed during the more rigorously performed trial were rationalized by the observation that the treatment interventions were not frequent enough during the intervention phase, to be effective. Playford (149) further rationalized these negative outcomes by considering the possibility that these interventions were "mistimed," suggesting that they were too late in the disease trajectories of the study subjects, and/or applied to a group of study subjects that were too severely impaired, such that the interventions were interpreted by these study subjects as trivial, intrusive, and distressing.

Nieuwboer et al. (2002) (150) investigation of physical therapy interventions in PD attempted to provide some guidelines to avoid "mistimed" application of treatments: a higher disease severity was negatively predictive of therapeutic benefits even in the context of the familiar home environment; compromised cognitive ability and older age were negatively predictive of ability to sustain the therapeutic benefits of treatment, particularly when transitioning from having in-hospital physical therapy to home. Their study, then, suggested that with more severe PD (not explicitly defined), rehabilitation efforts should be palliative and directed toward enhancing the interpersonal (caregivers) and physical environments of the individual. Moreover, for those who are older and/or cognitively impaired, and unlikely to respond positively to treatment, continuing rehabilitation on a trial basis, particularly during in-hospital to home transitions, may support achieving and sustaining any therapeutic effects in the meaningful or "ecological" home environment where more consistent and familiar contextual cues can be provided to guide optimal functioning. In those situations in which benefiting from rehabilitation interventions proves be unrealistic for the individuals with PD, the focus of treatment should be directed toward the caregivers through supporting their abilities for managing the care of those with PD.

These studies cited earlier (146–148) have observed quality of life as their major outcome variable as measured by multidimensional, ordinal measurement tools such as the SF-36, the SIP, and the Euroqol-5d. The influence of rehabilitation treatments on globally and multidimensionally measured quality of life was equivocal during these clinical trials. Other exploratory investigations have attempted to articulate what factors have more direct influence on quality of life for those who have PD, suggesting that some of these factors are more relevant for focused outcome measurement during clinical trials. Such interacting factors include: depression, pain, fatigue, self-perceived involvement in one's health and medical care, younger age of disease onset, and disease progression associated with mobility and ADL difficulties necessitating an increase in caregiver burden (30).

Depression in PD is common (20% prevalence cross-sectionally) and thought to be multifactorial in its basis including primary neurochemical imbalances and appropriate reaction to loss during disease progression (151,152). Pain in PD is viewed as an under-recognized but common problem affecting up to 50% of individuals, this reflects a higher prevalence than observed in the healthy elderly population (33%). While the pain experience of those who have PD can be categorized similarly to those who have other neurological disease processes (e.g., neuropathic, musculoskeletal, and visceral), their pain experience includes idiosyncratic syndromes, such as dystonia-induced pain associated with the use of dopaminergic agents (153,154). Moreover, during disease progression, there is an increase in musculoskeletal pain associated with degenerative arthritis, with a prevalence rate of up to 50%, higher than what is reported for the general elderly population (40%) (151). The interaction between neurologically-based involuntary movement and musculoskeletal pain continues to be unexplored. Fatigue in PD, another under-recognized problem, is associated with higher disease severity and level of disability (155). Fatigue in PD is also associated with, yet independent from, depression (156). A high self-perceived involvement in decision-making with one's medical care providers regarding treatment options appeared to make compliance with proposed treatment more likely (157). Younger individuals with PD, when compared to their older counterparts who have comparable disease severity and degree of disability, have been observed to be more depressed and have feelings of being more stigmatized by the disease; these emotional states may be explained by the necessity of the disease progression to induce unemployment/early retirement, with associated financial strain and marital discord (152). An increase in caregiver burden associated with declining functional status as the disease progresses is also associated with an increase in out of pocket medical and heath care expenditures, decreased perceived social support for the caregiver, poor psychological well-being of the caregiver, lower marital satisfaction for both the caregiver and the patient, and lower cognitive functioning of the individual with PD (151,158,159).

A series of nursing-based, patient-centered observational studies have qualitatively observed the decline in quality of life that occurs during the progression of PD. This has been articulated in a variety of ways including: being enslaved by illness; losing control; feeling insecure; having a lack of physical and social role competence; feeling misunderstood; feeling stigmatized; being afraid of passivity; and feeling socially uncomfortable (146,156). These observations, again, speak to alternative, patient-driven approaches for measuring quality of life. Such studies have proposed that to rectify such a negative disease experience and to maintain an optimal quality of life, individuals and caregivers take an adaptive, pragmatic, and proactive behavioral approach that is consistent with a rehabilitation philosophy (160). For example, Backer (161) has observed that "confrontative coping," that is, thinking what has to be done and setting up a plan of action that includes the use of rehabilitation interventions to operationalize the approach, is a more adaptive response to support optimal life quality. Such outcome measurement approaches that are informed by patient–caregiver experiences during clinical trials, driven by recognized risk factors, and guided by behavioral strategies that "modify" risk factors and "improve" patient–caregiver outcomes have not yet been rigorously performed.

Treatment of Locomotion and Postural Control Deficits by Physical Therapy

Several reviews of physical therapy clinical trials were ambivalent for supporting the efficacy of PD-specific interventions when compared to generic exercise interventions: sample sizes were small; randomization was poor; long-term outcomes were not observed; and physical therapy strategies were widely varied across the studies and eclectic within each study. Regarding this latter point, the state-of-art has not evolved such that standards of "best practice" have been defined. Exercise interventions are thought to be best applied during the on-medication state as they are considered adjunctive to dopaminergic and other types of neuromodulating interventions such as DBS (162–165). To extrapolate from these studies, when a reduction in parkinsonian motor signs is induced by DBS procedures, concurrently applied postsurgical rehabilitation interventions may be viewed as a useful adjunct to support improvements in functional abilities.

External Sensory Cueing

The best studied exercise based interventions to treat the gait and balance difficulties in PD are those that have used external sensory cueing strategies, more often visual (spatial) and auditory (temporal) (164). These strategies are based on hypotheses that propose that one of the fundamental deficits that underpin the locomotion and postural control deficits in PD is one of impaired "internal cueing" that may be mediated by the basal ganglia, directing cortical and supraspinal control of automatic motor behaviors. Thus, "external cueing" strategies have been studied as "bypass" strategies to compensate for impaired internal cueing. External cueing systems are thought to utilize different but interacting neural networks based in the cerebellum (166).

During locomotion, internal cues are thought to direct an appropriate sense of timing during automatic motor behaviors, as well as to activate and deactivate these automatic behaviors, across complex motor sequences. When internal cueing is impaired, as in PD, freezing of gait may become manifest during later stage presentation of the disease, when the environment demands switching from one submovement to another to achieve adequate motor task sequencing. External auditory cueing has been proposed as a compensatory strategy to treat deficits in internal cueing to facilitate improved timing within automatic motor behaviors, as well as switching across them. In contrast, external visual cues are thought to guide motor control using "on-line" feedback that guides accurate and goal directed motor activity to support upright stance that compensate for deficits in proprioceptive delivery in PD. For example, one rationalization as to why those who have PD assume a position of increased flexion throughout their limbs and trunk is that this may be compensatory to optimize proprioceptive feedback during walking and upright stance (164,167,168).

Motor programs are central templates of coordinated muscle commands that determine rational sequences of goal directed movements such as a reciprocal gait pattern. Sensory feedback controls motor programs in a manner of "error detection" that compares the ongoing experience of movement with the central reference pattern of the motor program. Sensory feedback provides data that allows for the recognition of divergence between the actual and expected movements. Compensatory movement sequences then occur. For example, to avoid an obstacle or to accommodate a change in the contour of a walking surface, the proprioceptive or visual information from the environment serve to modify the motor program to maintain upright stance as one moves forward in time and space. One's attentive resources are thought to determine the selection of sensory information within this model. Gait analyses studies have observed that there is less central delivery of proprioceptive feedback in PD, and that increased dependence on visual cueing is one among several neural strategies that are used to compensate for this (167–170).

Control of locomotion and posture have been viewed as being mediated by distinct, parallel, and interacting neural networks. The neural networks that control locomotion are thought to be more influenced by sensory feedback from distal lower limb motor groups, while the neural networks that control posture are thought to be more influenced by sensory feedback from proximal or axial muscle groups. Four components of postural control have been defined: (*i*) background antigravity muscle tone during quiet stance, (*ii*) centrally initiated motor programs that anticipate or plan postural adjustments to facilitate initiation of movements, (*iii*) centrally initiated motor programs that modify posture during voluntary movements, and (*iv*) compensatory postural reactions in response to external perturbations or postural stabilization responses. All four components have been observed to be impaired in PD; the initial two components have been observed to "normalize" in response to levodopa in the gait laboratory, while the latter two have not (171–173). Given the lack of normalization of these latter two postural components, an increasing role for physical therapy interventions that teach compensatory responses has been inferred. Rogers has pragmatically speculated that several strategies may be pursued but they require more rigorous study such as teaching "protective," rather than "corrective" balance responses that involve modified stepping (executing a faster initial step), grabbing of external supports and "arm rescue" responses that absorb the impact of falling (174). Several of these "protective" strategies explicitly utilize environmental cues.

Compensatory sensory systems (visual and auditory) aimed toward enhancing mobility performance have been explored during a series of gait laboratory and clinical studies that have compared outcomes during noncued and cued conditions, often comparing the performances of subjects with PD and control subjects. The applied visual cues have included floor stripes, timing lights, and mirrors; the auditory cues have included music and metronomes. Gait velocity and walking speed were consistently, but not universally, observed to be increased during the cued conditions in those with PD: visual cues were more frequently observed to increase stride length, while auditory cues were more frequently observed to increase cadence (164,166,169,175–184). When sensory cues were unpredictably or randomly presented to subjects with PD, they were observed to be detrimental, possibly displacing internal cues necessary for preinitiation of movement planning (182). When dual tasks paradigms (e.g., walking while carrying a tray with two cups) were applied during cued conditions, the sensory cueing did not increase walking speed as it did during the single task (walking only) condition. The sensory cueing (auditory) did, however, reverse the "interference effect" (i.e., decrease in step length) expected and observed during the noncued dual task condition when compared with the noncued single task condition. These findings support the hypothesis that external sensory cues are fundamentally enhancing attentional control during functional ambulation; enhanced attention directed toward an external cue may be compensating for a defective "internal timekeeper" in those with PD (184). Functional status was also observed to be improved in response to a physical therapy intervention that utilized a variety of cueing strategies over six weeks, and improvement was sustained three months later (178).

When criticizing these gait laboratory studies and clinical trials that have employed external sensory cueing strategies to enhance gait, Iansek and Morris (185) have observed that the reported increases in gait velocity as influenced by either increased stride length, increased cadence, or both are sometimes marginal even though reported as significant. These investigators (185) have hypothesized that the basic deficit in the control of gait in PD is one of stride length; cadence is viewed as intact in PD, and increasing cadence is a compensatory strategy to increase gait velocity. What is possible within this model is that a specific cue may be influencing either stride length or cadence, or both. However, these cues may not be essential, yet serve to direct an individual to use more attentional resources to increase stride length and/or cadence, and thus gait velocity. Other attention-enhancing strategies may be just as effective for increasing gait velocity. Woollacott and Shumway-Cook (186) have proposed that applying dual tasks paradigms is an effective model in which to investigate attentional control of gait and posture. Dual tasks paradigms, during which attention is divided between a primary task (walking) and a secondary task (e.g., talking, carrying something in the upper limbs), are thought to probe the attentional control of more complex cognitive tasks whether motoric or nonmotoric. Their review of this line of investigation, including their own work, has observed that the performance of a secondary task during locomotion or balance activities is deleterious to postural control in older adults. The exact nature of the attentional deficit remains elusive. When dual tasks paradigms have been applied during the investigation of gait and balance in PD, it has been observed that attentional deficits may underpin freezing of gait and slower gait velocity primarily because of shorter stride length.

Traditional Physical Therapy

More traditional approaches to exercise interventions in physical therapy employing a variety of strategies have demonstrated improved outcomes at least in response to the intervention phases of treatment. Sustaining improvements over the longer term continues to be challenging. It is assumed that continuing "to practice" a successful exercise regime beyond the intervention phase of treatment will maintain the observed gains over time, until medications become ineffective or the disease progresses to counteract the positive influence of exercise. Moreover, even if exercise interventions have demonstrated success, compliance with ongoing participation can be particularly challenging even in motivated patients for an array of reasons. Many individuals historically have not integrated regular exercise into their lives, thus starting to participate in later life may demand that they change who they have been constitutionally and culturally. Poor initiation in those who have PD can interfere with participating in any goal directed activity, including exercise. Strategies to provide external structure to bypass initiation problems must be individualized with the recognition that the development of effective strategies can sometimes be problematic. For example, when a spouse becomes the "exercise trainer," often nothing is accomplished; the exercise regime becomes another arena reinforcing tension within a longstanding relationship so that exercise can be experienced negatively and as something to be avoided. Moreover, many individuals or couples who live on limited incomes cannot afford to pay out of pocket for personal trainers to direct the exercise programs as a "neutral party" whether it be in the home, at a fitness center, or at a wellness program, much less be able to afford to join one of the latter options. Group exercise programs, while less expensive, may present a challenge for bradykinetic or cognitively impaired individuals to keep up with the group effort, and furthermore, these programs may be too generic to encompass the treatment of parkinsonian motor signs. Finally, many exercise regimes do not offer enough variety on a day-to-day basis, and individuals can become "bored" with the regime. Thus, to avoid repetition, it is essential from one day to the next to offer different sets of activities that encompass several components of therapeutic intervention (e.g., proximal lower limb strengthening, lower limb and trunk flexibility, gait enhancement activities, balance work and endurance work).

While it may be difficult to incorporate all of these components within a daily exercise routine, they can be included and structured into a routine across a weekly schedule that includes a different focus of exercise on a daily basis that can be carried out in different environments (home, fitness center, group exercise program, pool, etc.).

Several physical therapy clinical trials have applied a variety of psycho-educational and exercise interventions, comparing treatment and no treatment groups, in subjects with PD and control subjects. The intervention phases of treatment ranged from 1 to 20 weeks during these studies. When postintervention outcomes were observed, they were usually limited to less than six months after the end of the intervention phases. Outcome measurements included gait parameters, functional status, and quality of life. Outcomes were usually reported as improved at the end of the intervention phase of treatment, but not consistently sustained thereafter (187–196). Several of these trials applied novel treatments such as partial body weight-supported treadmill training, "polestriding," and structured treadmill training, and found these to be superior to traditional physical therapy approaches for increasing gait velocity and improving functional status (190–192,194).

Treatment of Deficits in Postural Control and Balance

Many of the discussed clinical trials have focused on observing gait parameters as the major outcome measures, and in doing so, have indirectly measured postural control during locomotion in those who have PD. When using such composite measures such as the ADL and the motor examination subscales of the UPDRS to measure outcomes, measurement of postural control and balance are embedded within them. Several open clinical trials have focused exclusively on observing postural control and balance (197–201). The components of postural control and balance that were observed as outcome measures in these studies included axially-controlled movements (moving form supine to sitting/sitting to supine, rolling in supine, moving from sitting to standing/standing to sitting), dynamic posturography, compensatory stepping in response to external provocations, and ability to sustain tandem stance. The exercise interventions that were used in these studies to enhance postural control and balance included upper and lower limb coordination and strengthening, spinal flexibility, postural correction, gait training and other sorts of functional mobility training, external provocations on stable and unstable surfaces, and endurance training. All observed outcomes were improved immediately after the intervention phases of treatment that ranged from 2 to 10 weeks (197–201), and up to two months after the intervention phases (200,201).

Falling

Falling is a common and expected consequence of the gait and balance difficulties associated with PD. It has been estimated that up to 70% of those who have PD fall annually, and 13% fall more than once weekly (202,203). Wielinski et al. (204) survey of 1092 individuals who have parkinsonism revealed that almost 55% had fallen at least once during the previous two years, and that 65% of these falls resulted in injuries; about 75% of these injuries required health care services, with fractures commonly reported (33%). These reports of falls in those who have PD, as well as associated major injuries, are approximately twice what has been reported in the general community-based elderly population, and higher than what has been reported in those with other neurological diseases (205,206). Falling risk factors for those who have PD have been defined, and to some extent prioritized. These risk factors both overlap with those that have been defined for the general elderly population (older age, polypharmacy, orthostasis, mobility impairments, balance impairments, visual impairments, affective disturbances including fear of falling, dementia) and are idiosyncratically associated with the disease process [disease severity; undesired effects of dopaminergic medication such as hallucinations, sleep disturbances, and dyskinesias; rigidity; bradykinesia; freezing of gait; impaired hand and foot agility; decreased arm swing during walking; inability to rise from a chair (202,203,207–211)]. The reduction of falling risks and episodes has not been directly observed during therapeutic clinical trials, and it can only be inferred based on the reduction of isolated risk factors such as impaired gait and balance as reported earlier. Multidimensional risk factor modification, as applied in the general elderly population, has been proposed as a rational model to decrease falling risks and episodes in those who have PD, but these clinical trials have not yet been executed (205,211–213).

Freezing of Gait

Motor blocks, or freezing of gait, continue to be poorly understood phenomena. They are reported to occur in up to 60% of individuals who have PD. They are associated with higher disease severity and become more apparent with disease progression. They have been categorized according to their common clinical occurrence: start hesitation (freezing during initiation of gait); gait arrests when approaching objects (e.g., when approaching a chair to sit down); gait arrest when in narrow spaces (e.g., doorways); gait arrests during turning; and hesitations when walking in open spaces. Motor blocks are viewed as sometimes refractory to dopaminergic agents and have been observed to worsen when these medications are on board, particularly after prolonged treatment. However, it has also been observed that motor blocks can decrease in frequency and duration when exposed to dopaminergic agents. Thus, distinguishing whether motor blocks occur in association with being "on"- or "off"-medications is emerging as an important clinical issue. Noradrenergic deficiency has been proposed as underpinning, in part, the pathophysiology of motor blocks, supported by the observation of decreased freezing episodes when subjects were exposed to deprenyl (a monoamine oxidase inhibitor), and re-emergence of predeprenyl freezing frequency in deprenyl wash-out during the Deprenyl and Tocopherol Antioxidative Therapy of Parkinsonism (DATATOP) trials (169,214–219). Motor blocks inconsistently can be interrupted with assistive devices that provide ongoing proprioceptive feedback such as wheeled walkers, sometimes in combination with "sensory-motor tricks," which when successful can be taught procedurally to individuals with PD and their caregivers. Such behavioral strategies include teaching these individuals not to actively disconnect their "glued feet" from the ground, but rather to allow the motor block to occur, momentarily relax, then reinitiate gait using a hip and knee hyperflexion maneuver to step out and over an imagined or real visual cue, for example, a self-triggered laser beam at ankle level generated from the wheeled walker or cane (220–222). Empirically, the presence of the sensory cue does not appear to be as essential as using the proximal leg flexors to reinitiate gait.

Treatment of Upper Limb Motor Control Deficits by Occupational Therapy

Murphy and Tickle-Degnen's (223) review of 16 studies involving occupational therapy-related interventions directed toward small samples of individuals who had PD was somewhat optimistic regarding the outcomes after a variety of interventions. Several studies incorporated external cueing strategies with observations of upper limb motor control during "nonecological" tasks that were not specifically related to functional motor tasks. For example, Platz et al. (224) studied the speed and accuracy of performing an upper limb aiming task in bradykinetic-predominant individuals who had PD under two training conditions: those in which auditory cueing was provided and those in which no cueing was provided. During training, there were no differences in improvements of performance speed between the cued and noncued training conditions. The findings of this study differed from what has been observed when cueing is incorporated into the gait and balance training for those who have PD. The lack of improvements in speed of movements during the training conditions in which cueing was provided was rationalized by the possibility that cueing may have been perceived by the subjects as a more complicated, and perhaps more distracting set of training conditions, demanding not only speed and accuracy as in the noncued training condition, but also an extra demand of synchronizing with the auditory cues. Thus, in this study, the external auditory cues did not appear to compensate for postulated impaired internal cueing, during upper limb motor tasks (224–226).

Rogers et al. (227) have also investigated the use of external sensory cues to compensate for the impaired basal ganglia's ability to internally cue automatic upper limb fine motor control during movement anticipation or preinitiation and during switching among automatic motor programs in sequential movements. These investigators applied a serial two-way reaction time task in which advanced information (visual cue) about the next movement was not provided until after the current movement was initiated, thus probing the ability to use advance information to guide movement. The subjects with PD and the control subjects differed significantly only when the cueing conditions were at the "high level," that is, those with PD displayed significant slowing of movement in comparison to the control subjects when the sequential sensory cues were more exact at guiding fine motor control. These findings suggest that those who have PD have limitations in the amount of advanced information they can process, or perhaps they can become overwhelmed when too much information is provided for guiding sequential movements. Fundamental deficits in attentional control associated with PD may be the best explanation for these findings.

In another study, Meshack et al. (228) studied the therapeutic use of weighted utensils and weighted wrist cuffs as a compensatory strategy in tremor-predominant individuals with PD: no differences in modifying the amplitude or frequency of tremor was observed. The study subjects were not actually observed during eating or other functional activities, but during tasks that were considered generic versions of such activities. The use of virtual reality has been viewed as a more "ecological" approach for treating upper limb motor control deficits in neurologically impaired individuals including those with PD. Not only does virtual reality provide external visual cueing, but demands the creation of motor plans during functional activities. By creation of a motor plan during a specific functional activity, it facilitates the appropriate selection of external cues that guide efficient and successful performance of that activity. Albani et al. (229) used a virtual reality training intervention that observed two individuals who had PD during the performance of three functional activities: opening a door, eating a meal while seated at a table, and turning on a faucet at the sink. While the use of virtual reality was successful in this study as a potential treatment strategy, it was not observed that these improvements translated into being useful in everyday life.

Treatment of Hypokinetic Dysarthria by Speech Therapy

The speech impairment in PD has been labeled hypokinetic dysarthria. Its salient components include impairments in phonation and articulation. Rigidity of respiratory muscles that support speech contributes to hypophonia, and impairments in vocal volume modification, and vocal phrasing. Individuals who have PD generally phonate at higher sound frequencies associated with rigid laryngeal motor control; they produce prolonged vowel sounds, and uncoordinated timing of phonation that includes delayed voice onset time associated with bradykinesia of laryngeal muscles. Associated with inadequate tongue elevation, individuals who have PD also articulate imprecise consonants, particularly those used phonetically for closure of phrases. Other components that contribute to hypokinetic dysarthria include impaired prosody or natural variations in pitch, and impaired intensity and rhythm during spontaneous speech production. Moreover, hypokinetic dysarthria has been conceptualized to include impaired sensory and perceptual components of speech that influence the feedback or monitoring systems that control the motoric components of speech.

Many of these impaired components of hypokinetic dysarthria have been reported to demonstrate variable improvements with the administration of dopaminergic agents (230–232). Given inconsistent reporting of improvements in speech after deep brain stimulation procedures, there is clearly a role for procedurally-based treatments to optimize vocal communication postsurgically. Critical reviews (231–234) of speech therapy interventions in individuals who have PD (but not after DBS) have concluded that there is equivocal evidence to support their efficacy: few acceptable studies had been completed; no standards of treatment exist; any reported therapeutic effects were not sustained beyond three months after the intervention phases of treatment.

Treatments for hypokinetic dysarthria fall into two broad categories: external strategies that employ orthotic (to enhance speech output) or prosthetic (to replace speech output) devices and behaviorally based treatments.

Orthotic devices that enhance speech output include voice amplifiers, delayed auditory feedback, wearable intensity biofeedback devices, and masking devices. Voice amplifiers improve vocal loudness but not intelligibility. Delayed auditory feedback devices and intensity wearable biofeedback devices improve loudness and intelligibility based on "on-line" sensory feedback when the devices are being worn. Masking devices induce the individual to increase vocal volume "to override" a concurrent background noise, thus increasing vocal volume. These types of orthotic devices have been observed to be effective based on a few small sample empirically based studies. Prosthetic devices that replace vocal communication in those individuals who have failed or who are likely to fail with the use of either orthotic devices or behaviorally based treatments because of severe dysarthria and/or hypophonia, include computer based augmentative communication devices. These usually require the use of a keyboard to enter what one wants to express, and speech output is expressed in written and/or vocal format. Their successful use requires relatively intact fine motor control to manipulate the keyboard, and relatively intact cognitive functions to learn how to use the device to support meaningful communication (231).

The best studied behaviorally based treatment for hypokinetic dysarthria is the Lee Silverman Voice Treatment (LSVT®). LSVT® is becoming viewed as efficacious in the short- and long-term (24 months) (235). It is an exercise-based treatment that proposes: (*i*) to increase strength and repetitive/sustained muscle endurance of the respiratory muscles in order to facilitate a greater respiratory effort to overcome rigid laryngeal muscles that create resistance to air flow for support of adequate vocal volume; (*ii*) to facilitate more complete vocal cord adduction by enhancing increases in subglottal air pressure and vocal cord vibration; and (*iii*) to "recalibrate" the internal sensory perception regarding the effort required to speak. LSVT aims to modify three features of hypokinetic dysarthria: (*i*) reduced vocal volume hypothesized to be induced by reduced amplitude of the neural drive to the muscles that control speech; (*ii*) impaired sensory perception of vocal volume that disallows accurate self-monitoring of vocal output; and (*iii*) difficulty with self-generated internal cueing to apply the appropriate degree of vocal effort and associated volume.

LSVT has been developed and rigorously studied by Ramig et al. (232,235–238). When performed appropriately, the speech therapist should have special certification in LSVT; it requires a commitment to intensive treatment for 50 minutes, four times weekly within a one-month time period; and it requires participation in daily "homework" during treatment and thereafter to maintain the observed gains during the intervention phase of treatment. When directly compared to treatment that has aimed to enhance vocal volume by facilitating increased respiratory effort alone, LSVT has been demonstrated to be superior because it additionally facilitates vocal cord adduction (235,236). It has also been observed that LSVT has "generalizability," with observed improvements beyond vocal volume to include prosody, intelligibility, facial expression, and swallowing (232,235,237). Clinical improvement after LSVT has also been studied in combination with dynamic brain imaging. Liotti et al. (238) observed changes in positron emission tomography (PET) of the brain in five right handed subjects with PD, before and after treatment with LSVT: After treatment, there was "normalization," or decreased cerebral activation, in the left motor, supplementary motor, and inferior lateral premotor cortices; and concurrently increased activation in the right anterior insular and dorsolateral prefrontal cortices, in the head of the caudate and putamen of the basal ganglia. These findings suggest that incorporation of LSVT strategies effect a change from functioning in a more cognitively conscious and effortful manner before treatment, to a more implicit or unconscious and automatic manner after treatment. Blumin et al. (239) endoscopically observed individuals with PD before treatment with DBS: 87% of their study patients demonstrated vocal cord bowing associated with self-reported speech difficulties. Such findings suggest that LSVT would be appropriate treatment whether DBS is offered or not.

Other related treatments have received more limited investigation to treat hypokinetic dysarthria in PD. These treatments usually incorporate some or all of the components of LSVT. For example, deSwart et al. (240) have compared Pitch Limiting Voice Treatment (PLVT), or "speak loud and low" treatments with LSVT, which has been coined "think loud, think shout" treatment. These investigators proposed that LSVT is too effortful and may result in pressured, highly pitched (high frequency vocalization), strained, "screaming" as the resulting vocal output. PLVT is viewed as similar to LSVT except that it guides individuals with PD not only to speak loudly, but "loud and low." deSwart et al. (240) have reported that PLVT is comparably therapeutic to LSVT, but that PLVT has the advantage of producing less pressured and effortful speech at more normalized vocal frequencies (240,241). Haneishi (242) has reported improvements in vocal volume and intelligibility in four patients who have PD using a music therapy voice protocol (MTVP) that had been developed for dysarthric individuals who have other neurological disorders. It is argued that singing naturally intensifies several components of speech production including volume, phrasing based on more efficient use of respiratory muscles, range of sound frequency, and prosody (pitch, volume, and rhythm). Moreover, singing also involves training of postural and facial muscles.

Kent et al. (243) have proposed clinical standards for assessing and treating dysarthria resulting from neurological disorders, including hypokinetic dysarthria. These investigators have developed the multi-dimensional voice program^{TM} (MDVP) which includes: (*i*) a standardized acoustic analysis that deconstructs speech production into 30 variables; (*ii*) standardized and high quality technology for voice recording; and (*iii*) age and gender matched normative data. Limited treatment application of MDVP to hypokinetic dysarthria in PD has demonstrated positive outcomes based on preliminary data. MDVP may best serve the need to standardize vocal assessments in those who have dysarthria associated with neurological diseases.

Caregiver Training

As a progressive neurodegenerative disease process, PD is characterized by an associated decline in functional abilities for everyday life activities. The fundamental concept that guides a rehabilitation philosophy during such loss is to allow the individual to maintain as much personal control, dignity, and meaning as possible within both interpersonal relationships and the physical environment. What one realistically "chooses" to participate in during everyday life demands defining priorities of what one can do by oneself versus what must be done by caregivers. Caregivers can be either "formal," that is, provide personal care services that are contracted and purchased, or "informal," that is, provide personal care services within the boundaries of filial, intimate or other relationships, usually without direct monetary exchange. Formal caregiver services are expensive, and typical health insurance plans do not provide coverage for personal care services over extended periods of time. Thus, most individuals with PD who become disabled depend on "informal" caregivers, broadly defined as spouses, children, grandchildren, extended family members, friends, neighbors, church community members, and volunteer organizations. In those who have deep brain stimulation procedures, the caregiver becomes essential for observing and validating the clinical experience of the individual with PD when being seen by health and medical providers, for managing medications and external monitoring devices that can modulate strength of stimulation, and for providing transportation during outpatient presurgical and postsurgical assessments, and thereafter. Moreover, caregivers are often expected to follow through with directing home-based exercise programs developed by rehabilitation therapists, this only adds to what is already expected of them. Needless to say, caregiving for those who have PD can be particularly challenging given several fundamental and idiosyncratic aspects of the disease process: poor initiation of goal directed activities, slow cognitive processing and motor control once participating in activities, and recurrent falling. Davey et al. (244) survey of spousal caregivers of recurrent fallers who had PD articulated that these caregivers had their own "fear of falling" syndrome regarding their spouses, and they often injured themselves when providing assistance to their spouses to arise from the floor. Pasetti et al. (245) investigation of informal caregivers for those who have PD realized that 58% were spouses and 37% were adult children; among these, 35% defined themselves as the only caregiver. Martinez-Martin et al. (246) investigation of the informal caregivers of individuals who have PD found that the functional status of the individual with PD was the main predictor of caregiver quality of life. Other investigators (247–249) have articulated an array of other factors that influence spousal caregiver burden for those who have PD. The "patient-associated factors" included psychiatric symptoms such as depression, hallucinations, agitation and confusion, and falling. The "caregiver-associated" factors included sleep disturbances, depression and level of satisfaction with their marital and sexual relationships.

Fernandez et al. (250) more specifically explored the factors that underpin depressive symptoms among spousal caregivers of those with PD: longer disease duration, was the strongest predictor of caregiver depression. As the disease progresses, increasing severity of cognitive impairment has been observed as fundamental in increasing the burden of care for those who have PD (251).

Caregiver "strain" is multifactorial and includes compromising health, increasing expenses, modifying the interpersonal homeostasis within relationships, losing sleep, disrupting domestic routines, disengaging from employment and leisure activities, preventing institutionalization, and developing fatigue and affective disturbances, including anxiety and depression. Realizing that "knowledge is power" for a patient–caregiver dyad, rehabilitation providers must be prepared to advise, emotionally support, counsel, and provide resource information for caregivers. Such processes occur during one-on-one interactions within traditional inpatient or outpatient care, or during support groups specifically designed for articulating a common ground among patient–caregiver dyads, as well as for generating "consumer-driven" understanding of, and solutions to, problematic and emotionally demanding situations. Collaboration among rehabilitation providers and psychologists appears essential for guiding the providers to utilize behavioral management approaches that can facilitate compliance with and efficacy of rehabilitation treatment interventions. Furthermore, such collaboration allows for direct psychotherapeutic services that help to prevent caregiver "burnout" both through the provision of emotional support and assistance in the development of behaviorally based strategies that support the productive management of the individual with PD (252).

Several investigator groups (253,254) have defined principles of "collaborative management" of chronic illness among health providers, caregivers and patients, and a "user-led pathway" that have been adapted for providing care to those who have neurodegenerative diseases such as PD. These principles can guide the practices of rehabilitation providers: (*i*) collaborative definition of problems that are patient–caregiver dyad driven, (*ii*) prioritizing problems for intervention, then planning treatments and setting goals of treatment that are realistic, and again driven by the patient–caregiver dyad, (*iii*) developing a continuum of formal support services that provide consultation and education for the patient–caregiver dyad to be as self-directed as possible in executing daily life rituals within a structured day, including such basic functions as eating, toileting, and taking medications, as well as participating in exercise, taking rest breaks, and going on community outings to see medical providers, to go shopping, to go to support groups, and so on, and (*iv*) monitoring for reinforcement of successful strategies and modification of interventions as disease progression occurs or when previously used strategies are no longer effective.

Several nursing investigators have identified successful coping strategies that can be taught and/or reinforced among caregivers of those with PD. These strategies have focused largely on cognitive-behavioral approaches aimed at counteracting caregiver depression, usually expressed as "learned helplessness" and "pessimism." Such approaches include: "learning optimism"; re-engaging with one's "inner locus of control" to counteract a sense of being controlled by "outer forces"; maintaining one's own life; encouraging the patient–caregiver dyad to stay active; and focusing on what is meaningful to the individual despite ongoing loss and frustration in handling loss during disease progression (255–257).

While the literature on caregiving in PD continues to evolve in the direction of more explicitly defining risk factors that underpin burden of care, caregiver "strain," and depression, and to offer theoretical and pragmatic solutions (primarily "psychoeducational" strategies) for modifying these risk factors and treating depression, the efficacy of these strategies in a therapeutic context continues to be untested. When taking a patient–caregiver dyad-driven approach to defining and prioritizing problems, it is clear that the "consumer" can effectively communicate the issues that are problematic. For example, in Davey et al. (244) study of fallers with PD, the caregivers articulated the lack of education about preventing falls, as well as a lack of education as to how to manage the consequences of falls, such as minimizing potential injury in assisting the faller to reachieve the sitting or standing positions. When rehabilitation treatments are directed toward optimizing the functional status of the individual with PD, it has been increasingly recognized by some investigators that outcome measurement should encompass parallel observations of the individual and the caregiver. For example, Trend et al. (147) investigation of multidisciplinary rehabilitation interventions performed at a day hospital setting measured functional status, affective status, and quality of life in the individuals with PD as direct outcomes of treatment; and caregiver strain, affective status, and quality of life as indirect outcomes of treatment. Observational studies are needed to assess caregivers' responses to interventions aimed toward teaching concrete skills that can facilitate their participation in the caregiver role (e.g., appropriate biomechanical methods to provide mobility assistance, aspiration prevention strategies for dysphagic individuals, behavioral management of difficult behaviors), and that are aimed toward reducing their caregiver "strain" risk factors, such as treating depression and managing sleep interruption (e.g., psychotherapy, support groups, anticholinergic agents/bedside urinals or condom drainage systems in men to manage night time urinary frequency, and incontinence that interrupt female caregivers' sleep). This line of investigation has recently been explored in other neurodegenerative patient–caregiver dyad populations, specifically Alzheimer's dementia (258–262). For example, Gitlin et al. (262–267) impressive body of work has observed occupational therapy interventions as part of the National Institutes of Health Resources for Enhancing Alzheimer's Caregiver Health (REACH) initiative. During this randomized controlled trial that longitudinally observed 127 caregivers assigned either to usual care or occupational therapy training groups, significant improvements in caregiver affect were reported at 12 months, and those skills that were reported as significantly improved at six months (at the end of the intervention phase) were sustained at 12 months. Other significant postintervention phase improvements that were sustained at 12 months included less need for providing assistance to the individual with dementia and fewer behavioral problems displayed in the individual with dementia. This line of investigation can serve as a model for caregiver training in PD.

Complementary and Alternative Treatments

It has been estimated that up to 40% of individuals who have PD use at least one type of complementary and alternative treatment; 12% have been reported to use five or more of these therapies. These estimates are higher than what has been reported for the general American population (about 30%). About 60% of those individuals with PD who have used complementary and alternative treatments, have done so without informing their primary or neurological care providers; their use is more common among those with PD who have a younger age of onset, who have higher levels of income and education, and who take a higher daily dose of dopaminergic agents. Complementary and alternative treatments include an array of therapies that are nutritionally based (vitamins, nutritional supplements, herbs, homeopathy); manual/biomechanical (massage, Pilates, yoga, Alexander technique, chiropractic, osteopathic); hypothesized as manipulative of "energy flow" (magnets, acupuncture/acupressure, Tai Chi, reflexology); spiritual (prayer, "faith healing"); psychological (biofeedback, hypnosis, relaxation); as well as art and music therapy. Vitamins and herbs (vitamins E and C, multivitamins, coenzyme Q10, Ginkgo biloba), massage, and acupuncture are most commonly reported to be used among those with PD (268,269). The potential efficacy of complementary and alternative treatments to treat PD has received little study, and reports of therapeutic effects are empiric. Among those treatments that have been subjected to rigorous investigation, the fat soluble antioxidant, vitamin E (2000 international units per day), has had no significant symptomatic or neuroprotective effect (268,270). Coenzyme Q10, another fat-soluble antioxidant, has been shown to be promising to stabilize functional status beyond one year (271). The reported postintervention improvements of "spa therapy" (thermal baths, drinking mineral water, relaxation, and exercise therapies) were not sustained six months later (269).

More relevant to exercise-based rehabilitation interventions, the Alexander technique has been reported to have therapeutic effects that were sustained over six months (272,273). Stallibrass and Chalmers (272) compared the Alexander technique, massage, and no treatment during a randomized clinical trial over 12 weeks: the Alexander technique was relatively comparable to massage, and significantly better than no treatment at stabilizing disability level. The study subjects who were treated with the Alexander technique qualitatively reported more improvements in posture, balance, gait, speech, and sitting ability; while those who were treated with massage reported more often a relaxation effect and a "higher sense of well-being." The effects of these treatments on pain relief were qualitatively comparable. The hypothesized physiological mechanism that underpins the Alexander technique is best characterized as "neuromuscular re-education" (272,273). Svircev et al. (274) compared neuromuscular massage and music relaxation therapy in a clinical trial that compared 32 subjects with PD, randomly assigned to each type of treatment: significant improvements were observed in those who received massage, as measured by the motor examination subscale of the UPDRS, after twice weekly treatments over four weeks.

SUMMARY AND CONCLUSIONS

1. Younger individuals were likely to have better outcomes after DBS procedures than older individuals; older individuals were more likely to need post-DBS rehabilitation services.
2. The cardinal clinical signs of PD that were levodopa responsive, improved by DBS, likely translate into parallel improvements in functional status and quality of life.
3. Vim-DBS appeared to be effective for decreasing tremor and improving handwriting up to five years after surgery; GPi-DBS appeared to be

more efficacious during the initial postsurgical year, with short-term improvements in clinical signs and functional status inconsistently sustained beyond one year.

4. The improvements in functional status and quality of life that occurred during the initial year after STN-DBS were generally sustained beyond one year. The motoric factors that contributed to these improvements appeared to be variable; gait has been more consistently reported as improved, while speech and postural control have not.

5. Cognition was usually reported as stable after DBS procedures particularly in those who were intact presurgically. Problematic mood and behavioral problems were rare after these procedures, and were considered treatable with neuromodulating agents.

6. Sensory cueing strategies have demonstrated promising results for improving gait and balance, but not upper limb motor control, for those who have PD.

7. LSVT® and similar treatments, have demonstrated promising results to treat hypokinetic dysarthria.

8. Caregiver involvement during rehabilitation interventions for those who have PD is essential, however, strategies for developing caregiver skills have received little investigation.

9. Complementary and alternative treatments are commonly used among those with PD, but few have received rigorous study.

REFERENCES

1. Lozano AM, Hamani C. The future of deep brain stimulation. J Clin Neurophysiol 2004; (21):68–69.
2. Breit S, Schulz JB, Benabid AL. Deep brain stimulation. Cell Tissue Research 2004; 318:275–288.
3. Ashkan K, Wallace B, Bell BA, et al. Deep brain stimulation of the subthalamic nucleus in Parkinson's disease 1993–2003: where are we 10 years on? Br J Neurosurg 2004; 18:19–34.
4. Deuschl G, Wenzelburger R, Kopper F, et al. Deep brain stimulation of the subthalamic nucleus for Parkinson's disease: As therapy approaching evidence-based standards. J Neurol 2003; 250(suppl 1):I/43–I/46.
5. Benebid AL. Deep brain stimulation for Parkinson's disease. Curr Opin Neurol 2003; 13:696–706.
6. Lozano AM, Mahant N. Deep brain stimulation surgery for Parkinson's disease: mechanisms and consequences. Parkinsonism Relat Disord 2004; 10:S49–S57.
7. Volkmann J. Deep brain stimulation for the treatment of Parkinson's disease. J Clin Neurophysiol 2004; 21:6–17.
8. Anderson VC, Burchiel KJ, Hogarth P, et al. Pallidal vs subthalamic nucleus deep brain stimulation in Parkinson disease. Arch Neurol 2005; 62:533–536.
9. Follett K, Weaver FM, Stern M, et al. VA Cooperative Study #468. A comparison of best medical therapy and deep brain stimulation of subthalamic nucleus and globus pallidus for the treatment of Parkinson's disease. Version 7, March 15, 2002; 1–102.

10. Lozano AM, Dostrovsky J, Chen R, et al. Deep brain stimulation for Parkinson's disease: disrupting the disruption. Lancet Neurol 2002; 1:225–231.
11. Krack P, Fraix V, Mendes A, et al. Postoperative management of subthalamic nucleus stimulation for Parkinson's disease. Mov Disord 2002; 17(suppl 3): S188–S197.
12. Lang AE. Subthalamic stimulation for Parkinson's disease—living better electrically? N Engl J Med 2003; 349:1888–1891.
13. Lang AE, Widner H. Deep brain stimulation for Parkinson's disease: patient selection and evaluation. Mov Disord 2002; 17(suppl 3):S94–S101.
14. Jaggi JL, Umemura A, Hurtig HI, et al. Bilateral stimulation of the subthalamic nucleus in Parkinson's disease: surgical efficacy and prediction of outcome. Stereotact Funct Neurosurg 2004; 82:104–114.
15. Charles PD, Van Blercom N, Krack P, et al. Predictors of effective bilateral subthalamic nucleus stimulation for PD. Neurology 2002; 59:932–934.
16. Welter ML, Houeto JL, Tezenas du Monteel S, et al. Clinical predictive factors of subthalamic stimulation in Parkinson's disease. Brain 2002; 125:575–583.
17. Robinson K, Cianci H, Noorigian J, et al. Functional outcome after subthalamic nuclear deep brain stimulation: six month follow-up. Mov Disord 2005; 20(suppl 10):S150.
18. Stewart RM, Desaloms JM, Sanghera MK. Stimulation of the subthalamic nucleus for the treatment of Parkinson's disease: postoperative management, programming, and rehabilitation. J Neurosci Nurs 2005; 37:108–114.
19. Fahn S, Elton RI. The UPDRS Development Committee, Unified Parkinson's Disease Rating Scale. In: Fahn S, Marsden CD, Calne D, Goldstein M, eds. Recent Developments in Parkinson's Disease, Vol. 2, Florham Park, NJ: McMillan Health Care Information, 1987:153–163, 293–304.
20. Hariz GM, Lindberg M, Hariz MI, et al. Does the ADL part of the Unified Parkinson's Disease Rating Scale measure ADL? An evaluation in patients after pallidotomy and thalamic deep brain stimulation. Mov Disord 2003; 18:373–381.
21. Capecci M, Ricciuti A, Burini D, et al. Functional improvement after subthalamic stimulation in Parkinson's disease: a non-equivalent controlled study with 12–24 month follow up. J Neurol Neurosurg Psychiatry 2005; 76:769–774.
22. Hariz MI. From functional neurosurgery to "interventional" neurology: survey of publications on thalamotomy, pallidotomy, and deep brain stimulation for Parkinson's disease from 1966 to 2001. Mov Disord 2003; 18:845–852.
23. Defebvre L, Blatt JL, Blond S, et al. Effect of thalamic stimulation on gait in Parkinson's disease. Arch Neurol 1996; 53:898–903.
24. Ondo W, Almaguer M, Janovic J, et al. Thalamic deep brain stimulation. Arch Neurol 2001; 58:218–222.
25. Lyons KE, Koller WC, Wilkinson SB, et al. Long term safety and efficacy of unilateral deep brain stimulation of the thalamus for parkinsonian tremor. J Neurol Neurosurg Psychiatry 2001; 71:682–684.
26. Putzke JD, Wharen RE, Wszolek ZK, et al. Thalamic deep brain stimulation for tremor-predominant Parkinson's disease. Parkinsonism Relat Disord 2003; 10:81–88.
27. Kumar R, Lozano AM, Sime E, et al. Long-term follow-up of thalamic deep brain stimulation for essential and parkinsonian tremor. Neurology 2003; 61:1601–1604.

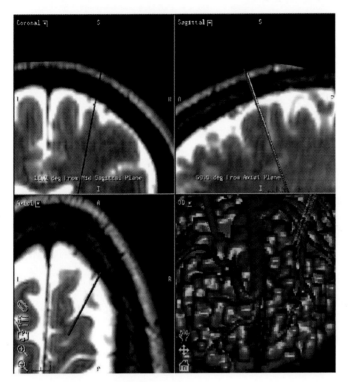

Figure 5-1 *See text page 73.*

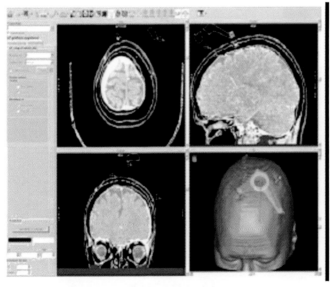

Figure 6-1 *See text page 85.*

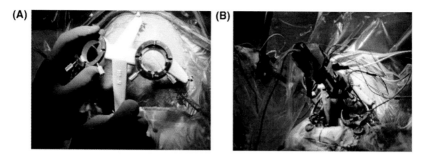

Figure 6-2 *See text page 86.*

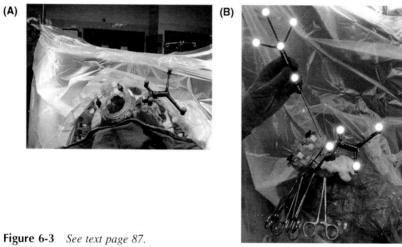

Figure 6-3 *See text page 87.*

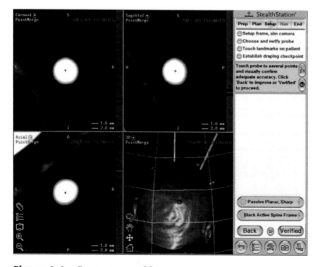

Figure 6-4 *See text page 88.*

28. Pinter MM, Murg M, Alesch F, et al. Does deep brain stimulation of the nucleus ventralis intermedius affect postural control and locomotion in Parkinson's disease. Mov Disord 1999; 14:958–963.
29. Speelman JD, Schuurman R, deBie RMA, et al. Stereotactic surgery for tremor. Mov Disord 2002; 17(suppl 3):S84–S88.
30. Diamond A, Jankovic J. The effect of deep brain stimulation on quality of life on movement disorders. J Neurol Neurosurg Psychiatry 2005; 76:1188–1193.
31. Tronnier VM, Fogel W, Kronenbuerger M, et al. Pallidal stimulation: as alternative to pallidotomy? J Neurosurg 1997; 87:700–705.
32. Kumar R, Lang AE, Lozano AM, et al. Deep brain stimulation of the globus pallidus pars interna in advanced Parkinson's disease. Neurology 2000; 55(suppl 6):S34–S39.
33. Loher TJ, Burgunder JM, Pohle T, et al. Long term pallidal deep brain stimulation in patients with advanced Parkinson disease: 1-year follow-up study. J Neurosurg 2002; 96:844–853.
34. Krystkowiak P, Blatt JL, Bourriez JL, et al. Chronic bilateral pallidal stimulation and levodopa do not improve gait in the same way in Parkinson's disease: a study using a video motion analysis system. J Neurol 2001; 248:944–949.
35. Defebvre LJ, Krystkowiak P, Blatt JL, et al. Influence of pallidal stimulation and levodopa on gait and preparatory postural adjustments in Parkinson's disease. Mov Disord 2002; 17:76–83.
36. Ghika J, Villemure JG, Fankhauser H, et al. Efficiency and safety of bilateral contemporaneous pallidal stimulation (deep brain stimulation) in levodopa-responsive patients with Parkinson's disease with severe motor fluctuations: a 2-year follow-up review. J Neurosurg 1998; 89:713–718.
37. Lyons KE, Wilkinson SB, Troster AI, et al. Long-term efficacy of globus pallidus stimulation for the treatment of Parkinson's disease. Stereotact Funct Neurosurg 2002; 79:214–220.
38. Durif F, Lemaire JJ, Debilly B, et al. Long-term follow-up of globus pallidus chronic stimulation in advanced Parkinson's disease. Mov Disord 2002; 17:803–807.
39. Visser-Vandewalle V, van der Linden C, Temel Y, et al. Long-term motor effect of unilateral pallidal stimulation in 26 patients with advanced Parkinson's disease. J Neurosurg 2003; 99:701–707.
40. Visser-Vandewalle V, Temel Y, van der Linden C, et al. Deep brain stimulation in movement disorders. The applications reconsidered. Acta Neurologica Belgique 2004; 104:33–36.
41. Volkmann J, Allert N, Voges J, et al. Long-term results of bilateral stimulation in Parkinson's disease. Ann Neurol 2004; 55:871–875.
42. Kumar R, Lozano AM, Kim YJ, et al. Double-blind evaluation of subthalamic nucleus deep brain stimulation in advanced Parkinson's disease. Neurology 1998; 51:850–855.
43. Katayama Y, Kasai M, Oshima H, et al. Subthalamic nucleus stimulation for Parkinson's disease: benefits observed in levodopa intolerant patients. J Neurosurg 2002; 96:213–221.
44. Simuni T, Jaggi JL, Mulholland H, et al. Bilateral stimulation of the subthalamic nucleus in patients with Parkinson's disease: a study of safety and efficacy. J Neurosurg 2002; 96:666–672.

45. Thobois S, Mertens P, Guenot M, et al. Subthalamic nucleus stimulation in Parkinson disease: clinical evaluation of 18 patients. J Neurol 2002; 249:529–534.

46. Vesper J, Klostermann F, Stockhammer F, et al. Results of chronic subthalamic nucleus stimulation for Parkinson's disease: a 1-year follow-up study. Surg Neurol 2002; 57:306–313.

47. Ostergaard K, Sunde N, Dupont E. Effects of bilateral stimulation of the subthalamic nucleus in patients with severe Parkinson's disease and motor fluctuations. Mov Disord 2002; 17:693–700.

48. Eriksen SK, Tuite PJ, Maxwell RE, et al. Bilateral subthalamic nucleus stimulation for the treatment of Parkinson's disease: results of six patients. J Neurosci Nurs 2003; 35:223–231.

49. Germano IM, Gracies JM, Weisz DJ, et al. Unilateral stimulation of the subthalamic nucleus in Parkinson disease: a double-blind 12-month evaluation study. J Neurosurg 2004; 101:36–42.

50. Jaggi JL, Umemura A, Hurtig HI, et al. Bilateral stimulation of the subthalamic nucleus in Parkinson's disease: surgical efficacy and prediction of outcome. Stereotact Funct Neurosurg 2004; 82:104–114.

51. Ford B, Winfield L, Pullman SL, et al. Subthalamic nucleus stimulation in advanced Parkinson's disease: blinded assessments at one year follow up. J Neurol Neurosurg Psychiatry 2004; 75:1255–1259.

52. Linazasoro G, Subthalamic deep brain stimulation for advanced Parkinson's disease: all that glitters is not gold. J Neurol Neurosurg Psychiatry 2003; 74:827.

53. Yokoyama T, Sugiyama K, Nishizawa, et al. Subthalamic nucleus for gait disturbances in Parkinson's disease. Neurosurgery 1999; 45:41–47.

54. Stolze H, Klebe S, Poepping, et al. Effects of bilateral subthalamic nucleus stimulation on parkinsonian gait. Neurology 2001; 57:144–146.

55. Ferrarin M, Rizzone M, Lopiano L, et al. Effects of subthalamic nucleus stimulation and L-dopa in trunk kinematics of patients with Parkinson's disease. Gait and Posture 2004; 19:164–171.

56. Krystkowiak P, Blatt JL, Bourriez JL, et al. Effects of subthalamic nucleus stimulation and levodopa treatment on gait abnormalities in Parkinson's disease. Arch Neurol 2003; 60:80–84.

57. Morris ME, Iansek R, Matyas TA, et al. Stride length regulation in Parkinson's disease: normalization strategies and underlying mechanism. Brain 1996; 119:551–568.

58. Bejjani BP, Gervais D, Arnulf I, et al. Axial parkinsonian symptoms can be improved: the role of levodopa and bilateral subthalamic stimulation. J Neurol Neurosurg Psychiatry 2000; 68:595–600.

59. Nilsson MH, Tornqvist AL, Rehncrona S. Deep brain stimulation in the subthalamic nuclei improves balance performance in patients with Parkinson's disease, when tested without anti-parkinsonian medications. Acta Neurologica Scandinavia 2005; 111:301–308.

60. Rocchi L, Chiari L, Horak FB. Effects of deep brain stimulation and levodopa on postural sway in Parkinson's disease. J Neurol Neurosurg Psychiatry 2002; 73:267–274.

61. Colnat-Coulbois S, Gauchard GC, Maillard L, et al. Bilateral subthalamic nucleus stimulation improves balance control in Parkinson's disease. J Neurol Neurosurg Psychiatry 2005; 76:780–787.

62. Wenzelburger R, Kopper F, Zhang BR, et al. Subthalamic nucleus stimulation for Parkinson's disease preferentially improves akinesia of proximal arm movements compared to finger movements. Mov Disord 2003; 18:1162–1169.
63. Taylor Tavares AL, Jefferis GS, Koop M, et al. Quantitative measurements of alternating finger tapping in Parkinson's disease correlate with UPDRS motor disability and reveal the improvement in fine motor control from medication and deep brain stimulation. Mov Disord 2005; 20(10):1286–1298.
64. Carella F, Genitrini S, Bressanelli M, et al. Acute effects of bilateral subthalamic nucleus stimulation on clinical and kinematic parameters in Parkinson's disease. Mov Disord 2001; 16:651–655.
65. Moretti R, Torre P, Antonello, et al. "Speech initiation hesitation" following subthalamic nucleus stimulation in a patient with Parkinson's disease. Eur Neurol 2003; 49:251–253.
66. Pinto S, Gentil M, Fraix V, et al. Bilateral subthalamic stimulation effects on oral force in Parkinson's disease. J Neurol 2003; 250:179–187.
67. Rousseaux M, Krystowiak P, Kozlowski O, et al. Effects of subthalamic nucleus stimulation on parkinsonian dysarthria and speech intelligibility. J Neurol 2004; 251:327–334.
68. Castelli L, Perozzo P, Genesia ML, et al. Sexual well being in parkinsonian patients after deep brain stimulation of the subthalamic nucleus. J Neurol Neurosurg Psychiatry 2004; 75:1260–1264.
69. Finazzi-Agro E, Peppe A. D'Amoco A, et al. Effects of subthalamic nucleus stimulation on urodynamic findings in patients with Parkinson's disease. J Urol 2003; 169:1388–1391.
70. Antonini A, Landi A, Mariani C, et al. Deep brain stimulation and its effect on sleep in Parkinson's disease. Sleep Med 2004; 5:211–214.
71. Iranzo A, Valldeoriola F, Santamaria J, et al. Sleep symptoms and polysomnographic architecture in advance Parkinson's disease after chronic bilateral subthalamic stimulation. J Neurol Neurosurg Psychiatry 2002; 72:661–664.
72. Cicolin A, Lopiano L, Zibetti M, et al. Effects of deep brain stimulation of the subthalamic nucleus on sleep architecture in parkinsonian patients. Sleep Med 2004; 5:207–210.
73. Lopiano L, Rizzone M, Bergamasco B, et al. Daytime sleepiness improvement following bilateral chronic electrical stimulation of the subthalamic nucleus in Parkinson's disease. Eur Neurol 2001; 46:49–50.
74. Monaca C, Ozsancak C, Jacquesson JM, et al. Effects of bilateral stimulation on sleep in Parkinson's disease. J Neurol 2002; 251:214–218.
75. Just H, Ostergaard K. Health-related quality of life in patients with advanced Parkinson's disease treated with deep brain stimulation of the subthalamic nuclei. Mov Disord 2002; 17:539–545.
76. Lagrange E, Krack P, Moro E, et al. Bilateral subthalamic nucleus stimulation improves health-related quality of life. Neurology 2002; 59:1976–1978.
77. Erola T, Karinen P, Heikkinen E, et al. Bilateral subthalamic nucleus stimulation improves health-related quality of life in parkinsonian patients. Parkinsonism Relat Disord 2005; 11:89–94.
78. Hariz MI. Complications after deep brain stimulation surgery. Mov Disord 2002; 17(suppl 3):S162–S166.

79. Lyons KE, Pahwa R. Deep brain stimulation in Parkinson's disease. Curr Neurol Neurosci Rep 2004; 4:290–295.

80. Macia F, Perlemoine C, Coman I, et al. Parkinson's disease patients with bilateral deep brain stimulation gain weight. Mov Disord 2004; 19:206–212.

81. Moro E, Scerrati M, Romito LM, et al. Chronic subthalamic nucleus stimulation reduces medication requirements in Parkinson's disease. Neurology 1999; 53: 85–90.

82. Rodriguez-Oroz MC, Obeso JA, Gorospe A, et al. Bilateral deep brain stimulation of the subthalamic nucleus in Parkinson's disease. Neurology 2000; 55(suppl 6):45–51.

83. Tavella A, Bergamasco B, Bosticco E, et al. Deep brain stimulation of the subthalamic nucleus in Parkinson's disease: long term follow-up. Neurological Science 2002; 23:S111–S112.

84. Vingerhoets FJ, Villemure JG, Temperli P, et al. Subthalamic DBS replaces levodopa in parkinson's disease: two-year follow-up. Neurology 2002; 58:396–401.

85. Figueiras-Mendez R, Regidor I, Riva-Meana C, et al. Further supporting evidence of beneficial subthalamic stimulation in Parkinson's patients. Neurology 2002; 58:469–470.

86. Valldeoriloa F, Pilleri M, Tolosa E, et al. Bilateral subthalamic stimulation monotherapy in advanced Parkinson's disease: long-term follow-up of patients. Mov Disord 2002; 17:125–132.

87. Mesnage V, Houeto JL, Welter ML, et al. Parkinson's disease: neurosurgery at an earlier stage? J Neurol Neurosurg Psychiatry 2005; 73:778.

88. Romito LMA, Scerrati M, Contarino MF, et al. Long-term follow up of subthalamic nucleus stimulation in Parkinson's disease. Neurology 2002; 58:1546–1550.

89. Herzog J, Volkmann J, Krack P, et al. Two year follow-up of subthalamic deep brain stimulation in Parkinson's disease. Mov Disord 2003; 18:1332–1337.

90. Pahwa R, Wilkinson SB, Overman J, et al. Bilateral subthalamic stimulation in patients with Parkinson disease: long-term follow up. J Neurosurg 2003; 99:71–77.

91. Krack P, Batir A, Van Blercom N, et al. Five-year follow-up of bilateral stimulation of the subthalamic nucleus in advanced Parkinson's disease. N Engl J Med 2003; 349:1925–1934.

92. Kleiner-Fisman G, Fisman DN, Sime E, et al. Long-term follow up of bilateral deep brain stimulation of the subthalamic nucleus in patients with advanced Parkinson disease. J Neurosurg 2003; 99:489–495.

93. Romito LM, Scerrati M, Contarino F, et al. Bilateral high frequency subthalamic stimulation in Parkinson's disease: long-term neurological follow-up. J Neurosurg 2003; 47:119–128.

94. Krause M, Fogel W, Mayer P, et al. Chronic inhibition of the subthalamic nucleus in Parkinson's disease. Journal of Neurological Sciences 2004; 219:119–124.

95. Rodriguez-Oroz MC, Zamabide I, Guridi J, et al. Efficacy of deep brain stimulation of the subthalamic nucleus in Parkinson's disease 4 years after surgery: double blind and open label evaluation. J Neurol Neurosurg Psychiatry 2004; 75:1382–1385.

96. Visser-Vandewalle V, van der Linden C, Temel Y, et al. Long-term effects of bilateral subthalamic nucleus stimulation in advanced Parkinson disease: a four year follow-up study. Parkinsonism Relat Disord 2005; 11:157–165.

97. Lezcano E, Gomez-Estaban C, Zarranz JJ, et al. Improvements in quality of life in patients with advanced Parkinson's disease following bilateral deep-brain stimulation in subthalamic nucleus. Eur J Neurol 2004; 11:451–454.

98. Russmann H, Ghika J, Villemure JG, et al. Subthalamic nucleus deep brain stimulation in Parkinson disease: patients over age 70 years. Neurology 2004; 63:1952–1954.
99. Maurer C, Mergner T, Xie J, et al. Effect of chronic bilateral subthalamic nucleus stimulation (STN) on postural control in Parkinson's disease. Brain 2003; 126:1146–1163.
100. The Deep Brain Stimulation for Parkinson's Disease Study Group. Deep-brain stimulation of the subthalamic nucleus or the pars interna of the globus in Parkinson's disease. New England Journal of England 2001; 345:956–963.
101. Allert N, Volkmann J, Dotse S, et al. Effects of bilateral pallidal or subthalamic stimulation on gait in advanced Parkinson's disease. Mov Disord 2001; 16:1076–1085.
102. Rocchi L, Chiari L, Cappello A, et al. Comparison between subthalamic nucleus and globus pallidus internus stimulation for postural performance in Parkinson's disease. Gait and Posture 2004; 19:172–183.
103. Follett KA. Comparison of pallidal and subthalamic deep brain stimulation for the treatment of levodopa-induced dyskinesias. Neurosurg Focus 2004; 17:14–19.
104. Alberts JL, Elder CM, Okun MS, et al. Comparison of pallidal and subthalamic stimulation on force control in patients with Parkinson's disease. Motor Control 2004; 8:484–499.
105. Scotto di Luzio AE, Ammannati F, Marini P, et al. Which target for DBS in Parkinson's disease? Subthalamic nucleus versus globus pallidus internus. Neuro Sci 2001; 22:87–88.
106. Robertson LT, Horak FB, Anderson VC, et al. Assessments of axial motor control during deep brain stimulation in parkinsonian patients. Neurosurgery 2001; 48:544–551.
107. Farrell A, Theodoros D, Ward E, et al. Effects of neurosurgical management of Parkinson's disease on speech characteristics and oromotor function. J Speech Lang Hear Res 2005; 48:5–20.
108. Rodriguez-Oroz MC, Obeso JA, Lang AE, et al. Bilateral deep brain stimulation in Parkinson's disease: a multicentre study with 4 year follow-up. Brain 2005; 128(10):2240–2249.
109. Dujardin K, Blairy S, Defebvre L, et al. Subthalamic nucleus stimulation induces deficits in decoding emotional facial expressions in Parkinson's disease. J Neurol Neurosurg Psychiatry 2004; 75:202–208.
110. Witt K, Pulkowski U, Herzog J, et al. Deep brain stimulation of the subthalamic nucleus improves cognitive flexibility but impairs response inhibition in Parkinson's disease. Arch Neurol 2004; 61:697–700.
111. Pillon B. Neuropsychological assessment for management of patients with deep brain stimulation. Mov Disord 2002; 17:S116–S122.
112. Alegret M, Junque C, Valldeoriola F, et al. Effects of bilateral subthalamic stimulation on cognitive function in Parkinson's disease. Arch Neurol 2002; 58:1223–1227.
113. Hershey T, Revilla FJ, Wernle A, et al. Stimulation of STN impairs aspects of cognitive control in PD. Neurology 2004; 62:1110–1114.
114. Brusa L, Pierantozzi M, Peppe A, et al. Deep brain stimulation (DBS) attentional effects parallel those of l-dopa treatment. J Neural Transm 2001; 108:1021–1027.
115. Gironell A, Kulisevsky J, Rami L, et al. Effects of pallidotomy and bilateral subthalamic stimulation on cognitive function in Parkinson disease. J Neurol 2003; 250:917–923.

116. Field JA, Troster AI. Cognitive outcomes after deep brain stimulation for Parkinson's disease: a review of initial studies and recommendation for future research. Brain Cogn 2000; 42:268–293.

117. Funkiewiez A, Ardouin C, Caputo E, et al. Long term effects of bilateral subthalamic stimulation on cognition function, mood, and behavior in Parkinson's disease. J Neurol Neurosurg Psychiatry 2003; 250:917–923.

118. Daniele A, Albanese A, Contarino MF, et al. Cognitive and behavioral effects of chronic stimulation of the subthalamic nucleus in patients with Parkinson's disease. J Neurol Neurosurg Psychiatry 2003; 74:175–182.

119. Anderson KE, Mullins J. Behavioral changes associated with deep brain stimulation surgery for Parkinson's disease. Curr Neurol Neurosci Rep 2003; 3:306–313.

120. Dujardin K, Defebvre L, Krystkowiak P, et al. Influence of chronic bilateral stimulation of the subthalamic nucleus on cognitive function in Parkinson's disease. J Neurol 2001; 248:603–611.

121. Morrison CE, Borod JC, Perrine K, et al. Neuropsychological functioning following bilateral subthalamic nucleus stimulation in Parkinson's disease. Arch Clin Neuropsych 2004; 19:165–181.

122. Moretti R, Torre P, Antonello RM, et al. Neuropsychological changes after subthalamic nucleus stimulation: a 12 month follow-up in nine patients with Parkinson's disease. Parkinsonism Relat Disord 2003; 10:73–79.

123. Zanini S, Melatini A, Capus L, et al. Language recovery following subthalamic nucleus stimulation in Parkinson's disease. Cognitive Neuroscience and Neuropsychology 2003; 14:511–516.

124. Whelan B-M, Murdoch BE, Theodoros DG, et al. Beyond verbal fluency: investigating the long-term effects of bilateral subthalamic (STN) deep brain stimulation (DBS) on language function in two cases. Neurocase 2005; 11:93–102.

125. Whelan B-M, Murdoch BE, Theodoros DG, et al. Defining a role for the subthalamic nucleus within operative theoretical models of subcortical participation in language. J Neurol Neurosurg Psychiatry 2003; 74:1543–1550.

126. Mayberg HS, Lozano AM. Penfield revisited? Understanding and modifying behavior by deep brain stimulation for PD. Neurology 2002; 59:1298–1299.

127. Houeto JL, Mesnage V, Mallet L, et al. Behavioural disorders, Parkinson's disease and subthalamic stimulation. J Neurol Neurosurg Psychiatry 2002; 72:701–707.

128. Piasecki SD, Jefferson JW. Psychiatric complications of deep brain stimulation for Parkinson's disease. J Clin Psychiatry 2004; 65:845–849.

129. Perozzo P, Rizzone M, Beramasco RB, et al. Deep brain stimulation of the subthalamic nucleus in Parkinson's disease: comparison of pre- and postoperative neuropsychological evaluation. J Neurol Sci 2001; 192:9–15.

130. Okun MS, Green J, Saben R, et al. Mood changes with deep brain stimulation of STN and GPi: results of a pilot study. J Neurol Neurosurg Psychiatry 2003; 74:1584–1586.

131. Schneider F, Habel U, Volkmann J, et al. Deep brain stimulation of the subthalamic nucleus enhances emotional processing. Arch General Psychiat 2003; 60:296–302.

132. Berney A, Vingerhoets F, Perrin A, et al. Effect on mood of subthalamic DBS for Parkinson's disease. Neurology 2002; 59:1427–1429.

133. Doshi PK, Chhaya N, Bhatt MH. Depression leading to attempted suicide after bilateral subthalamic nucleus stimulation for Parkinson's disease. Mov Disord 2002; 17:1084–1100.

134. Romito LM, Raja M, Daniele A, et al. Transient mania with hypersexuality after surgery for high-frequency stimulation of the subthalamic nucleus in Parkinson's disease. Mov Disord 2002; 17:1371–1374.

135. Pluck GC, Brown RG. Apathy in Parkinson's disease. J Neurol Neurosurg Psychiatry 2002; 72:636–642.

136. Sensi M, Eleopra R, Cavallo MA, et al. Explosive behavior related to bilateral subthalamic stimulation. Parkinsonism Relat Disord 2004; 10:247–251

137. Perozzo P, Rizzone M, Bergamasco B, et al. Deep brain stimulation of the subthalamic nucleus: behavioral modifications and familiar relations. Neurological Sciences 2001; 22:81–82.

138. Montgomery EB. Rehabilitative approaches to Parkinson's disease. Parkinsonism Relat Disord 2004; 10:S43–S47.

139. Kreb HI, Hogan N, Hening W, et al. Procedural learning in Parkinson's disease. Exp Brain Res 2001; 141:425–437.

140. Agostino R, Curra A, Solkati G, et al. Prolonged practice is a scarce benefit in improving motor performance in Parkinson's disease. Mov Disord 2004; 11:1285–1293.

141. Sutoo D, Akiyama K. Regulation of brain function by exercise. Neurobiol Dis 2003; 13:1–14.

142. Tillerson JL, Caudle WM, Reveron ME, et al. Exercise induces behavioral recovery and attenuates neurochemical deficits in rodent models of Parkinson's disease. Neuroscience 2003; 119:899–911.

143. Gage H, Storey L. Rehabilitation for Parkinson's disease: a systematic review of available evidence. Clin Rehabil 2004; 18:463–482.

144. Movement Disorder Society. Physical and occupational therapy in Parkinson disease. Mov Disord 2002; 17(suppl 4):

145. Deane KHO, Ellis-Hill C, Jones D, et al. Systemic review of paramedical therapies for Parkinson's disease. Mov Disord 2002; 17:984–991.

146. Sunvisson H, Ekman SL. Environmental influences on the experiences of people with Parkinson's disease. Nurs Inq 2001; 8:41–50.

147. Trend P, Kaye J, Gage H, et al. Short-term effectiveness of intensive multidisciplinary rehabilitation for people with Parkinson's disease and their carers. Clin Rehabil 2002; 16:717–725.

148. Wade DT, Gage H, Owen C, et al. Multidisciplinary rehabilitation for people with parkinson's disease: a randomized controlled study. J Neurol Neurosurg Psychiatry 2003; 74:158–162.

149. Playford ED. Multidisciplinary rehabilitation for people with Parkinson's disease. J Neurol Neurosurg Psychiatry 2003; 74:148–149.

150. Nieuwboer A, DeWeerdt W, Dom R, et al. Prediction of outcome of physiotherapy in advanced Parkinson's disease. Clin Rehabil 2002; 16:886–893.

151. Schenkman M, Zhu CW, Cutson TM, et al. Longitudinal evaluation of economic and physical impact of Parkinson's disease. Parkinsonism and Related Disorders 2001; 8:41–50.

152. Schrag A, Hovris A, Morley D, et al. Young-versus older-onset Parkinson's disease: impact of disease and psychosocial consequences. Mov Disord 2003; 18:1250–1256.

153. Mott S, Kenrick, M, Dixon M, et al. Pain as a sequela of Parkinson's disease. Australian Family Physicians 2004; 33:663–664.

154. Quittenbaum BH, Grahn B. Quality of life and pain in Parkinson's disease: as controlled cross-sectional study. Parkinsonism and Related Disorders 2004; 10:129–136.

155. Herlofson K, Larsen JP. The influence of fatigue on health-related quality of life in patients with Parkinson's disease. Acta Neurologica Scandanavia 2003; 107:1–6.

156. Capp-Ahlgren M, Lannerheim L, Dehlin O. Older Swedish women's experience of living with symptoms related to Parkinson's disease. J Adv Nurs 2002; 39:87–95.

157. Grosset KA, Grosset DG. Patient-perceived involvement and satisfaction in Parkinson's disease: effect on therapy and quality of life. Mov Disord 2005; 20:616–619.

158. Edwards NE, Scheetz PS. Predictors of burden for caregivers of patients with Parkinson's disease. J Neurosci Nurs 2002; 34:184–190.

159. Thommessen B, Aarsland D, Braekus A, et al. The psychosocial burden on spouses of the elderly with stroke, dementia and Parkinson's disease. International Journal of Geriatric Psychiatry 2002; 17:78–84.

160. Fleming V, Tolson D, Schartau E. Changing perceptions of womanhood: living with Parkinson's disease. International Journal of Nursing Studies 2004; 41:515–524.

161. Backer JH. Stressors, social support, coping and health dysfunction in individuals with Parkinson's disease. Journal of Gerontological Nursing 2000; 26:6–16.

162. Deane KHO, Jones D, Ellis-Hill C, et al. Physiotherapy for Parkinson's disease: a comparison of techniques (Review). The Cochrane Database of Systematic Reviews 2001; Issue 1, Article number: CD002815. DOI: 12/1002/14651858.CD002815.

163. Cees JT, deGoede PT, Samyra HJ, et al. The effects of physical therapy Parkinson's disease: a research synthesis. Arch Phys Med Rehab 2001; 82:509–515.

164. Rubinstein TC, Giladi N, Hausdorff JM. The power of cueing to circumvent dopamine deficits: a review of physical therapy treatment of gait disturbances in Parkinson's disease. Mov Disord 2002; 17:1148–1160.

165. Ebersbach G, Wissel, J Poewe, W. Parkinson's disease and other Mov Disord. In: Selzer ME, Clarke S, Cohen LG, Duncan PW, Gage FH, eds. Textbook of Neural Repair and Rehabilitation, Vol. II, Cambridge, U.K.: Cambridge University Press, 2006:560–578.

166. Azulay JP, Mesure S, Amblard B, et al. Visual control of locomotion. Brain 1999; 122:111–120.

167. Dietz V. Neurophysiology of gait disorders: present and future applications. Electroencephalog Clin Neurophysiol 1997; 103:333–355.

168. Dietz V. Gait disorders in spasticity and Parkinson's disease. Advances in Neurology 2001; 87:143–154.

169. Stolze H, Kuhtz-Buschbeck JP, Drucke H, et al. Comparative analysis of the gait disorder of normal pressure hydrocephalus and Parkinson's disease. J Neurol Neurosurg Psychiatry 2001; 70:298–297.

170. Ziv I, Avraham M, Dabby R, et al. Early occurrence of manual motor blocks in Parkinson's disease: a quantitative assessment. Acta Neurologia Scandinavia 1999; 99:106–111.

171. Frank JS, Horak FB, Nutt J. Centrally initiated postural adjustments in parkinsonian patients on and off levodopa. Journal of Neurophysiology 2000; 84:2440–2448.

172. Horak FB, Frank J, Nutt J. Effects of dopamine on postural control in parkinsonian subjects: scaling, set, and tone. J Neurophysiol 1996; 75:2380–2396.

173. Steiger MJ, Thompson PD, Marsden CD. Disordered axial movement in Parkinson's disease. J Neurol Neurosurg Psychiatry 1996; 61:645–648.
174. Rogers MW. Disorders of posture, balance, and gait in Parkinson's disease. Gait and Balance Disorders 1996; 12:825–845.
175. Miller RA, Thaut MH, McIntosh GC, et al. Components of EMG symmetry and variability in parkinsonism and healthy elderly gait. Electroencephalography and Neurophysiology 1996; 101:1–7.
176. Ziljlstra W, Rutgers AW, Van Weerden TW. Voluntary and involuntary adaptation of gait in Parkinson's disease. Gait and Posture 1998; 7:53–63.
177. Lewis GN, Byblow WD, Walt SE. Stride length regulation in Parkinson's disease: the use of extrinsic, visual cues. Brain 2000; 123:2077–2090.
178. Marchese R, Diverio M, Zucchi F, et al. The role of sensory cues in the rehabilitation of parkinsonian patients: a comparison of two physical therapy protocols. Mov Disord 2000; 15:879–883.
179. Fernandez del Olmo M, Cudeiro J. Temporal variability of gait in Parkinson disease: effects of a rehabilitation programme based on rhythmic sound cues. Parkinsonism Relat Disord 2005; 11:25–33.
180. Freedland RL, Festa C, Sealy M, et al. The effects of pulsed auditory stimulation on various measurements in persons with Parkinson disease. NeuroRehabilitation 2002; 17:81–87.
181. Howe TE, Lovgreen B, Cody FWJ, et al. Auditory cues can modify the gait of persons with early-stage Parkinson's disease: a method for enhancing parkinsonian walking performance? Clin Rehabil 2003; 17:363–367.
182. Dibble DE, Nicholson DE, Shultz B, et al. Sensory cueing effects on maximal speed gait initiation in persons with Parkinson's disease and healthy elders. Gait and Posture 2004; 19:215–225.
183. Suteerawattananon M, Morris GS, Etnyre BR, et al. Effects of visual and auditory cues on gait in individuals with Parkinson's disease. Journal of Neurological Sciences 2004; 219:63–69.
184. Rochester L, Hetherington V, Jones D, et al. The effect of external rhythmic cues (auditory and visual) on walking during a functional task in homes of people with Parkinson's disease. Arch Phys Med Rehabil 2005; 86:999–1006.
185. Iansek R, Morris M. Rehabilitation of gait in Parkinson's disease. J Neurol Neurosurg Psychiatry 1997; 63:556.
186. Woollacott M, Shumway-Cook A. Attention and the control of posture and gait: a review of an emerging area of research. Gait and Posture 2002; 16:1–14.
187. Muller V, Mohr B, Rosin R, et al. Short term effects of behavioral treatment on movement initiation and postural control in Parkinson's disease: a controlled clinical trial. Mov Disord 1997; 12:306–314.
188. Behrman AL, Teitelbaum P, Cauraugh JH. Verbal instructional sets to normalize the temporal and spatial gait variables in Parkinson's disease. J Neurol Neurosurg Psychiatry 1998; 65:580–582.
189. Lokk J. The effects of mountain exercise in parkinsonian persons—a preliminary study. Arch Gerontol Geriat 2000; 31:19–25.
190. Miyai I, Fujimoto Y, Ueda Y, et al. Treadmill training with body weight support: its effect on Parkinson's disease. Arch Physical Med Rehabil 2000; 81:849–852.

191. Miyai I, Fujimoto Y, Yamamoto H, et al. Long term effect of body weight-supported treadmill training in Parkinson's disease: a randomized controlled trial. Arch Phys Med Rehabil 2002; 83:1370–1373.
192. Baastile J, Langbein WE, Weaver F, et al. Effect of exercise on perceived quality of life of individuals with Parkinson's disease. J Rehabil Res Dev 2000; 37:529–534.
193. Bergen JL, Toole T, Elliot, et al. Aerobic exercise intervention improves aerobic capacity and movement initiation in Parkinson's disease patients. NeuroRehabilitation 2002; 17:161–168.
194. Pohl M, Rockstroh, Ruckriem S, et al. Immediate effects of speed-dependent treadmill training on gait parameters in early Parkinson's disease. Arch Phys Med Rehabil 2003; 84:1760–1766.
195. Pellecchia MT, Grasso A, Biancardi LG, et al. Physical therapy in Parkinson's disease: an open long-term rehabilitation trial. J Neurol 2004; 251:595–598.
196. Ellis T, deGoede CJ, Feldman RG et al. Efficacy of a physical therapy program in patients with Parkinson's disease: a randomized controlled trial. Arch Phys Med Rehabil 2005; 86:626–632.
197. Viliani T, Pasquetti P, Magnolfi S, et al. Effects of physical training on straightening-up processes in patients with Parkinson's disease. Disabil Rehabil 1999; 21:68–73.
198. Toole T, Hirsch MA, Forkink A, et al. The effects of a balance and strength training program on equilibrium in parkinsonism: a preliminary study. NeuroRehabilitation 2000; 14:165–174.
199. Hirsch MA, Toole T, Maitland CG, et al. The effects of balance training and high resistance training on persons with idiopathic Parkinson's disease. Arch Phys Med Rehabil 2003; 84:1109–1117.
200. Jobges M, Heuschkel G, Pretzel C, et al. Repetitive training of compensatory steps: a therapeutic approach for postural instability in Parkinson's disease. J Neurol Neurosurg Psychiatry 2004; 75:1682–1687.
201. Stankovic I. The effect of physical therapy on balance of patients with Parkinson's disease. International Journal of Rehabilitation Research 2004; 27:53–57.
202. Koller WC, Glatt S, Vetere–Overfield B, et al. Falls in Parkinson's disease. Clin Neuropharmacol 1989; 12:98–105.
203. Wood BH, Biclough JA, Bowron A, et al. Incidence and prediction of falls in Parkinson's disease: a prospective multidisciplinary study. J Neurol Neurosurg Psychiatry 2002; 72:721–725.
204. Wielinski CL, Erickson-Davis C, Wichman R, et al. Falls and injuries resulting from falls among patients with Parkinson's disease and other parkinsonian syndromes. Mov Disord 2005; 20:410–415.
205. Tinetti ME. Preventing falls in the elderly. The N Engl J Med 2003; 349:42–49.
206. Stolze H, Klebe S, Zechlin S, et al. Falls in frequent neurological diseases—prevalence, risk factors and aetiology. J Neurol 2004; 251:79–84.
207. Ashburn A, Stack E, Pichering RM, et al. A community-dwelling sample of people with Parkinson's disease: characteristic of fallers and non-fallers. Age and Ageing 2001; 30:47–52.
208. Gray P, Hildebrand K. Fall risk factors in Parkinson's disease. J Neurosci Nurs 2000; 32:222–228.
209. Paulson GW, Schafer K, Hallum B. Avoiding mental changes and falls in older Parkinson's patients. Geriatrics 1986; 41:59–67.

210. Bloem BR, Grimbergen YA, Cramer M, et al. Prospective assessment of falls in Parkinson's disease. J Neurol 2002; 248:950–958.
211. Robinson KM, Dennison AC, Roalf D, et al. Falling risk factors in Parkinson's disease. NeuroRehabilitation 2005; 20:169–182.
212. Gillespie LD, Gillespie WJ, Robertson MC, et al. Interventions for preventing falls in elderly people (Cochrane Review). The Cochrane Library 2004; 4:1–29.
213. Grimbergen YAM, Munneke M, Bloem BR. Falls in Parkinson's disease. Curr Opin Neurol 2004; 17:405–415.
214. Lamberti P, Armenise S, Castaldo V, et al. Freezing of gait in Parkinson's disease. Eur Neurol 1997; 38:297–301.
215. Giladi N, Treves A, Simon ES, et al. Freezing of gait in patients with advanced Parkinson's disease. J Neural Transm 2001; 108:53–61.
216. Giladi N, McDermott MP, Fahn S, et al. The Parkinson Study Group. Freezing of gait in PD: prospective assessment in the DATATOP cohort. Neurology 2001; 56:1712–1721.
217. Schaafsma JD, Balash Y, Gurevich T, et al. Characterization of freezing of gait subtypes and the response of each to levodopa in Parkinson's disease. Eur J Neurol 2003; 10:391–398.
218. Bleom BR, Hausdorff JM, Visser JE, et al. Falls and freezing of gait in Parkinson's disease: a review of two interconnected, episodic phenomena. Mov Disord 2004; 19:871–884.
219. Hausdorff JM, Schaafsma JD, Balash Y, et al. Impaired regulation of stride variability in Parkinson's disease subjects with freezing of gait. Exp Brain Res 2003; 149:187–194.
220. Cubo E, Moore CG, Leurgans S, et al. Wheeled and standard walkers in Parkinson's disease patients with gait freezing. Parkinsonism Relat Disord 2003; 10:9–14.
221. Kompoliti K, Goetz CG, Leugans S, et al. "On" freezing in Parkinson's disease: resistance to visual cue walking devices. Mov Disord 2000; 15:309–312.
222. Bunting-Perry LK, Robinson KM, Noorigian J, et al. The efficacy of visual cues to treat patients with Parkinson's disease experiencing freezing of gait (FOG) episodes: a pilot study. Mov Disord 2005; 20(suppl 10):S81.
223. Murphy S, Tickle-Degnen L. The effectiveness of occupational therapy-related treatments for persons with Parkinson's disease: a meta-analytic review. Am J Occup Ther 2001; 55:385–392.
224. Platz T, Brown RG, Marsden CD. Training improves the speed of aimed movements in Parkinson's disease. Brain 1998; 121:505–514.
225. Brown RG, Marsden CD. Internal versus external cues and control of attention in Parkinson's disease. Brain 1988; 111:323–345.
226. Rosin R, Topka H, Dichgans J. Gait initiation in Parkinson's disease. Mov Disord 1997; 12:682–690.
227. Rogers MA, Phillips JG, Bradshaw JL, et al. Provision of external cues and movement sequencing in Parkinson's disease. Motor Control 1998; 2:125–132.
228. Meschak RP, Norman KE. A randomized controlled trial of the effects of weights on amplitude and frequency of postural hand tremor in people with Parkinson's disease. Clin Rehabil 2002; 16:481–492.
229. Albani G, Pignatti R, Bertella L, et al. Common daily activities in the virtual environment: a virtual study in parkinsonian patients. Neurological Science 2002; 23:S49–S50.

230. Goberman AM, Coelho C. Acoustic analysis of parkinsonian speech I: speech characteristics and L-dopa therapy. NeuroRehabilitation 2002; 17:237–246.

231. Schulz GM. The effects of speech therapy and pharmacologic treatments on voice and speech in Parkinson's disease: a review of the literature. Current Medicinal Chemistry 2002; 9:1359–1366.

232. Ramig LO, Fox C, Sapir W. Parkinson's disease: speech and voice disorders and their treatment with Lee Silverman Voice Treatment. Semin Speech Lang 2004; 25:169–180.

233. Movement Disorder Society. Speech therapy in Parkinson's disease. Mov Disord 2002; 17(suppl 4):S163–S166.

234. Deane KHO, Whurr R, Playford ED, et al. Speech and language therapy for dysarthria in Parkinson's disease: a comparison of techniques (review). The Cochrane Database of Systematic Review 2001; Issue 2, Article number:CD0022814. DOI:12.1002/14651858.CD002814 (on-line publication).

235. Ramig LO, Sapir S, Countryman S, et al. Intensive voice treatment (LSVT) for patients with Parkinson's disease: a 2 year follow up. J Neurol Neurosurg Psychiatry 2001; 71:493–498.

236. Baumgartner CA, Sapir S, Ramig LO. Voice quality changes following phonatory-respiratory effort treat (LSVT) versus respiratory effort treatment in individuals with Parkinson disease. J Voice 2001; 15:105–114.

237. Spielman Jl, Borod JC, Ramig LO. The effects of intensive voice treatment on facial expressiveness in Parkinson disease. Cogn Behav Neurol 2003; 16:177–188.

238. Liotti M, Ramig LO, Vogel D, et al. Hypophonia in Parkinson's disease. Neural correlates of voice treatment revealed by PET. Neurology 2003; 60:432–440.

239. Blumin JH, Pcolinsky DE, Atkins JP. Laryngeal findings in advanced Parkinson's disease. Ann Oto Rhinol Laryngol 2004; 113:253–258.

240. deSwart BJM, Willemse SC, Maassen BAM, et al. Improvement of voicing in patients with Parkinson's disease by speech therapy. Neurology 2003; 60:498–500.

241. Liotti M, deSwart BJM, Sanne MA, et al. Improvement of voicing in patients with Parkinson's disease by speech therapy. Neurology 2003; 61:1316–1317 (Letter to the editor).

242. Haneishi E. Effects of a music therapy voice protocol on speech intelligibility, vocal acoustic measures, and mood of individuals with Parkinson's disease. J Music Ther 2001; 38:273–290.

243. Kent RD, Vorperian HK, Kent JF, et al. Voice dysfunction in dysarthria: application of the Multi-Dimensional Voice Program™. J Commun Disord 2003; 36:281–306.

244. Davey C, Wiles R, Ashburn A, et al. Falling in Parkinson's disease: the impact on informal caregivers. Disabil Rehabil 2004; 26:1360–1366.

245. Pasetti C, Rossi Ferrario S, Fornara R, et al. Caregiving and Parkinson's disease. Neurological Science 2003; 24:203–204.

246. Martinez-Martin P, Benito-Leon J, Alonso F, et al. Quality of life of caregivers in Parkinson's disease. Qual Life Res 2005; 14:463–472.

247. Aarsland D, Larsen JP, Karlsen K, et al. Mental symptoms in Parkinson's disease are important contributors to caregiver distress. Int J Geriatr Psychiatry 1999; 14:866–874.

248. Happe S, Berger K, on behalf of the FAQT Study Investigators. The association between caregiver burden and sleep disturbances in partners of patients with Parkinson's disease. Age and Ageing 2002; 31:349–354.

249. Schrag A, Hovris A, Morley D, et al. Caregiver-burden in Parkinson's disease is closely associated with psychiatric symptoms, falls and disability. Parkinsonism Relat Disord 2006; 12:35–41.

250. Fernandez HH, Tabamo REJ, David RR, et al. Predictors of depressive symptoms among spouse caregivers in Parkinson's disease. Mov Disord 2001; 16:1123–1125.

251. Thommessen B, Aarsland D, Braekhus A, et al. The psychosocial burden of spouses of the elderly with stroke, dementia and Parkinson's disease. Int J Geriatr Psychiatry 2002; 17:78–84.

252. Bhatia S, Gupta A. Impairments in activities of daily living in Parkinson's disease: implications for management. NeuroRehabilitation 2003; 1:209–214.

253. Von Korff M, Gruman J, Schaefer J, et al. Collaborative management of chronic illness. Ann Intern Med 1997; 127:1097–1102.

254. Holloway M. Traversing the network: a user-led Care Pathway approach to the management of Parkinson's disease in the community. Health Soc Care Community 2005; 14:63–73.

255. Habermann B. Spousal perspective of Parkinson's disease in middle life. J Adv Nurs 2000; 31:1409–1415.

256. Lyons KS, Stewert BJ, Archbold PG, et al. Pessimism and optimism as early warning signs for compromised health for caregivers of patients with Parkinson's disease. Nurs Res 2004; 53:354–362.

257. Andersen S. Patient perspective and self-help. Neurology 1999; 52(7):S26–S28.

258. Gerdner LA, Buckwalter KC, Reed D. Impact of a psychoeducational intervention on caregiver responses to behavioural problems. Nurs Res 2002; 51:363–374.

259. Suhr J, Anderson S, Tranel D. Progressive muscle relaxation in the management of behavioural disturbances in Alzheimer's disease. Neuropsychol Rehabil 1999; 9:31–44.

260. Clare L, Wilson BA, Carer G, et al. Depression and anxiety in memory clinic attendees and their carers: implications for evaluating the effectiveness of cognitive rehabilitation interventions. J Geriatr Psychiatry 2002; 17:962–967.

261. Quayhagen MP, Quayhagen M. Testing of a cognitive intervention for dementia caregiver dyads. Neuropsychol Rehabil 2001; 11:319–332.

262. Gitlin LN, Hauck WW, Dennis MP, et al. Maintenance of effects of the home environmental skill-building program for family caregivers and individuals with Alzheimer's disease and related disorders. Journal of Gerontology: Medical Sciences 2005; 60A:368–374.

263. Gitlin LN, Winter S, Dennis MP, et al. Strategies used by families with Alzheimer's disease and related disorders: psychometric analysis of the task management strategy index (TMSI). Gerontologist 2002; 42:61–69.

264. Gitlin LN, Belle SH, Burgio LD, et al. Effect of multicomponent interventions on caregiver burden and depression: the REACH multisite initiative at 6-month follow-up. Psychol Aging 2003; 18:361–374.

265. Gitlin LN. Conducting research on home environments: lessons learned and new directions. Gerontologist 2003; 43:628–637.

266. Gitlin LN, Roth DL, Burgio LD, et al. Caregiver appraisals of functional dependence in individuals with dementia and associated caregiver upset: psychometric properties of a new scale and response patterns by caregiver and care recipient characteristics. J Aging Health 2005; 17:148–171.

267. Gitlin LN, Winter L, Corcoran M, et al. Effects of the home environmental skill-building on the caregiver-care recipient dyad: 6-month outcomes from the Philadelphia REACH initiative. Gerontologist 2003; 43:532–546.
268. Rajendran PR, Thompson RE, Reich SG. The use of alternative therapies by patients with Parkinson's disease. Neurology 2001; 57:790–794.
269. Brefel-Courbon C, Desboeuf K, Thalamas C, et al. Clinical and economic analysis of spa therapy in Parkinson's disease. Mov Disord 2003; 18:578–584.
270. The Parkinson Study Group. Effects of Tocopherol and deprenyl on the progression of disability in early Parkinson's disease. N Engl J Med 1993, 32:176–183.
271. The Medical Letter, Inc. Coenzyme Q10. The Medical Letter (Issue 1229) 2006; 48:19–20.
272. Stallibrass C, Sissons P, Chalmers C. Randomized controlled trial of the Alexander Technique for idiopathic Parkinson's disease. Clin Rehabil 2002; 16:695–708.
273. Ernst E, Canter PH. The Alexander Technique: a systematic review of controlled clinical trials. Forsch Komplementarmed Klass Naturheilkd 2003; 10:325–329.
274. Svircev A, Craig LH, Juncos JL. A pilot study examining the effects of neuromuscular therapy on patients with Parkinson's disease. J Am Osteopath Assoc 2005; 105:26.

12

Deep Brain Stimulation of the Subthalamic Nucleus: Clinical Outcome

Casey H. Halpern and Howard I. Hurtig

Departments of Neurology and Neurosurgery, Penn Neurological Institute at Pennsylvania Hospital, Hospital of the University of Pennsylvania, Philadelphia, Pennsylvania, U.S.A.

Deep brain stimulation (DBS) has proven to be an effective surgical therapy for patients with advanced Parkinson's disease (PD) who continue to respond to dopaminergic therapy, but face disabling complications such as dyskinesias and motor fluctuations. Tremor, rigidity, bradykinesia, and levodopa-related dyskinesia appear to be most responsive (1,2), whereas axial signs and symptoms, including postural instability, as well as speech and swallowing, are more resistant to DBS.

Recent evidence from a large nonrandomized and one small randomized clinical trial shows that DBS of either the globus pallidus internus (GPi) or subthalamic nucleus (STN) produces equivalent clinical benefit in carefully selected patients with PD (3,4). A meta-analysis of 31 STN and 14 GPi studies demonstrated similar findings with no significant difference in beneficial effect on motor function or activities of daily living (ADLs), regardless of the DBS target (5). However, medication dosages were reduced by 50% following STN DBS, whereas no change in required dosage was seen in patients who had undergone GPi DBS. Although GPi DBS may be effective treatment for motor symptoms and ADLs, only bilateral STN DBS has been shown to provide sufficient improvement to permit decreasing the dosage of antiparkinsonian medication (6,7). Moreover, GPi DBS has been associated with more adverse effects, eventual loss of benefit, subsequent higher doses of medication, and even subsequent reimplantation of electrodes into the STN (8). Recently, STN has gained general acceptance as the preferred target for DBS in treating most motor symptoms of PD, but without supporting level 1 (randomized controlled trial) data. The 2006 Report of the Quality Standards Subcommittee of the American Academy of Neurology recommends STN DBS as a treatment option in PD to improve motor function and reduce dyskinesia, motor fluctuations, and reliance on adjunctive medication. According to this report, there is insufficient evidence to make any recommendations regarding GPi DBS in PD patients (9).

Bilateral STN DBS has evolved to become standard of care for surgical treatment of PD, but unilateral STN DBS is sometimes used in patients with marked asymmetry in clinical signs. The complication rate and cost are lower than with a bilateral procedure, but it may be less effective (10). Two studies have addressed this question with conflicting conclusions. Germano et al. (2004) reported unilateral STN DBS on 12 patients who were potential candidates for bilateral STN DBS (11). In 10 of the 12 patients, the benefit associated with the unilateral procedure was sufficient to avoid a second operation, and benefits were confirmed by double-blind testing. Kumar et al. (1999) compared unilateral with bilateral STN stimulation by turning off one of the stimulators in 10 bilaterally implanted patients (12). Unilateral stimulation provided a 25% reduction in off-period parkinsonism, whereas bilateral DBS was associated with a 55% improvement (10).

We performed a literature search for studies of bilateral DBS of the STN in PD with the following minimum inclusion criteria for each study: (*i*) at least 10 subjects followed for 6 months after surgery, (*ii*) change in UPDRS as an outcome measure, (*iii*) other evaluations of ADLs, dyskinesia, and (*iv*) reported levodopa equivalent daily dosing pre- and postoperatively. Twenty-five studies met our inclusion criteria (3,13–36) (Table 1). One 12 month follow-up series of 60 PD patients found a significant correlation between motor improvement, according to the UPDRS III (motor) score,[a] and quality of life, as measured by the PD Quality of Life (QOL) scale ($r = 0.7$; $p < 0.001$) (29). A recent long-term follow-up study of 71 PD patients who underwent bilateral STN DBS reported sustained improvement in QOL for a mean of 38 months (36). STN DBS may also improve mood, social functioning, and involvement in hobbies (17). Some studies have reported that patients who had depended on a caregiver for ADLs before STN DBS were independent postoperatively. Few studies report complete discontinuation of medication (15,37). Speech may be more sensitive to dopaminergic therapy. However, STN DBS combined with low dose dopaminergic therapy may offer significant benefit, despite worsening speech seen in some patients with bilateral DBS (38).

---

[a]The Unified Parkinson's Disease Rating Scale (UPDRS) is a 42 item scale that rates severity on a 0–4 continuum (0 = normal, 4 = severe). The UPDRS has three categories: mentation, behavior, and mood (UPDRS I); activities of daily living (UPDRS II); and complications of treatment (UPDRS IV).

Table 1 Literature Review of Clinical Outcome of Bilateral STN DBS in Patients with Parkinson's Disease[a]

Series	N	Mean follow-up period (months)	Improvement motor (%)[c]	Improvement ADL (%)[d]	Reduction dyskinesia (%)[e]	Reduction LEDD (%)[f]
DBS for PD study group (3)	96	6	52[i]	44[i]	58[i]	37[i]
Jaggi et al. (13)	28	12	42[j]	38[l]	71[j]	49[l]
Krack et al. (14)	49	60	54[i]	49[i]	58[i]	63[i]
Volkman et al. (15)	16	12	60[k]	56[i]	90[i]	63[i]
Molinuevo et al. (16)	15	6	66[i]	72	81[i]	80[i]
Lagrange et al. (17)	60	12	55[i]	55[i]	40[i]	48[i]
Krause et al. (18)	24	30	38[g]	17[g]	69[b]	30[g]
Vingerhoets et al. (19)	20	21	45[i]	37[h]	92[i]	79[b]
Simuni et al. (20)	12	12	47[i]	42[k]	64[i]	55[h]
Lezcano et al. (21)	11	24	51[i]	59[i]	NA[c]	55[i]
Rodriguez-Oroz et al. (22)	49	46	50[l]	43[e]	72[g]	34[i]
Rodriguez-Oroz et al. (23)	10	48	40[g]	61[g]	53[h]	50[h]
Patel et al. (24)	16	12	61[i]	41[g]	67[b]	48[h]
Visser-Vandewalle et al. (25)	20	54	43[i]	59[k]	79[h]	47[g]
Kleiner-Fisman et al. (26)	25	30	39[i]	26[i]	50[h]	36[i]
Herzog et al. (27)	20	24	57[i]	43[b]	85[i]	68[b]
Thobois et al. (28)	18	6	55[i]	53[i]	76[i]	66[h]
Martinez-Martin et al. (29)	17	6	63[i]	72[i]	78[h]	64[b]
Valldeoriola et al. (30)	16	18	58[b]	62[b]	73[i]	47[b]
Schubach et al. (31)	37	60	54[g]	40[g]	67[h]	58[h]
Ford et al. (32)	30	12	30[l]	34[g]	60[i]	30[i]
Romito et al. (33)	31	26	56[i]	NA	100[b]	55[g]
Tavella et al. (34)	47	24	63[g]	55[g]	90[g]	81[g]

(Continued)

Table 1   Literature Review of Clinical Outcome of Bilateral STN DBS in Patients with Parkinson's Disease[a] (*Continued*)

Series	N	Mean follow-up period (months)	Improvement motor (%)[c]	Improvement ADL (%)[d]	Reduction dyskinesia (%)[e]	Reduction LEDD (%)[f]
Erola et al. (35)	24	12	31[g]	19[g]	53[h]	19[i]
Lyons and Pahwa (36)	71	38	36[g]	32[g]	NA	53[g]
Total or average	666	25	50	47	71	53

[a]We report the longest period of follow-up in each study.
[b]Significance not reported.
[c]Motor evaluated using UPDRS III.
[d]ADL evaluated using UPDRS II or Activities of Daily Living Scale of Schwab-England.
[e]Dyskinesia evaluated with UPDRS 32–33, 32–35 or the Abnormal Involuntary Movement Scale.
[f]LEDD, all dopaminergic therapies.
[g]p < 0.05.
[h]p < 0.01.
[i]p < 0.001.
[j]p < 0.002.
[k]p < 0.005.
[l]p < 0.0001.

Abbreviations: ADL, activities of daily living; DBS, deep brain stimulation; STN, subthalamic nucleus; NA, not available/applicable; LEDD, levodopa equivalent daily dose; PD, Parkinson's disease.

NEUROPSYCHOLOGICAL EFFECTS OF STN DBS

There is only one report in the literature that uses a clinically matched disease control group to evaluate cognitive change following DBS (39). When comparing the presurgical baseline to stimulation-on conditions, this study reported delayed verbal recall and decline in verbal fluency. Other reports of neuropsychological scores in category and lexical fluency, thought disorders, and apathy have shown significant change for the worse postoperatively (40). Verbal fluency was shown to diminish one year after surgery, but remained stable at three years (40). Decline in verbal fluency, has been shown to be one of the few consistent findings in studies of cognition following STN DBS (39). Interestingly, verbal impairment was shown to significantly correlate with increasing apathy postoperatively (40). Apathy has been inversely correlated with decreasing doses of levodopa in the postoperative period (40). However, a recent study demonstrated that long term bilateral STN DBS does not significantly alter baseline neuropsychological function, and suggests fluctuations in behavior could be modified pharmacologically and by stimulation parameters (14). Because of the high prevalence of mild cognitive impairment in advanced PD, these patients are vulnerable and subject to decompensation in the aftermath of neurosurgical intervention. Therefore, careful evaluation of neuropsychologic function is a mandatory component of preoperative evaluation in these patients in order to exclude those who lack sufficient cognitive reserve to endure the procedure and postoperative period.

EFFECTS OF STN DBS ON MOOD

The reported adverse effects on mood include inappropriate laughter (41), depression (42), mania (43), and aggression (44). Mania and hypomania are rare perioperative complications and may be explained by additive psychotropic effects of STN DBS and dopaminergic treatment (45). Tapering long acting dopamine agonists before surgery may decrease the risk of mania following surgery (46). In contrast, depression tends to appear weeks after surgery and may be related to decreased dopaminergic treatment and the loss of a possible antidepressant effect associated with levodopa (45). Depressive episodes did not recur in patients with a diagnosis of major depressive disorder preoperatively, but rather developed in patients who had no previous history. Such chronic adaptive changes may not be directly due to stimulation (47). On the contrary, behavioral changes may be a consequence of stimulating an untargeted neighboring neural structure (47). One case report documented aggressive outbursts in both the "on" and "off" drug states, with complete resolution occurring days after DBS was turned off (46). Thus, worsening of mood may occur postoperatively, and close follow-up is necessary for appropriate early therapeutic intervention (48). Krack et al. (2003) proposed multifactorial etiologies to explain such disturbances, including pre-existing psychiatric illness, surgery-related stress,

Table 2 Literature Review of Complication Rates in Patients with Parkinson's Disease Following Bilateral STN DBS

Series[a]	N	Diagnosis	Postoperative adverse events[b]	Device-related complications[c]	Treatment-related side effects[d]	Neuropsychological, cognitive, mood effects	Urinary retention
DBS for PD Study Group (3)	102	PD	25	5	7		
Krack et al.[e] (14)	49	PD	28	2	56	7	
Volkman et al. (15)	57	PD	6	2	32	7	
Molinuevo et al. (16)	15	PD			2	3	
Lagrange et al. (17)	60	PD	5			3	
Krause et al. (18)	24	PD	1	1	12		
Vingerhoets et al. (19)	20	PD	3	1		3	
Simuni et al. (20)	12	PD	5				
Lezcano et al. (21)	12	PD	6	1	7	4	1
Rodriguez-Oroz et al. (22)	49	PD	6	6	26	15	
Rodriguez-Oroz et al. (23)	10	PD	1		2	1	
Patel et al. (24)	16	PD			3		
Visser-Vandewalle et al. (25)	20	PD	8				

Study	n[a]						
Kleiner-Fisman et al. (26)	25	PD	6	2	12	17	
Herzog et al. (27)	20	PD	9	2	7	9	
Thobois et al. (28)	18	PD	2		3	11	
Martinez-Martin et al. (29)	17	PD			5	3	
Valldeoriola et al. (30)	26	PD			7	5	
Schupbach et al. (31)	37	PD	7	2	44	20	2
Ford et al. (32)	30	PD	11		30		
Romito et al. (33)	31	PD			17	2	
Umemura et al.[f] (50)	109	PD	15			2	

[a] Values are total number of cases reported.
[b] Postoperative adverse events infection, skin erosion, irritation, subcutaneous hematoma, confusion, intracranial hemorrhage, seizure, delirium, and ballism.
[c] Device-related complications: diminished battery life, malfunction or malposition requiring lead, or IPG adjustment or replacement.
[d] Treatment-related side effects (related to dopaminergic treatment, subthalamic stimulation, or both): paresthesiae (inconsistently reported), dyskinesia, dystonia, eyelid-opening apraxia, diplopia apraxia, diplopia, dysarthria (some studies reported the combination of dysarthria with hypophonia and word-finding difficulties), dysphagia, weight gain, hyperhydrosis, hypersalivation, afaxia, mild paresis, restless leg, and somnolence.
[e] First three postoperative months.
[f] Includes adverse events reported in Jaggi et al. (15) found in Table 2.
Abbreviations: DBS, deep brain stimulation; PD, Parkinson's disease.

alterations in social life, lower dose of dopaminergic therapy, and unrealistic patient expectations (14).

COMPLICATIONS

The overall rate of complications for STN DBS is generally low, although a recent large series of 81 consecutive patients (160 STN DBS procedures) reported a 26% rate of hardware-related problems (49). Transient adverse effects such as eyelid-opening apraxia, dyskinesia, and paresthesia occurring often when the stimulators are adjusted during the procedure or in the follow-up period have been reported (48). Overall, most side effects are reversible by adjusting stimulation parameters (48). Rare deaths have been reported from pulmonary emboli, myocardial infarction, stroke, intracerebral hemorrhage, and suicide. Table 2 summarizes complications reported in 22 studies that met our inclusion criteria for systematic review (3,14–33,50). Some reports that met our inclusion criteria for review were excluded from Table 2 because adverse effects were not completely documented.

REFERENCES

1. Bejjani BP, Gervais D, Arnulf I, et al. Axial parkinsonian symptoms can be improved: the role of levodopa and bilateral subthalamic stimulation. J Neurol Neurosurg Psychiatry 2000; 68:595–600.
2. Yokoyama T, Sugiyama K, Nishizawa S, Yokota N, Ohta S, Uemura K. Subthalamic nucleus stimulation for gait disturbance in Parkinson's disease. Neurosurgery 1999; 45:41–47, discussion 47–49.
3. The deep-brain stimulation for Parkinson's disease study group. Deep-brain stimulation of the subthalamic nucleus or the pars interna of the globus pallidus in Parkinson's disease. N Engl J Med 2001; 345:956–963.
4. Anderson VC, Burchiel KJ, Hogarth P, Favre J, Hammerstad JP. Pallidal vs subthalamic nucleus deep brain stimulation in Parkinson disease. Arch Neurol 2005; 62:554–560.
5. Weaver F, Follett K, Hur K, Ippolito D, Stern M. Deep brain stimulation in Parkinson disease: a meta-analysis of patient outcomes. J Neurosurg 2005; 103(6):956–967.
6. Siegfried J, Lippitz B. Bilateral chronic electrostimulation of ventroposterolateral pallidum: a new therapeutic approach for alleviating all parkinsonian symptoms. Neurosurgery 1994; 35:1126–1129.
7. Krack P, Pollak P, Limousin P, et al. Opposite motor effects of pallidal stimulation in Parkinson's disease. Ann Neurol 1998; 43:180–192.
8. Houeto JL, Bejjani PB, Damier P, et al. Failure of long-term pallidal stimulation corrected by subthalamic stimulation in PD. Neurology 2000; 55:728–730.
9. Pahwa R, Factor SA, Lyons KE, et al. Practice parameter: treatment of Parkinson disease with motor fluctuations and dyskinesia (an evidence-based review): Report of the Quality Standards Subcommittee of the American Academy of Neurology. Neurology 2006; 66:983–995.
10. Kumar R, Lozano AM, Sime E, Halket E, Lang AE. Comparative effects of unilateral and bilateral subthalamic nucleus deep brain stimulation. Neurology 1999; 53: 561–566.

11. Germano IM, Gracies JM, Weisz DJ, Tse W, Koller WC, Olanow CW. Unilateral stimulation of the subthalamic nucleus in Parkinson disease: a double-blind 12-month evaluation study. J Neurosurg 2004; 101(1):36–42.

12. Benabid AL, Pollak P, Gervason C, et al. Long-term suppression of tremor by chronic stimulation of the ventral intermediate thalamic nucleus. Lancet 1991; 337:403–406.

13. Jaggi JL, Umemura A, Hurtig HI, et al. Bilateral stimulation of the subthalamic nucleus in Parkinson's disease: surgical efficacy and prediction of outcome. Stereotact Funct Neurosurg 2004; 82(2):104–114.

14. Krack P, Batir A, Nadège VB, et al. Five-year follow-up of bilateral stimulation of the subthalamic nucleus in advanced parkinson's disease. N Engl J Med 2003 349; 20:1925–1934.

15. Volkmann J, Allert N, Voges J, Weiss PH, Freund HJ, Sturm V. Safety and efficacy of pallidal or subthalamic nucleus stimulation in advanced PD. Neurology 2001; 56(4):548–551.

16. Molinuevo JL, Valldeoriola F, Tolosa E, et al. Levodopa withdrawal after bilateral subthalamic stimulation in advanced Parkinson's disease. Arch Neurol 2000; 57(7):983–988.

17. Lagrange E, Krack P, Moro E, et al. Bilateral subthalamic nucleus stimulation improves health-related quality of life in PD. Neurology 2002; 59:1976–1978.

18. Krause M, Fogel W, Mayer P, Kloss Tronnier V. Chronic inhibition of the subthalamic nucleus in Parkinson's disease. J Neurol Sci 2004; 219:119–124.

19. Vingerhoets FJG, Villemure JG, Temperli P, Pollo C, Pralong E, Ghika J. Subthalamic DBS replaces levodopa in Parkinson's disease. Neurology 2002; 58:396–401.

20. Simuni T, Jaggi J, Mulholland H, et al. Bilateral stimulation of the subthalamic nucleus in patients with Parkinson disease: a study of efficacy and safety. J Neurosurg 2002; 96:666–672.

21. Lezcano E, Gomez JC, Lambarri I, et al. Bilateral subthalamic nucleus deep-brain stimulation (STN-DBS) in Parkinson's disease: initial experience in Cruces Hospital. Neurologia 2003; 18(4):187–195.

22. Rodriguez-Oroz MC, Obeso JA, Lang AE, et al. Bilateral deep brain stimulation in Parkinson's disease: a multicentre study with 4 years follow-up. Brain 2005; 128:2240–2249.

23. Rodriguez-Oroz MC, Zamarbide I, Guridi J, Palmero MR, Obeso JA. Efficacy of deep brain stimulation of the subthalamic nucleus in Parkinson's disease 4 years after surgery: double blind and open label evaluation. J Neurol Neurosurg Psychiatry 2004; 75(10):1382–1385.

24. Patel NK, Plaha P, O'Sullivan K, McCarter R, Heywood P, Gill SS. MRI directed bilateral stimulation of the subthalamic nucleus in patients with Parkinson's disease. J Neurol Neurosurg Psychiatry 2003; 74(12):1631–1637.

25. Visser-Vandewalle V, van der Linden C, Temel Y, et al. Long-term effects of bilateral subthalamic nucleus stimulation in advanced Parkinson disease: a four year follow-up study. Parkinsonism Relat Disord 2005; 11(3):157–165.

26. Kleiner-Fisman G, Fisman DN, Sime E, Saint-Cyr JA, Lozano AM, Lang AE. Long-term follow up of bilateral deep brain stimulation of the subthalamic nucleus in patients with advanced Parkinson disease. J Neurosurg 2003; 99(3):489–495.

27. Herzog J, Volkmann J, Krack P, et al. Two-year follow-up of subthalamic deep brain stimulation in Parkinson's disease. Mov Disord 2003; 18(11):1332–1337.

28. Thobois S, Mertens P, Guenot M, et al. Subthalamic nucleus stimulation in Parkinson's disease: clinical evaluation of 18 patients. J Neurol 2002; 249(5):529–534.

29. Martinez-Martin P, Valldeoriola F, Tolosa E, et al. Bilateral subthalamic nucleus stimulation and quality of life in advanced Parkinson's disease. Mov Disord 2002; 17(2):372–377.

30. Valldeoriola F, Pilleri M, Tolosa E, Molinuevo JL, Rumia J, Ferrer E. Bilateral subthalamic stimulation monotherapy in advanced Parkinson's disease: long-term follow-up of patients. Mov Disord 2002; 17(1):125–132.

31. Schupbach WM, Chastan N, Welter ML, et al. Stimulation of the subthalamic nucleus in Parkinson's disease: a 5 year follow up. J Neurol Neurosurg Psychiatry 2005; 76(12):1640–1644.

32. Ford B, Winfield L, Pullman SL, et al. Subthalamic nucleus stimulation in advanced Parkinson's disease: blinded assessments at one year follow up. J Neurol Neurosurg Psychiatry 2004; 75(9):1255–1259.

33. Romito LM, Contarino MF, Ghezzi D, Franzini A, Garavaglia B, Albanese A. High frequency stimulation of the subthalamic nucleus is efficacious in Parkin disease. J Neurol 2005; 252(2):208–211.

34. Tavella A, Bergamasco B, Bosticco E, et al. Deep brain stimulation of the subthalamic nucleus in Parkinson's disease: long-term follow-up. Neurol Sci. 2002; 23(suppl 2):S111-S112.

35. Erola T, Heikkinen ER, Haapaniemi T, Tuominen J, Juolasmaa A, Myllyla VV. Efficacy of bilateral subthalamic nucleus (STN) stimulation in Parkinson's disease. Acta Neurochir (Wien) 2006; 148:389–394.

36. Lyons KE, Pahwa R. Long-term benefits in quality of life provided by bilateral subthalamic stimulation in patients with Parkinson disease. J Neurosurg 2005; 103(2): 252–255.

37. Limousin P, Krack P, Pollak P, et al. Electrical stimulation of the subthalamic nucleus in advanced Parkinson's disease. N Engl J Med 1998; 339:1105–1111.

38. Gentil M, Pinto S, Pollak P, Benabid AL. Effect of bilateral stimulation of the subthalamic nucleus on parkinsonian dysarthria. Brain Lang 2003; 85:190–196.

39. Morrison CE, Borod JC, Perrine K, et al. Neuropsychological functioning following bilateral subthalamic nucleus stimulation in Parkinson's disease. Arch Clin Neuropsychol 2004; 19(2):165–181.

40. Funkiewiez A, Ardouin C, Caputo E, et al. Long term effects of bilateral subthalamic nucleus stimulation on cognitive function, mood, and behavior in Parkinson's disease. J Neurol Neurosurg Psychiatry 2004; 75:834–839.

41. Krack P, Kumar R, Ardouin C, et al. Mirthful laughter induced by subthalamic nucleus stimulation. Mov Disord 2001; 16:867–875.

42. Kumar R, Krack P, Pollak P. Transient acute depression induced by high-frequency deep brain stimulation. N Engl J Med 1999; 341:1003–1004.

43. Kulisevsky J, Berthier ML, Gironell A, Pascual-Sedano B, Molet J, Parés P. Mania following deep brain stimulation for Parkinson's disease. Neurology 2002; 59: 1421–1424.

44. Bejjani BP, Houeto JL, Hariz M, et al. Aggressive behavior induced by intraoperative stimulation of the triangle of Sano. Neurology 2002; 59:1425–1427.

45. Funkiewiez A, Ardouin C, Krack P, et al. Acute psychotropic effects of bilateral subthalamic nucleus stimulation and levodopa in Parkinson's disease. Mov Disord 2003; 18:524–530.

46. Sensi M, Eleopra R, Cavallo MA, et al. Explosive-aggressive behavior related to bilateral subthalamic stimulation. Parkinsonism and Related Disorders 2004; 10:247–251.
47. Berney A, Vingerhoets F, Perrin A, et al. Effects on mood of subthalamic DBS for Parkinson's disease: a consecutive series of 24 patients. Neurology 2002; 59: 1427–1429.
48. Krack P, Fraix V, Mendes A, Benabid AL, Pollak P. Postoperative management of subthalamic nucleus stimulation for Parkinson's disease. Mov Disord 2002; 17(suppl 3):S188–S197.
49. Lyons KE, Wilkinson SB, Overman J, Pahwa R. Surgical and hardware complications of subthalamic stimulation. Neurology 2004; 63:612–616.
50. Umemura A, Jaggi JL, Hurtig HI, et al. Deep Brain stimulation for movement disorders: morbidity and mortality in 109 patients. J Neurosurg 2003; 98(4):779–784.

13

Deep Brain Stimulation for Parkinson's Disease: Motor Outcomes

Tanya Simuni

Parkinson's Disease and Movement Disorders Center, Northwestern University, Feinberg School of Medicine, Chicago, Illinois, U.S.A.

Frances M. Weaver

Midwest Center for Health Services Research and Policy Studies and Research, Spinal Cord Injury Quality Enhancement Research Initiative, Hines VA Hospital, and Department of Neurology and Institute for Healthcare Studies, Northwestern University, Chicago, Illinois, U.S.A.

INTRODUCTION

Deep brain stimulation (DBS) of the subthalamic nucleus (STN) is now considered the procedure of choice for surgical treatment of patients with advanced Parkinson's disease (PD) complicated by motor fluctuations. The procedure was pioneered a little over a decade ago and quickly replaced ablative surgical techniques for management of PD (pallidotomy and thalamotomy). Following the first published case report of DBS for PD in 1995 (1), many papers have been written regarding the efficacy, effectiveness, and adverse events resulting from DBS. As of today more than 50 articles have been published analyzing the impact of DBS surgery on motor function in PD. These include DBS of the STN or the globus pallidum interna (GPi). Despite the large number of publications, most of these studies were designed as pre–post intervention nonrandomized observational studies that involved relatively small number of patients and constitute level IV evidence. Based on the most recent review published by the American Academy of Neurology (AAN), there are four Class III studies (defined as controlled trials with independent assessment of objective outcome measures) of STN and one of GPi DBS (72). Observational data are very important as a first step in the analysis of the efficacy of any new intervention, but large-scale randomized controlled studies are necessary to establish the long-term efficacy of the procedure in the overall management of PD. Such studies are under way. Weaver, Follett, Hur, and Reda (Chapter 18) review in detail the requirements for the design of vigorous scientific trials for surgical intervention in PD, the standard outcome measures used in such trials, and briefly review current trials. This chapter will summarize the available data on the short- and long-term impact of STN DBS on motor function in PD, and discuss limited data on the comparison between STN and GPi surgical targets. The adverse effects of the procedure are discussed in Chapter 7.

MOTOR OUTCOME MEASURES IN PARKINSON'S DISEASE CLINICAL TRIALS

Motor function is the primary outcome examined in studies of DBS for PD. A Committee on the Core Assessment Program for Intracerebral Transplantation (CAPIT and CAPSIT-PD) (2,3) recommended the core methodology for the clinical assessment of the efficacy of the surgical intervention in PD. CAPIT protocol is considered the "gold" standard, however, only a limited number of studies have used it in the entirety. The most consistently reported outcome measure in STN DBS trials is the Unified PD Rating Scale (UPDRS), Part III (motor subscale) (69). The score for motor function ranges from 0 to 104, with higher scores indicating greater impairment. The 14 items on the scale are rated by a trained observer, usually a movement disorders neurologist. Observations of the efficacy of DBS can be made under various conditions including a medication-off state (e.g., patient refrains from taking PD medications for 12 hours, usually overnight prior to the evaluation), and medication-on state (e.g., patient takes PD medication and is assessed in the best "on"-state usually an hour after the dose (CAPIT) (2). STN DBS is most effective for the improvement of PD symptoms in the medication-off state. The most frequently reported effect of DBS is the comparison of the UPDRS scores prior to surgery in the off-medications state, and then at multiple points after surgery in stimulation on, medication-off state. The effect is reported as the percent improvement over the baseline medication-off state score.

Other measures of motor function are also reported, although there is significant variation across published studies on the scope of reported data. These measures include subcomponents of the motor scale including tremor, rigidity, akinesia or bradykinesia, postural stability, and gait. Benefit of surgery is also assessed by the impact on the activities of daily living (ADL), as measured by UPDRS ADL (Part II) score, and Schwab and England Scale. One of the most functionally important outcome measures is the effect of STN DBS on the motor fluctuations and dyskinesia reported based on Part IV of the UPDRS and/or from PD motor function diaries completed by the patients.

Most published studies summarize 6 to 12 months postsurgery results. There are a limited number of reports of long-term (up to five years) outcomes. The majority of STN DBS surgeries are performed with bilateral electrode implantation; however, there is limited body of literature on the efficacy of unilateral DBS.

Unilateral Deep Brain Stimulation Studies

A review of the DBS for PD literature revealed only a few publications of unilateral stimulation of either the STN or GPi in PD that reported motor outcomes (Table 1). These studies had small sample sizes and were designed as pretest, post-test studies comparing UPDRS motor scores off-medication at baseline, and UPDRS off-medication/on-stimulation at post-test. Most

Table 1 Motor Outcomes of Unilateral Deep Brain Stimulation Studies (Globus Pallidum Interna and Subthalamic Nucleus)

Author	Publication	N	Average age	% Male	Baseline UPDRS off-meds	Post-UPDRS off-meds	% Change[a]
Gpi							
Gross (1997) (4)	J Neurosurg	7	53.4	100	53.4	39.4	26
Vingerho et al. (1999) (5)	JNNP	20	55	75	33	17	48
Kumar (2000) (6)	Neurology	5			38.9	25.8	37
Loher (2002) (7)	J Neurosurg	9	65.1	66	57.2	35.2	38
Merello (1999) (8)	Mov Disord	13	57.4	69	28.5	20.3	30
Summary							36
STN							
Kumar (1999) (9)	Neurology	10	65.9	50	45	34.7	23
Linazasoro (2003) (10)	Mov Disord	8	64.6	50	47.7	27.1	43
Germano (2004) (11)	J Neurosurg	12	64	83	42	31.1	26
Summary							31

[a]Mean calculated based on baseline score and % improvement.
Abbreviations: Gpi, globus pallidum interna; STN, subthalamic nucleus; UPDRS, unified Parkinson's disease rating scale.

assessed motor function at six months postsurgery. In all studies reported in Table 1, motor function improved significantly following unilateral DBS stimulation, regardless of the target. The average reduction of UPDRS motor score was 30%. The limited number of unilateral studies suggests that physicians quickly moved to bilateral stimulation as a more effective procedure, once the initial data demonstrated that stimulation was safe and effective.

Bilateral Subthalamic Nucleus Deep Brain Stimulation

STN DBS surgery was pioneered by Dr. Benabid and colleagues in France (12). Limousin et al. published the first data of that group on bilateral simulation of the STN for patients with PD in 1995 (1). The study included three patients. Two patients underwent staged procedures, whereas the third underwent simultaneous bilateral electrode implantation. Targets were determined using microelectrode recordings. Motor function using the UDPRS motor subscale were assessed prior to surgery in the off-medication stage, and at three months after surgery with medication-off and with stimulation-on and -off. The average improvement in motor function for these patients was 65.2%.

Limousin reported the experience of the same group with the first 20 patients who underwent bilateral STN DBS (13). The mean age of the cohort of patients in that study was 56 ± 8, which is younger than the general PD population. The data were reported for 3 and 12 months postsurgery. Patients were evaluated in four conditions: medications off and on, and stimulation off and on. The outcomes were reported as the degree of change compared to preoperative assessment. At 12 months postsurgery, the patients experienced mean 60% reduction in UPDRS motor scores in the medications-off condition with stimulation. Improvement was seen in all cardinal manifestations of PD: rigidity, bradykinesia, and tremor, as well as axial symptoms of gait and postural stability in the medications-off state. In the medications-on state, the benefit was much less robust though still statistically significant; a 10% reduction in the motor UPDRS scores with stimulation. The benefit was seen for rigidity but not for bradykinesia subscores. UPDRS Part II, ADL scores were reduced on average by 60% in the medications-off state with no further improvement in the medications-on state. Improvement in Part II UPDRS correlated with the change in Schwab and England ADL scores. Hoehn and Yahr (H&Y) staging changed from 4.6 ± 0.5 in the medications-off state before surgery to 2.8 ± 0.6 with stimulation, and remained unchanged in the medications-on state at 12 months postoperatively. There was 73% reduction in the duration of off-time based on UPDRS Part IV scores, though the study did not report data from PD patient motor diaries. Patients experienced significant reduction of off-period dystonia. There was significant reduction of severity and frequency of dyskinesia that was attributed to the reduction of PD medications based on the observation that postoperative levodopa challenge resulted in the same degree of dyskinesia as preoperatively. Stimulation parameters remained relatively stable for the duration of follow-up, and stimulation was well tolerated. This was a pivotal study, as it summarized the initial experience with STN DBS that was subsequently confirmed by the other groups. The study also helped to establish the clinical parameters that predict the best surgical outcomes.

This key study was followed in the next 10 years by dozens of papers describing the outcomes of bilateral STN DBS (Table 2). A recent meta-analysis reviewed all publications that reported motor outcomes of bilateral STN and GPi DBS through September 2003 (14). The review excluded studies that did not have data on pre–postoperative UPDRS motor scores. The publication included cumulative data on 565 patients that underwent bilateral STN DBS procedure and 136 patients with bilateral GPi DBS target. The meta-analysis reported on two measures of motor function: UPDRS motor and ADL subscales, reviewing short-term outcomes (six months) (14). The review included 31 papers with STN as the target, of which eight studies included both STN and GPi targets. All papers reported UPDRS motor scores off-medication at baseline and off-medication/on-stimulation at approximately six months following surgery. Motor function improved significantly; the average percent improvement in UPDRS motor scores was 54.3%. Motor findings were consistent across the surgical centers, despite variability in surgical technique and use of intraoperative microelectrode recording. Results of the procedure were not affected by the sample size or mean patient age, suggesting that DBS had a robust positive effect on motor function regardless of these factors. The paper did not analyze the impact of stimulation on the motor function in medications-on state; however, there is a consensus that STN DBS does not have a significant impact on the motor function in the medications-on state.

The meta-analysis also included an examination of UPDRS ADL scores when they were available. Sixteen papers reported ADL scores for STN target. ADL scores improved by approximately 40% in the medications-off state. Meta-regression analyses pointed out, however, that the effect size for ADL improvement was significantly smaller for studies with small sample sizes, more recent studies (e.g., after the year 2000), and for studies in which the mean age of study participants was greater than 55.

The largest Class III study published to date was conducted by the Deep Brain Stimulation for Parkinson's Disease Study Group (30). This multi-site prospective study included 134 patients with advanced PD: 96 underwent bilateral DBS of the STN, and 38 patients had bilateral DBS of the GPi. The choice of the surgical target was based on the preference and experience of the investigator. The primary outcome measure was the change in UPDRS motor score stimulation-on versus -off at six months postsurgery. Evaluation was performed in a double-blind crossover manner (stimulation-on vs. -off). The STN group experienced a median improvement of 49% in their motor scores with stimulation in the medications-off state. In addition to the blinded assessment, the patients had unblinded evaluations performed preoperatively and at one, three, and six months postsurgery. These assessments included UPDRS

Table 2 Bilateral Subthalamic Nucleus Deep Brain Stimulation Studies: Short-Term (6 to 12 Months) Outcome Data. Unified Parkinson's Disease Rating Scale Part III Data Are Reported for the Medications-Off State

First author	Year	Country	N	Mean age	% Male	Follow-up (months)	Mean baseline UPDRS motor	Follow-up UPDRS motor[a]	% Change
Studies published between 1995 and September 2003									
Limousin (1)	1995	France	3	52	100	3	58.3 ± 7.6	20.3 ± 16.2	65.2
Limousin (15)	1997	France	6	53 ± 4	67	na	53[b]	22 ± 8	58
Krack (16)	1997	France	15	60 ± 8	60	na	63.0 ± 15.0	28.0 ± 15.0	55.6
Krack (17)	1998	France	8	51 ± 10	63	6	57.5 ± 14.5	17.1 ± 8.2	70.3
Limousin (13)	1998	France	24	56 ± 8	45	12			60
Brown (18)	1999	France, Spain	6	53	67	8.3 (ave)	63.3 ± 11.3	21.7 ± 8.3	65.7
Burchiel (19)	1999	USA	6	62.8 ± 12	70[c]	12	49.0 ± 12	27.4[b]	44
Moro (20)	1999	Italy	7	57.4 ± 5.5	14	1,3,6,12	67.6 ± 9.9	43.5 ± 11.5	35.7
Figueiras-Mendez (21)	1999	Spain	1	68	100	3	51.0	37.0	27.5
Pinter (22)	1999	Austria	9	56.8 ± 9.6	67	3	60.0 ± 14.3	27.8 ± 5.8	53.7
Molinuevo (23)	2000	Spain	15	60.9 ± 6.8	67	6	49.6 ± 14.0	16.9 ± 7.0	65.9
Houeto (24)	2000	France	23	53 ± 2	70	6	51.7 ± 14.4	17.1[c]	66.9
Pillon (25)	2000	France	48	55.7 ± 7.5	56	3	55.4 ± 12.8	18.1 ± 11.8	67.3
Pillon (25)	2000	France	15	53.5 ± 9.7	67	6	56.1 ± 17.9	19.4 ± 20.4	65.4
Rodriguez-Oroz (26)	2000	Spain	15	59.9 ± 7.03	80	3,6,12	56 ± 16.42[b] (se = 4.2392)	22.4[b]	60
Krause (27)	2001	Germany	12	58.7	na	3,6,12	57.9 ± 4.6	34.6 ± 6.0	40.2
Broggi (28)	2001	Italy	17	59 ± 6.06	65	8.2 (ave)	52.07 ± 17.49	32.93 ± 12.99	36.2
Lopiano (29)	2001	Italy	20	61.2	60	3,12	58	25.7	55.7
Parkinson's Disease Study Group (30)	2001	Multiple countries, USA	96	59 ± 15.1	62	6	54.0 ± 15.1	25.7 ± 14.1	52.4
Volkmann (31)	2001	Germany	16	60.2 ± 9.8	na	6	56.4 ± 11.62	18.6 ± 14.12	37.8
Beric (70)	2001	USA	23	58	70	6	33	11	66.6

Study	Year	Country	N						
Vesper (32)	2002	Germany	38	55.6	68	1,6,12	48.3	26.8	44.5
Figueiras-Mendez (33)	2002	Spain	22	57 ± 12	64	12,24	49	18	63.3
Vingerhoets (34)	2002	Swiss	20	63 ± 8	70	3,6,12,24	48.8 ± 14.6	27.1 ± 10.9	44.5
Ostergaard (35)	2002	Denmark	26	59 ± 8	81	3,12	51.3 ± 21.1	20.1 ± 13.6	60.8
Simuni (36)	2002	USA	12	58 ± 11	83	3,6,12	43.5 ± 3.6	25.5 ± 2.8	41.4
Iansek (37)	2002	Australia	105	54.1 ± 12.6	60	6,12	29.5 ± 13.9	18.20 ± 10.94	38.3
Thobois (38)	2002	France	18	56.9 ± 6	50	6,12	44.9 ± 13.4	20.2 ± 10	55
Bronte-Stewart (71)	2003	USA	19	59.4 ± 9.3	na	6,12	40.4 ± 11.7	8.1 ± 5.0	80
Varma (39)	2003	England	7	61.0 ± 8.1	100	6	74.29 ± 10.134	36.57 ± 14.68	61
Kleiner-Fisman (40)	2003	Canada	25	57.2 ± 11.7	60	12	50.1 ± 12.3	24.6 ± 7.3	50.9
Chen (41)	2003	China	7	57.3 ± 8.8	86	6	65.7 ± 21.7	32.8 ± 20.1	53
Summary (N = 31)			565	57.8	66				54.3
Studies published from September 2003 to December 2005									
Krack (42)	2003	France	49	55 ± 7.5	49	12,36,60	55.7 ± 11.9	19 ± 11	66
Pahwa (43)	2003	USA	33	58.5		12,24			38.1[b]
Herzog (44)	2003	Germany	48	60 ± 6	62	6,12,24	44.2 ± 13.9	21.7 ± 11.5	50.9
Jaggi (45)	2004	USA	39			12			42[b]
Anderson (46), STN vs. GPi	2005	USA	10 STN	61 ± 9	62	12	51 ± 13	27 ± 11	48
			10 GPi						39
Capecci (47)	2005	Italy	23	59.5 + 7.5	52	12,24	38.3 ± 11.6	17.9 ± 11.7	47
Erola (48)	2005	Finland	29			12			31.4
Hilker (49)	2005	Germany, Netherlands	30	59.8 + 7.2	63	16 (12–36)	42.9 ± 11.4	20.4 ± 8.4	52
Summary (N = 8)			261						46.9

[a] Reported for 6 to 12 months outcome data, or the closest value if 6 to 12 months data was not available.

[b] Calculated based on other information available.

[c] All studies that reported P-levels were significant at $P < 0.05$ or better. Fourteen studies did not provide P-values.

Abbreviations: ave, average; Gpi, globus pallidum interna; na, not applicable; SE, standard errors; STN, subthalamic nucleus.

subscores, dyskinesia rating, and PD patient motor diaries. Compared to baseline, patients had mean 51.3% improvement with stimulation in medications-off state and 25.8% in the medications-on state at six months. ADL scores also improved in the medications-off state (43.7%), but no changes were noted for the on-medication state. The patients experienced a 47% increase in the duration of on-time without dyskinesia based on the PD motor diaries. The mean dyskinesia score improved by 58% and the mean PD medication dose reduction was 38%.

Several studies ($n = 8$) have been published since the meta-analysis of bilateral DBS was completed in 2003 (Table 2). Some of the studies included long-term data on the patients who were previously reported in the earlier publications (16,45). The size of the reported cohorts ranged from 10 to 49. The duration of follow-up ranged between 6 and 60 months but most of the studies reported at least 12 months of DBS experience. The average reduction of UPDRS motor score with stimulation 12 months postoperatively was 46.9% with the range between 31% and 66%. The conclusions of the recent studies were consistent with the earlier observations. However, even recently published data are mostly based on the open label pre–post intervention comparisons of the motor outcome measures with no control groups. The only randomized study published to date compared the efficacy of STN versus GPi target and will be discussed later (46). One other randomized study was recently published which compared efficacy of unilateral pallidotomy with bilateral STN DBS (50). Predictably, STN DBS was unequivocally superior to unilateral pallidotomy in all motor outcome measures at six months follow-up. The STN group had a 49% reduction of motor UPDRS scores when compared with 21% in the pallidotomy group. The utility of these data are limited as presently it is well established that majority of the patients require bilateral intervention for adequate control of bilateral PD symptoms. Furthermore, ablative surgery is used only in limited situations today.

Another important outcome measure of the efficacy of STN DBS intervention is change in the amount of motor fluctuations and dyskinesia experienced by patients with PD. The most commonly used method to capture the 24-hour pattern of motor functioning in PD is the use of patient self-reported diaries (51). The diaries are used to identify five categories of motor function: asleep, off, on without dyskinesia, on with nontroublesome dyskinesia, and on with troublesome dyskinesia. At 30-minute intervals, the patient marks off which of the five categories best reflect his or her physical functioning for the prior 30 minutes. Good time is defined as the sum of 30-minute increments in which the patient was either on without dyskinesia or on with nontroublesome dyskinesia; while the bad time is the sum of the off-periods and on with troublesome dyskinesias periods. Motor diaries are frequently used in studies of medications for PD and much less frequently for surgical trials. Germano and colleagues (11) used PD diaries as part of the assessment of the efficacy of unilateral STN stimulation in PD over 12 months. The percent of medication on time without troubling dyskinesias increased from 46% to 56% following unilateral DBS and the mean daily sleep time increased by an average of 30 minutes. Two studies reported on the change in percent of off-time using motor diaries for individuals undergoing bilateral STN and GPi DBS (30,52). In both studies and for both target sites, off-time decreased, while on-time without troublesome dyskinesia increased following DBS.

Another important outcome measure of the efficacy of the surgical intervention in PD is the impact of the procedure on the use of PD medications. Most trials report medication use as levodopa equivalence dose that is calculated by converting the dosages of all dopaminergic medications to a single value. The formula varies slightly across sites, but it is less relevant as the value that is important is the percent reduction of the dose compared to the preoperative level. All studies report reduction of the dose of dopaminergic therapy with STN stimulation (34,72). The amount of reduction of PD medications varies between 20% and 70%, with a small minority of the patients being able to stop PD medications completely (72). Improvement of dyskinesia with STN DBS surgery is attributed to the reduction of the dose of dopaminergic medications (20,34). STN stimulation per se is not believed to be effective for suppression of dyskinesia based on the observation that postoperative levodopa challenge at the preoperative dose resulted in the same degree of dyskinesia as preoperatively (13). However, there are a few case reports of the direct dyskinesia suppressing effect of DBS stimulation. The benefit was attributed to the more dorsal location of the stimulated contact in STN (21,53).

Presently, there is published data on nearly 1000 patients who have undergone bilateral STN DBS. Despite wide variability in the scope of publications, the data are very consistent regarding the short-term efficacy of the intervention and can be summarized as following:

- STN DBS is effective for the improvement of PD motor disability.
- The benefit of stimulation is most robust in the medications-off state and marginal in the medications-on state.
- Stimulation reduces motor fluctuations.
- Stimulation reduces dyskinesia as the result of reduction of medications intake.
- The best predictor of the motor benefit of surgery is preoperative performance in the medications-on state and the "delta" (difference) between the UPDRS scores in the medications-on versus -off state. The larger the "delta" the greater is the expected benefit of stimulation.

Long-Term Results of Subthalamic Nucleus Deep Brain Stimulation

There is much less information on the long-term impact of STN DBS on PD motor disability, although in the past two years, several new publications report on long-term (greater than 12 months) outcomes. The published long-term outcome data remains in the format of pre–post intervention observations. Analysis of the long-term outcomes is limited not only by the design of the studies, but also the progressive nature of PD which makes it impossible in the absence of a medically treated control group to separate the impact of surgery from disease progression. Table 3 summarizes the findings from studies that evaluated the long-term outcomes of surgery on PD motor disability. We restricted data analysis to the studies that reported at least 48 months data and included UPDRS motor scores pre- and postoperatively for each data point. The Grenoble group who pioneered STN DBS surgery was the first to publish the long-term outcome data for DBS. Krack et al. (42) reported the five-year outcome data on the first 49 patients who underwent STN DBS surgery between 1993 and 1997. Outcome measures were the same as reported by Limousin (13) for the original cohort. Patient outcomes were reported for preoperative evaluation, and one and five years postoperatively. Consistent with the previous reports in the medications-off state, UPDRS motor scores improved 66% from baseline to one year and by 54% from baseline to five years postsurgery, UPDRS ADL scores improved by 66% at one year and 49% at five years. Painful dystonia resolved in the majority of patients at one year and the benefit persisted for five years. Compared to baseline at five years postsurgery, STN DBS resulted in persistent improvement of tremor (75%), rigidity (71%), and bradykinesia though to a less degree (49%). At five years, gait and postural stability were still better than baseline and did not change significantly compared to one year. Speech improved at one year but declined to the baseline level by five years. STN DBS did not have any impact on UPDRS motor and ADLs scores

Table 3 Long-Term Subthalamic Nucleus Deep Brain Stimulation Outcome Data: Data Reported for Unified Parkinson's Disease Rating Scale Part II Motor Scores in Stimulation-On, Medications-Off State

First author	Year	Country	N	Follow-up (months)	UPDRS-off % change at 1 year[a]	UPDRS-off % change at last follow-up (3–5 yrs)
Krack (42)	2003	France	49	60	66	54
Visser Vandewalle (54)	2005	Netherlands	20	48	55[b]	43
Rodriquez-Oroz (52)	2005	Multiple countries, Spain	49	36–48	57	50
Ostergaard (55)	2005	Denmark	22	48	65	55
Schupbach (56)	2005	France	30	60	59[c]	54
Total/average			170		60.4	51.2

[a]Percentage change is reported as the difference compared with baseline.
[b]Evaluation was performed three months postoperatively.
[c]Evaluation was performed at six months postoperatively.
Abbreviations: UPDRS, unified Parkinson's disease rating scale.

in the medications-on state, which is consistent with earlier reports. Between the first and the fifth year, tremor and rigidity scores did not change in the medications-on state, however, scores for bradykinesia, speech, postural stability, and freezing of gait worsened resulting in worsening of the total motor UPDRS score and ADLs score. Compared to baseline, the duration and severity of dyskinesia reduced by 71% and 58%, respectively, and the benefit persisted up to five years. Patients were able to reduce the dose of PD medications by 59% on average at one year, and did not require further dose escalation by five years. At five years, 11 of 42 patients were not taking levodopa, and three others were not taking any dopaminergic therapy. The investigators concluded that DBS had persistent benefit for the reduction of dyskinesia and painful dystonia. Further, motor benefit was most robust for tremor and rigidity and less so for akinesia. Worsening of akinesia, speech, postural stability, and gait in the medications-on state at five years was attributed to the natural progression of PD disability.

Rodriguez-Oroz et al. (52) reported the long-term data on the original cohort of patients enrolled in the multicenter DBS study the short-term results of which were discussed previously (30). The original cohort included 96 patients who underwent STN DBS and 38 who underwent GPi DBS. A total of 69 patients from the original cohort (49 STN and 20 GPi) were followed for a long term (mean follow-up was 3.8 years). The assessment battery was similar to the one reported by the Grenoble group, but also included the Goetz dyskinesia scale (57) and Global Assessment scale. The primary outcome measure was the change in the UPDRS motor score off-medications with stimulation at the last evaluation (minimum of three years) compared to baseline. STN DBS resulted in 50% reduction of UPDRS motor score compared to the baseline in the medications-off state and no change in the medications-on state. Similar to the Grenoble findings, stimulation improved all subscores of the motor and ADL scales in the off-medications state with the exception of speech. Compared to the one-year findings, UPDRS motor and ADL scores declined by the three- to four-year follow-up point, specifically in speech, gait, and postural stability. The benefit of stimulation for tremor, rigidity, and dyskinesia persisted long term. PD medication intake was reduced by 41% at one year and remained stable at three to four years. These findings are very similar to the Grenoble experience and support the universal nature of the findings considering the multi center and multinational nature of the protocol. Both studies demonstrate long-lasting benefit of STN DBS, however, the patients experience worsening of specifically axial symptoms of PD (speech, posture, and gait) that is attributed to the progression of PD. This study included evaluation of patients in the medications-off and stimulation-off state, three to four years postsurgery: the UPDRS motor scores in that condition did not differ from baseline scores. At the first glance, lack of escalation of PD disability in the drug and stimulation "naïve" condition would argue for a neuroprotective effect of DBS, but the authors legitimately caution against such a quick conclusion. They attributed the finding to the potential long duration effect of medications and stimulation at the time of the assessment. In other words, these patients may not have gotten to a true off-medication/off-stimulation status at the time of assessment.

Ostergaard and Sunde (55) reported four-year outcome data on 22 patients treated with bilateral STN DBS in Denmark. In addition to the standard outcome measures, they also included PD patient motor diaries. The results were consistent with the previously reported data: UPDRS motor score was reduced by 65% one year postsurgery in the medications-off state, and the benefit persisted long term. Similar to the other studies, worsening of gait, postural stability, and speech were noted between one- and four-year assessment. Deterioration of those parameters was seen in the medications-on state as well. This group also evaluated the patients in the medications and stimulation-off setting four years after surgery and demonstrated no decline in UPDRS motor scores compared to the baseline. They attributed lack of decline to the medications and stimulation's long-lasting effect, similar to the other groups.

Finally, Schupbach et al. (56) reported five-year outcomes of STN DBS surgery in the cohort of 37 patients who underwent surgery between 1996 and 1999 in Paris, France. Of the original cohort, 30 patients were available for the five-year follow-up. That group reported a 59% reduction in UPDRS motor scores with stimulation in the medications-off state at six months postsurgery compared to baseline with long-term persistent benefit (54%), but noted decline in the axial PD symptoms. Dyskinesia was reduced by 79% and motor fluctuations by 67% at five years compared to the baseline scores. The PD medication dose requirement was reduced by 64% at six months and 58% at five years compared to baseline. UPDRS ADL scores were reduced by 67% in the medications-off state at six months, and 40% by five years postsurgery, the decline in ADLs between one and five years was statistically significant.

In conclusion, there is a limited but growing amount of published data on the long-term outcomes of bilateral STN DBS. The duration of published studies ranged between 36 and 60 months, with average follow-up of 51 months. All the published studies included standard evaluation based on the CAPIT protocol. However, none of the studies were controlled randomized protocols. All the studies reached similar conclusions that can be summarized as following:

- The benefit of STN DBS for improvement of PD motor disability persists long term.
- STN DBS is effective for the improvement of PD motor disability in the medications-off state.
- STN DBS is effective for reduction of dyskinesia and motor fluctuations, but does not provide additional benefit in the medications-on state.
- STN DBS provides persistent long-term improvement for tremor, rigidity, and less so for bradykinesia.
- STN DBS results in the reduction of PD medications intake by an average of 50%.

- Axial symptoms of PD (speech, gait, and postural stability) worsen long term. The decline is likely due to the progression of PD.

The longest reported duration of post-STN DBS outcome observations is five years. Although it is a significant time-period for the procedure that is hardly 10-years-old, it is still insufficient to establish the impact of this intervention on the course of the disease that can span more than two decades, especially considering the fact that surgical patients usually represent the younger subset of PD patient population. Continuous follow-up of the surgical cohort and accumulation of long-term data is necessary. At present, decline in PD axial symptoms at three- to five-years postsurgery is attributed to the naturally progressive course of PD disability. However, in the absence of a medically treated control group, that conclusion remains an unproven hypothesis. Historical controls are of limited value as it is challenging to match them by the disease severity, duration, and medications intake. Although designing long-term controlled PD surgical trials is expensive and difficult, from the ethical standpoint of declining patients the procedure that is known to be effective at least for a short term, such studies are necessary to establish the role of DBS surgery in the long-term management of PD.

At the beginning of the STN DBS era, the PD research and clinical communities were not only excited by the efficacy of intervention for management of PD motor disability, but also hopeful that the procedure potentially could turn out to be neuroprotective. The anticipation was based on the hypothesis that STN DBS reduces the glutaminegric outflow from STN nucleus that could be contributing to further degeneration of nigrostriatal structures (58,59). As of today, there is no evidence of neuroprotective effect of STN DBS. Some studies demonstrated no change in UPDRS motor scores in the medications-off–stimulation-off state as far as five years compared to the preoperative evaluation (30,55,56). The expected rate of progression of PD motor disability is 10% annual increase in PD motor scores early in the course of the disease though the curve can flatten out in more advanced disease (60–62). While it is tempting to attribute lack of change to the neuroprotective effect of the intervention, the more likely explanation is the long duration effect of medications and stimulation that outlast the standard 12 hours "defined medications-off" period. It already has been established in the ELLDOPA study that the long duration response to levodopa can last more than two weeks (63). The long duration response to dopamine agonists and other PD medications has not been systematically studied. The latency of the effect of DBS is not well established but also can be prolonged. Hilker et al. (49) has recently published F-dopa positron emission tomography (PET) study of 30 patients with successful STN DBS. PET scans were performed preoperatively and 16 ± 6 months postsurgery. The average reduction of PD motor symptoms was 52% consistent with other reported cohorts. PET data demonstrated 9.5% to 12% annual rate of decline of tracer uptake in the putamen. These data are in agreement with the rate of decline of tracer-binding reported in medically treated PD patients. The rate of decline of F-dopa uptake was shown to correlate with the rate of progression of PD disability and is considered to be the surrogate marker of the progression of PD (64). Hilker et al. is the first study to report the rate of F-dopa uptake decline in the cohort of patients with successful STN DBS. Based on these results, STN DBS provides effective control of PD motor disability but does not have an impact on the rate of progression of dopaminergic cell loss. That conclusion correlates with the long-term STN DBS outcome data demonstrating long-term worsening of the axial symptoms of PD, considered to be the markers of disease progression, despite otherwise successful DBS.

COMPARISON BETWEEN GLOBUS PALLIDUM INTERNA AND SUBTHALAMIC NUCLEUS DEEP BRAIN STIMULATION

The other target of DBS for PD used less frequently is the GPi. Studies of GPi stimulation also have reported improved motor function and time spent in the "on"-state (Table 4). Although STN has become the preferred surgical target for PD patients, there is paucity of studies comparing the two. GPi stimulation can directly suppress dyskinesia independent from the reduction of the dose of PD medications. Actually, one consistent difference between outcomes of STN versus GPi DBS is the lack of reduction of the dose of PD medications with the GPi target (46). GPi may be a more forgiving target with respect to the development of adverse events but due to its larger size, may also be more difficult to target for maximal benefit in motor symptoms (65). Secondly, since the GPi is a much larger target than the STN and there are few structures lateral and anterior to the GPi that can affect nonmotor function, it might be associated with less side effects on behavior, mood, and cognitive function (46).

A recent meta-analysis comparing bilateral STN to GPi stimulation found that motor function improvement was comparable in both groups (14). The meta-analysis included 31 STN and 14 GPi studies published prior to 2004. Motor function improved significantly following stimulation for both targets (54% for STN; 40% for GPi), with effect sizes of 2.59 and 2.04, respectively. STN and GPi subjects had comparable improvement in motor function following surgery after controlling for baseline characteristics ($P = 0.094$). As discussed before, medication requirements were significantly reduced for STN, but did not change for GPi subjects (14). The first randomized trial of STN and GPi DBS was published in 1999 (19), and a follow-up was published in 2005 (46). This study included 10 GPi and 13 STN subjects followed for up to 12 months. Off-medication UPDRS motor scores improved after 12 months of DBS in both GPi and STN groups (39% and 48%; $P = 0.40$), whereas levodopa dosage was decreased by 38% in the STN group versus 3% in the GPi group ($P = 0.08$). The authors concluded that stimulation of either site improves many of the features of PD and that it is too early to exclude GPi as a target for DBS in persons with PD. However, given the small sample size, a larger

Table 4 Bilateral Globus Pallidum Interna Deep Brain Stimulation Studies[a]

First author	Year	Country	N	Mean age	% Male	Follow-up period (mos)	Mean baseline UPDRS motor	Follow-up UPDRS motor[b]	% Change
Pahwa (66)	1997	USA	3[a]	57	100	3	48 ± 12.77	15.3 ± 11.78	68.1
Limousin (15)	1997	France	6	50	83	na	43	26 ± 11	40
Krack (17)	1998	France	5	51	80	6	53.6 ± 10.4	32.5 ± 12.4	39.4
Ghika (67)	1998	Swiss	6	55	na	3,6,12,15,18,24	66.0	31.0	53.0
Brown (18)	1999	France, Spain	6	50.7	67	8.3 (ave)	54.2 ± 9.2	27.2 ± 12.0	49.8
Burchiel (19)	1999	USA	4	46.5	70	12	67.0 ± 24	40.87	39
Durif (68)	1999	France	6	64	33	6	36 ± 2	23 ± 5	36.1
Pillon (25)	2000	France	8	52.5	75	3	55.4 ± 8.5	37.1 ± 13.3	33.0
Pillon (25)	2000	France	5	55.2	60	6	41.6 ± 14.1	27.0 ± 12.5	35.1
Kumar (6)	2000	Canada, France, Spain	22	52.7	68	6	53.4 ± 3.3	37.1 ± 3.8	31
Krause (27)	2001	Germany	6	58.5	na	6	43.8 ± 8.2	39.2 ± 4.9	10.5
Volkmann (31)	2001	Germany	11	56.6	na	6	52.5 ± 14.16	22.9 ± 15.48	56.4
Parkinson's Disease Study Group (30)	2001	Multiple countries, USA	38	55.7	71	6	50.8 ± 11.6	33.9 ± 12.3	33.3
Loher (7)	2002	Swiss, Germany	106	64.6	50	3,12	63.4 ± 17.4	40.3 ± 10.3	36.4
Summary, N = 14			136	55.0	69	6 mos (median)			40.1

[a]All studies that reported *P*-values were significant at *P* < 0.05 or better except Durif 1999 (*P* = 0.27). Six studies did not provide *P*-values.
[b]The six-month assessment was used or the closest assessment in time to six months.
Abbreviations: ave, average; na, not applicable; UPDRS, unified Parkinson's disease rating scale.
Source: From Ref. 14.

randomized trial with additional outcomes and longer follow-up is warranted to better understand the impact of both targets on physical and cognitive functioning, as well as quality of life in persons with advanced PD.

The AAN Quality Standards Subcommittee has recently published an evidence-based review on treatment of PD with motor fluctuations and dyskinesia that contains a section on surgical treatment (72). The Committee commented on the paucity of the Class III evidence, but concluded that based on the available data "STN DBS is possibly effective in improving motor function and reducing motor fluctuations, dyskinesia, and anti-parkinsonian medications usage in PD patients. Adverse events may limit application of this therapy . . . data are insufficient to determine efficacy of GPi DBS."

CONCLUSIONS

DBS surgery is now an accepted and widely used procedure for management of patients with advanced PD complicated by motor fluctuations. The criteria for patient selection and short-term efficacy of DBS are reasonably well established. DBS is undoubtedly the most effective intervention in the history of PD surgery. The preferred target of choice is STN though there is paucity of controlled studies confirming its superiority over GPi as a target. STN DBS is effective for the management of PD motor disability in the medications-off state, as well as reduction of motor fluctuations and dyskinesia. The benefit of stimulation persists long-term, though the patients experience worsening in axial PD motor symptoms (speech, gait, and postural control), likely as the reflection of the progressive nature of PD, but controlled studies are lacking to prove that concept.

The future research of DBS in PD should:

- Establish the mechanism of action of DBS.
- Establish comparative efficacy of STN versus GPi DBS target.
- Collect long-term data on the efficacy of STN DBS for the motor and nonmotor manifestations of PD.
- Establish the long-term impact of STN DBS on PD disability compared to the medically treated cohort
- Simplify the surgical and programming algorithm.

REFERENCES

1. Limousin P, Pollak P, Benazzouz A, et al. Effect of parkinsonian signs and symptoms of bilateral subthalamic nucleus stimulation. Lancet 1995; 345(8942):91–95.
2. Langston JW, Widner H, Goetz CG, et al. Core assessment program for intracerebral transplantations (CAPIT). Mov Disord 1992; 7(1):2–13.
3. Defer GL, Widner H, Marie RM, Remy P, Levivier M. Core assessment program for surgical interventional therapies in Parkinson's disease (CAPSIT-PD). Mov Disord 1999; 14(4):572–584.

4. Gross C, Rougier A, Guehl D, Boraud T, Julien J, Bioulac B. High-frequency stimulation of the globus pallidus internalis in Parkinson's disease: a study of seven cases. J Neurosurg 1997; 87(4):491–498.

5. Vingerhoets G, Lannoo E, van der Linden C, et al. Changes in quality of life following unilateral pallidal stimulation in Parkinson's disease. J Psychosom Res 1999; 46(3):247–255.

6. Kumar R, Lang AE, Rodriguez-Oroz MC, et al. Deep brain stimulation of the globus pallidus pars interna in advanced Parkinson's disease. Neurology 2000; 55(12 suppl 6):S34–S39.

7. Loher TJ, Burgunder JM, Pohle T, Weber S, Sommerhalder R, Krauss JK. Long-term pallidal deep brain stimulation in patients with advanced Parkinson disease: 1-year follow-up study. J Neurosurg 2002; 96(5):844–853.

8. Merello M, Nouzeilles MI, Kuzis G, et al. Unilateral radiofrequency lesion versus electrostimulation of posteroventral pallidum: a prospective randomized comparison. Mov Disord 1999; 14(1):50–56.

9. Kumar R, Lozano AM, Sime E, Halket E, Lang AE. Comparative effects of unilateral and bilateral subthalamic nucleus deep brain stimulation. Neurology 1999; 53(3):561–566.

10. Linazasoro G, Van Blercom N, Lasa A. Unilateral subthalamic deep brain stimulation in advanced Parkinson's disease. Mov Disord 2003; 18(6):713–716.

11. Germano IM, Gracies JM, Weisz DJ, Tse W, Koller WC, Olanow CW. Unilateral stimulation of the subthalamic nucleus in Parkinson disease: a double-blind 12-month evaluation study. J Neurosurg 2004; 101(1):36–42.

12. Benabid AL, Pollak P, Louveau A, Henry S, de Rougemont J. Combined (thalamotomy and stimulation) stereotactic surgery of the VIM thalamic nucleus for bilateral Parkinson disease. Appl Neurophysiol 1987; 50(1–6):344–346.

13. Limousin P, Krack P, Pollak P, et al. Electrical stimulation of the subthalamic nucleus in advanced Parkinson's disease. N Engl J Med 1998; 339(16):1105–1111.

14. Weaver F, Follett K, Hur K, Ippolito D, Stern M. Deep brain stimulation in Parkinson disease: a metaanalysis of patient outcomes. J Neurosurg 2005; 103(6):956–967.

15. Limousin P, Greene J, Pollak P, Rothwell J, Benabid AL, Frackowiak R. Changes in cerebral activity pattern due to subthalamic nucleus or internal pallidum stimulation in Parkinson's disease. Ann Neurol 1997; 42(3): 283–291.

16. Krack P, Pollak P, Limousin P, Benazzouz A, Benabid AL. Stimulation of subthalamic nucleus alleviates tremor in Parkinson's disease. Lancet 1997; 350(9092):1675.

17. Krack P, Pollak P, Limousin P, et al. Subthalamic nucleus or internal pallidal stimulation in young onset Parkinson's disease. Brain 1998; 121(Pt 3):451–457.

18. Brown RG, Dowsey PL, Brown P, et al. Impact of deep brain stimulation on upper limb akinesia in Parkinson's disease. Ann Neurol 1999; 45(4):473–488.

19. Burchiel KJ, Anderson VC, Favre J, Hammerstad JP. Comparison of pallidal and subthalamic nucleus deep brain stimulation for advanced Parkinson's disease: results of a randomized, blinded pilot study. Neurosurgery 1999; 45(6):1375–1382; discussion 1382–1384.

20. Moro E, Scerrati M, Romito LM, Roselli R, Tonali P, Albanese A. Chronic subthalamic nucleus stimulation reduces medication requirements in Parkinson's disease. Neurology 1999; 53(1):85–90.

21. Figueiras-Mendez R, Marin-Zarza F, Antonio Molina J, et al. Subthalamic nucleus stimulation improves directly levodopa induced dyskinesias in Parkinson's disease. J Neurol Neurosurg Psychiatry 1999; 66(4):549–550.

22. Pinter MM, Alesch F, Murg M, Seiwald M, Helscher RJ, Binder H. Deep brain stimulation of the subthalamic nucleus for control of extrapyramidal features in advanced idiopathic Parkinson's disease: one year follow-up. J Neural Transm 1999; 106(7–8):693–709.

23. Molinuevo JL, Valldeoriola F, Tolosa E, et al. Levodopa withdrawal after bilateral subthalamic nucleus stimulation in advanced Parkinson disease. Arch Neurol 2000; 57(7):983–988.

24. Houeto JL, Damier P, Bejjani PB, et al. Subthalamic stimulation in Parkinson disease: a multidisciplinary approach. Arch Neurol 2000; 57(4):461–465.

25. Pillon B, Ardouin C, Damier P, et al. Neuropsychological changes between "off" and "on" STN or GPi stimulation in Parkinson's disease. Neurology 2000; 55(3):411–418.

26. Rodriguez-Oroz MC, Gorospe A, Guridi J, et al. Bilateral deep brain stimulation of the subthalamic nucleus in Parkinson's disease. Neurology 2000; 55(12 suppl 6):S45–S51.

27. Krause M, Fogel W, Heck A, et al. Deep brain stimulation for the treatment of Parkinson's disease: subthalamic nucleus versus globus pallidus internus. J Neurol Neurosurg Psychiatry 2001; 70(4):464–470.

28. Broggi G, Franzini A, Ferroli P, et al. Effect of bilateral subthalamic electrical stimulation in Parkinson's disease. Surg Neurol 2001; 56(2):89–94, discussion 94–96.

29. Lopiano L, Rizzone M, Perozzo P, et al. Deep brain stimulation of the subthalamic nucleus: selection of patients and clinical results. Neurol Sci 2001; 22(1):67–68.

30. Parkinson's Disease Study Group. Deep-brain stimulation of the subthalamic nucleus or the pars interna of the globus pallidus in Parkinson's disease. N Engl J Med 2001; 345(13):956–963.

31. Volkmann J, Allert N, Voges J, Weiss PH, Freund HJ, Sturm V. Safety and efficacy of pallidal or subthalamic nucleus stimulation in advanced PD. Neurology 2001; 56(4):548–551.

32. Vesper J, Klostermann F, Stockhammer F, Funk T, Brock M. Results of chronic subthalamic nucleus stimulation for Parkinson's disease: a 1-year follow-up study. Surg Neurol 2002; 57(5):306–311; discussion 311–313.

33. Figueiras-Mendez R, Regidor I, Riva-Meana C, Magarinos-Ascone CM. Further supporting evidence of beneficial subthalamic stimulation in Parkinson's patients. Neurology 2002; 58(3):469–470.

34. Vingerhoets FJ, Villemure JG, Temperli P, Pollo C, Pralong E, Ghika J. Subthalamic DBS replaces levodopa in Parkinson's disease: two-year follow-up. Neurology 2002; 58(3):396–401.

35. Ostergaard K, Sunde N, Dupont E. Effects of bilateral stimulation of the subthalamic nucleus in patients with severe Parkinson's disease and motor fluctuations. Mov Disord 2002; 17(4):693–700.

36. Simuni T, Jaggi JL, Mulholland H, et al. Bilateral stimulation of the subthalamic nucleus in patients with Parkinson disease: a study of efficacy and safety. J Neurosurg 2002; 96(4):666–672.

37. Iansek R, Rosenfeld JV, Huxham FE. Deep brain stimulation of the subthalamic nucleus in Parkinson's disease. Med J Aust 2002; 177(3):142–146.

38. Thobois S, Mertens P, Guenot M, et al. Subthalamic nucleus stimulation in Parkinson's disease: clinical evaluation of 18 patients. J Neurol 2002; 249(5):529–534.

39. Varma TR, Fox SH, Eldridge PR, et al. Deep brain stimulation of the subthalamic nucleus: effectiveness in advanced Parkinson's disease patients previously reliant on apomorphine. J Neurol Neurosurg Psychiatry 2003; 74(2):170–174.

40. Kleiner-Fisman G, Fisman DN, Sime E, Saint-Cyr JA, Lozano AM, Lang AE. Long-term follow-up of bilateral deep brain stimulation of the subthalamic nucleus in patients with advanced Parkinson disease. J Neurosurg 2003; 99(3):489–495.

41. Chen CC, Lee ST, Wu T, Chen CJ, Chen MC, Lu CS. Short-term effect of bilateral subthalamic stimulation for advanced Parkinson's disease. Chang Gung Med J 2003; 26(5):344–351.

42. Krack P, Batir A, Van Blercom N, et al. Five-year follow-up of bilateral stimulation of the subthalamic nucleus in advanced Parkinson's disease. N Engl J Med 2003; 349(20):1925–1934.

43. Pahwa R, Wilkinson SB, Overman J, Lyons KE. Bilateral subthalamic stimulation in patients with Parkinson disease: long-term follow-up. J Neurosurg 2003; 99(1):71–77.

44. Herzog J, Volkmann J, Krack P, et al. Two-year follow-up of subthalamic deep brain stimulation in Parkinson's disease. Mov Disord 2003; 18(11):1332–1337.

45. Jaggi JL, Umemura A, Hurtig HI, et al. Bilateral stimulation of the subthalamic nucleus in Parkinson's disease: surgical efficacy and prediction of outcome. Stereotact Funct Neurosurg 2004; 82(2–3):104–114.

46. Anderson VC, Burchiel KJ, Hogarth P, Favre J, Hammerstad JP. Pallidal vs subthalamic nucleus deep brain stimulation in Parkinson disease. Arch Neurol 2005; 62(4):554–560.

47. Capecci M, Ricciuti RA, Burini D, et al. Functional improvement after subthalamic stimulation in Parkinson's disease: a non-equivalent controlled study with 12–24 month follow-up. J Neurol Neurosurg Psychiatry 2005; 76(6):769–774.

48. Erola T, Karinen P, Heikkinen E, et al. Bilateral subthalamic nucleus stimulation improves health-related quality of life in Parkinsonian patients. Parkinsonism Relat Disord 2005; 11:89–94.

49. Hilker R, Portman AT, Voges J, et al. Disease progression continues in patients with advanced Parkinson's disease and effective subthalamic nucleus stimulation. J Neurol Neurosurg Psychiatry 2005; 76(9):1217–1221.

50. Esselink RA, de Bie RM, de Haan RJ, et al. Unilateral pallidotomy versus bilateral subthalamic nucleus stimulation in PD: a randomized trial. Neurology 2004; 62(2):201–207.

51. Hauser RA, Deckers F, Lehert P. Parkinson's disease home diary: further validation and implications for clinical trials. Mov Disord 2004; 19(12):1409–1413.

52. Rodriguez-Oroz MC, Obeso JA, Lang AE, et al. Bilateral deep brain stimulation in Parkinson's disease: a multicentre study with 4 years follow-up. Brain 2005; 128(Pt 10):2240–2249.

53. Alterman RL, Shils JL, Gudesblatt M, Tagliati M. Immediate and sustained relief of levodopa-induced dyskinesias after dorsal relocation of a deep brain stimulation lead. Case report. Neurosurg Focus 2004; 17(1):E6.

54. Visser-Vandewalle V, van der Linden C, Temel Y, et al. Long-term effects of bilateral subthalamic nucleus stimulation in advanced Parkinson disease: a four-year follow-up study. Parkinsonism Relat Disord 2005; 11(3):157–165.

55. Ostergaard K, Aa Sunde N. Evolution of Parkinson's disease during 4 years of bilateral deep brain stimulation of the subthalamic nucleus. Mov Disord 2005.

56. Schupbach WM, Chastan N, Welter ML, et al. Stimulation of the subthalamic nucleus in Parkinson's disease: a 5-year follow-up. J Neurol Neurosurg Psychiatry 2005; 76(12):1640–1644.

57. Goetz CG, Stebbins GT, Shale HM, et al. Utility of an objective dyskinesia rating scale for Parkinson's disease: inter- and intrarater reliability assessment. Mov Disord 1994; 9(4):390–394.

58. Rodriguez MC, Obeso JA, Olanow CW. Subthalamic nucleus-mediated excitotoxicity in Parkinson's disease: a target for neuroprotection. Ann Neurol 1998; 44(3 suppl 1): S175–S188.

59. Obeso JA, Rodriguez-Oroz MC, Rodriguez M, et al. Pathophysiologic basis of surgery for Parkinson's disease. Neurology 2000; 55(12 suppl 6):S7–S12.

60. The Parkinson Study Group. Effects of tocopherol and deprenyl on the progression of disability in early Parkinson's disease. N Engl J Med 1993; 328(3):176–183.

61. Jankovic J, Kapadia AS. Functional decline in Parkinson disease. Arch Neurol 2001; 58(10):1611–1615.

62. Jankovic J, McDermott M, Carter J, et al. Variable expression of Parkinson's disease: a base-line analysis of the DATATOP cohort. The Parkinson Study Group. Neurology 1990; 40(10): 1529–1534.

63. Fahn S, Oakes D, Shoulson I, et al. Levodopa and the progression of Parkinson's disease. N Engl J Med 2004; 351(24):2498–2508.

64. Marek K, Jennings D, Seibyl J. Imaging the dopamine system to assess disease-modifying drugs: studies comparing dopamine agonists and levodopa. Neurology 2003; 61(6 suppl 3):S43–S48.

65. Vitek JL. Deep brain stimulation for Parkinson's disease. A critical re-evaluation of STN versus GPi DBS. Stereotact Funct Neurosurg 2002; 78(3–4):119–131.

66. Pahwa R, Wilkinson S, Smith D, Lyons K, Miyawaki E, Koller WC. High-frequency stimulation of the globus pallidus for the treatment of Parkinson's disease. Neurology 1997; 49(1):249–253.

67. Ghika J, Villemure JG, Fankhauser H, Favre J, Assal G, Ghika-Schmid F. Efficiency and safety of bilateral contemporaneous pallidal stimulation (deep brain stimulation) in levodopa-responsive patients with Parkinson's disease with severe motor fluctuations: a 2-year follow-up review. J Neurosurg 1998; 89(5):713–718.

68. Durif F, Lemaire JJ, Debilly B, Dordain G. Acute and chronic effects of anteromedial globus pallidus stimulation in Parkinson's disease. J Neurol Neurosurg Psychiatry 1999; 67(3):315–322.

69. Fahn S, Elton RL, Members of the UPDRS Development Committee. Unified Parkinson's Disease Rating Scale. In Fahn S, Marsden CD, Goldstein M, eds. Recent Developments in Parkinson's Disease, Vol. 2. Florham Park, NJ: Macmillan Health Care Information, 1987:153–164.

70. Beric A, Kelly PJ, et al. Six-month clinical outcome of bilateral subthalamic deep brain stimulation in Parkinson's disease. Stereotact Funct Neurosurg 2001; 77:146.

71. Bronte-Stewart H, Courtney T, McGuire K, et al. Bilateral Subthalamic Nucleus Deep Brain Stimulation (B-STN DBS) Changes the Expected Course of Advanced Parkinson's Disease (PD). American Academy of Neurology 55th Annual Meeting 2003; P02.059.

72. Pahwa R, Factor SA, Lyons KE, et al. Practice parameter: treatment of Parkinson's disease with motor fluctuations and dyskinesia (an evidence based review). Neurology 2006; 66:983–995.

14

Subthalamic Nucleus Deep Brain Stimulation and Nonmotor Symptoms of Parkinson's Disease

David J. Houghton

*Department of Neurology, Hospital of the University of Pennsylvania,
Philadelphia, Pennsylvania, U.S.A.*

Galit Kleiner-Fisman

*Parkinson's Disease Research, Education, and Clinical Center (PADRECC),
Veterans Affairs Medical Center, University of Pennsylvania,
Philadelphia, Pennsylvania, U.S.A.*

INTRODUCTION

Parkinson's Disease and Motor Symptoms

Dating back to 1817 and his first descriptions of six patients with the "shaking palsy," James Parkinson established the common motor symptoms of parkinsonism consisting of resting tremor, decreased motor control, stooped posture, and gait abnormalities (1). Today, clinicians still diagnose idiopathic Parkinson's disease (PD) based on the presence of four cardinal motor features: bradykinesia, tremor, rigidity, and postural instability (U.K. Parkinson's Disease Society Brain Bank Clinical Diagnostic Criteria) (2). Bradykinesia and one other symptom listed are considered sufficient to make a diagnosis of probable PD.

Parkinson's Disease and Nonmotor Symptoms

Our understanding of PD has expanded to include numerous nonmotor symptoms that may accompany the classic motor features. Though Parkinson described

219

nonmotor symptoms such as sleep disturbances, constipation, speech impairment, dysphagia, sialorrhea, fatigue, and delirium in his original treatise (1), the recognition and wide acceptance of nonmotor symptoms as part of the spectrum of disease has occurred only recently. The commonly identified nonmotor symptoms of PD are listed in Table 1.

Nonmotor symptoms are highly prevalent in PD. In one recent study, ninety-nine PD patients were asked whether they experienced fatigue, anxiety, depression, sleep disorders, or sensory symptoms. Nearly 90% endorsed at least one such complication (3).

Cognitive impairment, a frequent occurrence, may affect over three-fourths of PD patients during the course of disease (4), and over 40% of patients have dementia after four years (5,6). More than half of all PD patients experience

Table 1   Nonmotor Symptoms in Parkinson's Disease

Cognitive impairment/mood
  Dementia
  Psychosis
  Depression
  Anxiety
Autonomic disorders
  Cardiovascular reflexes (orthostasis, bradycardia, etc.)
  Gastroparesis and constipation
  Sialorrhea
  Dysphagia
  Hyperhidrosis and seborrhea
  Temperature dysregulation
  Urologic dysfunction
  Sexual dysfunction
Disorders of smell
Speech disorders
  Hypophonia
  Dysarthria
Sleep disorders
  Insomnia
  Excessive daytime sleepiness (EDS)
  Circadian rhythm disorder
  REM behavioral disorder (RBD)
  Restless legs syndrome (RLS)/periodic leg movements disorder (PLMD)
  Fatigue
Weight loss/gain
Sensory
  Pain
  Tightness
  Tingling
  Burning

dysautonomic symptoms including urinary problems, constipation, dysfunction (7). Furthermore, just as PD patients suffer motor fluctuatio disease progresses, nonmotor fluctuations can occur. In one survey of no fluctuations, dysautonomic fluctuations affected up to 64% of PD patients with moderate-to-severe PD (mean H and Y "off" = 3.8) while sensory fluctuations affected 54% (8). More than one-quarter of these patients felt that the nonmotor fluctuations were more troublesome than the motor fluctuations they experienced.

Emerging Recognition of Nonmotor Symptoms

The well-established and widely-used Unified Parkinson's Disease Rating Scale (UPDRS), developed in 1987 (9), is a relatively sensitive instrument to assess motor symptom severity, but it does not adequately address nonmotor symptoms (10). Similarly, it has been shown that even movement disorder specialists fail to recognize such features in their patients more than 50% of the time (11). In acknowledgment of this, the UPDRS is being revised to incorporate a wide spectrum of nonmotor symptoms pertaining to altered cognition, mood, dysautonomia, sleep, and the implication of these on daily function (12). In addition, the American Academy of Neurology has recently published evidence-based practice parameters for the treatment of cognitive and psychiatric nonmotor symptoms in PD (13). With wider recognition, nonmotor symptoms have greater bearing on the surgical treatments for PD.

Pathophysiology of Motor and Nonmotor Symptoms and Subthalamic Nucleus Deep Brain Stimulation

The classic Albin-Delong anatomic model of basal ganglionic function (14,15) has some limitations, but it remains useful in conceptualizing the origin of the motor symptoms in PD. These symptoms, particularly bradykinesia and rigidity, are attributed to the loss of dopaminergic neurons originating in the substantia nigra and projecting to the striatum, accompanied by the presence of Lewy bodies in the surviving neurons. This dopamine-mediated system is usually responsive to treatment with levodopa and dopamine agonists; success with medication predicts success with subthalamic nucleus deep brain stimulation (STN-DBS) (16).

Conversely, nonmotor symptoms may be mediated by both dopaminergic and nondopaminergic neurotransmitter systems that become increasingly affected as the disease progresses. There is good experimental evidence of cognitive, autonomic, and sensory functions affected by dopaminergic pathology in the basal ganglia (17,18,19). In addition, Lewy body inclusions have been found in the nondopaminergic neurons of the substantia innominata, the mesocortico-limbic system, nucleus basalis of Meynert, locus ceruleus, midline raphe nucleus, dorsal motor nucleus (DMN) of the vagus, and hypothalamus. The sympathetic, parasympathetic, and enteric nervous systems are also involved. Such pathological changes of central nondopaminergic neurons, as well as peripheral sympathetic, parasympathetic, and enteric neurons, likely lead to some of the nonmotor symptoms of PD (Table 2) (20). Given the dual involvement of dopaminergic and nondopaminergic neurons in nonmotor symptoms of PD, such symptoms are relatively refractory to dopaminergic medications. As such, many nonmotor, nondopaminergic symptoms do not benefit from STN-DBS. However, clinical experience reveals this is not universal; some nonmotor symptoms improve while others worsen following surgery. It should also be noted that worsening of symptoms may occur due to the progression of disease as opposed to a direct result of the surgery.

Response of Motor and Nonmotor Symptoms to Deep Brain Stimulation

Numerous case series and cohort studies have been published evaluating outcomes of STN-DBS in PD patients including a recent meta-analysis and summary of outcomes (16). The overall clinical experience supports a robust improvement in motor symptoms following STN-DBS. Results from this meta-analysis of 34 studies found UPDRS motor scores to improve by approximately 50% over the ensuing six months to five years. Significant reduction in

Table 2 Extra-nigral Sites of Cell Loss and Presence of Lewy Bodies in Parkinson's Disease: Neurotransmitter Involvement and Possible Anatomical Localization of Nonmotor Symptom(s)

Location	Neurotransmitter	Nonmotor symptoms
Mesocorticolimbic system	Dopamine	Neuropsychiatric
Nucleus basalis of Meynart	Acetylcholine	Cognitive
Locus ceruleus	Norepinephrine	Cognitive; neuropsychiatric; sleep; sensory/pain
Midline raphe nucleus	Serotonin	Neuropsychiatric Sleep
Hypothalamus	Dopamine, Norepinephrine Acetylcholine, GABA	Dysautonomias; sleep; fatigue; weight gain
Parasympathetic nuclei Dorsal motor nucleus of the vagus Pedunculopontine nucleus Edinger-Westphal nucleus	Acetylcholine	Dysautonomias; sleep
Sympathetic	Acetylcholine, norepinephrine	Dysautonomias
Parasympathetic	Acetylcholine	Dysautonomias
Enteric	Acetylcholine, Norepinephrine, Dopamine	Dysautonomias

dyskinesia, off-time, and dopaminergic medication requirement following surgery was also reported. Though literature regarding impact of STN-DBS on quality of life is limited, available data suggest an overall benefit; in these studies, assessments were generally based upon physical aspects of functions rather than nonmotor symptoms (16,21). This emphasizes the importance of assessing the consequences of STN-DBS on nonmotor functions as well as on motor function.

This chapter will discuss evidence for the efficacy of STN-DBS for nonmotor symptoms in PD, including disorders of autonomic function, olfaction, speech, sleep, weight, and sensation. Cognitive and psychiatric nonmotor symptoms will be addressed separately in chapters 15 and 16.

AUTONOMIC DISORDERS

The term "autonomic disorders" or "dysautonomias" refers to a broad category of nonmotor symptoms in PD. These include symptomatic orthostasis, urinary and bowel dysfunction, sexual dysfunction, sialorrhea, temperature dysregulation, and swallowing problems. Such symptoms likely involve neuronal loss in the areas of the hypothalamus, parasympathetic nuclei, and autonomic ganglia and plexi of the peripheral nervous system. Additionally, Lewy bodies have been found in the hypothalamus, sympathetic system (intermediolateral nucleus from T1 to L2 and sympathetic ganglia), parasympathetic system (dorsal, vagal, and sacral parasympathetic nuclei), adrenal medulla, and the plexi of the gut, heart, and pelvis (22). The impact of dysautonomias and their response to STN-DBS are discussed subsequently.

Cardiovascular Reflexes

Epidemiology

PD patients often experience heart rate and blood pressure variability, clinically manifested as orthostatic and/or postprandial hypotension (23,24). Orthostatic hypotension occurs in 20% to 50% of patients with PD (25–27), while the true prevalence of postprandial hypotension in PD is unknown (28).

Pathophysiology

Both orthostatic and postprandial cardiovascular changes may involve central and peripheral dysregulation of projections between the nigrostriatal pathway and the arterial baroreceptor reflex. Centrally, stimulation of the substantia nigra pars compacta has been shown to release dopamine into the striatum causing hypertension and tachycardia in animal models (29). Treatment with levodopa and dopamine agonists may also exacerbate orthostasis (30–32), while receptor blockage with haloperidol (a dopamine antagonist) blunts this effect (33). Peripherally, cardiovascular sympathetic denervation occurs in most PD patients as well, with the loss being most dramatic in those with orthostatic hypotension. Finally, postprandial effects may arise from excess release of vasodilatory gut peptides (28).

Impact of Subthalamic Nucleus-Deep Brain Stimulation

According to the classical model of basal ganglia function in PD, there is increased excitatory output from the STN resulting in increased inhibitory output from the thalamus (14); this is postulated to reduce the compensatory tachycardic response to postural changes required to prevent symptomatic orthostasis (18).

The effect of STN-DBS on cardiovascular function has been evaluated during and after surgery. Sauleau et al. (34) directly monitored objective intraoperative autonomic side effects in 17 patients undergoing STN-DBS for PD. In fifteen of these patients (88%), tachycardia arose within seconds of stimulation, while hypertension lagged by approximately one minute. Return to baseline occurred within a few minutes following discontinuation of stimulation. Kaufmann et al. (35) noted that high-frequency STN-DBS caused tachycardia six months after surgery, suggesting that the immediate trend towards tachycardia after STN-DBS may persist. Conversely, Holmberg et al. (30) investigated cardiovascular autonomic function in 11 patients with bilateral STN-DBS for advanced PD and found no lasting effect after surgery. Five of 11 (45%) patients showed significant orthostatic hypotension and pathological heart rate variability with deep breathing at enrollment; there was no significant change in these functions at one-year follow-up.

As such, available data suggest that STN-DBS may cause transient tachycardia and hypertension though the long-term clinical significance of this is unknown.

Gastroparesis and Constipation

Epidemiology

Gastroparesis and constipation were recognized as features of PD by Dr. Parkinson (1) and remain frequent complications of the disease. Collectively, early satiety, abdominal fullness, nausea, vomiting, and constipation have been identified in up to 48% of PD patients (36). Edwards et al. (37) found 51% of PD patients with constipation (less than three bowel movements per week) and 64% with defecatory dysfunction (stooling with straining or incomplete evacuation). Constipation alone also increases in severity and frequency as PD progresses (37,38).

Pathophysiology

The presence of Lewy bodies in the myenteric plexi of the esophagus and colon supports a primarily peripheral mechanism for these symptoms of dysmotility. Nausea and vomiting may also arise from central involvement of the dorsal motor nucleus of the vagus. These symptoms have shown variable responses to levodopa replacement (37,39). One study by Hardoff et al. (36) proposed that levodopa may initially further slow gastric emptying, while long-term treatment resulted in improved motility as a result of increasing intestinal dyskinesia. Use of central dopamine agonists to improve motility have been disappointing, and nausea can be further exacerbated by levodopa or dopamine agonists due to unwanted stimulation of peripheral dopamine receptors. The addition of peripheral dopamine antagonists (i.e., domperidone) improves gastric emptying in PD and alleviates nausea (40,41).

Impact of Subthalamic Nucleus-Deep Brain Stimulation

There is no data available regarding the effects of STN-DBS on gastric dysmotility. However, given the relatively unreliable response to dopaminergic replacement therapy described above, it is unlikely that STN-DBS would markedly affect gastroparesis or constipation.

Sialorrhea

Epidemiology

Sialorrhea occurs in 70% to 80% of PD patients (42,43). It is typically an early feature of the disease, initially occurring at night as wetting of the pillow, and progressing to daytime drooling as the disease advances. It may occur in combination with dysphagia. Eadie and Tyrer (42) reported drooling in 86% of PD patients with swallowing difficulties and in 44% of patients without swallowing difficulties.

Pathophysiology

Sialorrhea may be both a motor and a nonmotor symptom of PD. Management of secretions depends on two processes: salivary production and salivary control. Pathophysiologically, salivary production involves central and peripheral dopaminergic activity (43a) as well as parasympathetic cholinergic activity at the glandular level. Salivary production may actually be lessened in PD patients (44), but lingual and facial bradykinesia worsen salivatory control and lead to drooling (42,45). Sialorrhea may cause serious medical consequences (i.e., choking and aspiration pneumonia) as well as embarrassing social situations.

Impact of Subthalamic Nucleus-Deep Brain Stimulation

No published STN-DBS studies have evaluated sialorrhea as a primary outcome. Two reports of increased sialorrhea have been published as adverse effects (46,47). One of these may have been complicated by worsened cognition contributing to reduced control of secretions. Esselink (48) reported increased drooling at six months of follow-up in three out of 20 PD patients that underwent STN-DBS. It is not clear that this is an effect of DBS; other factors, such as natural progression of disease or modification of medication regimens, may have influenced this outcome. Dry mouth or improved salivary control has not been reported after STN-DBS.

Dysphagia

Epidemiology

Dysphagia is a relatively common and treatment-resistant manifestation of PD, affecting approximately 50% of patients with mild-to-moderate disease (Hoehn and Yahr stage $= 2-3$) (37). The prevalence of dysphagia rises as disease duration progresses (42,49). Up to 30% of PD patients have accompanying signs of aspiration (coughing, choking, and nocturnal dyspnea) (49,50). Evaluating two cohorts of PD patients with similar severity, Ali et al. (51) found at least one objective indicator of pharyngeal dysfunction in 12 out of 12 patients with subjective dysphagia (mean H & Y $= 2.58$), as well as in six out of seven patients without subjective dysphagia (mean H & Y $= 2.43$), indicating that swallowing abnormalities are more prevalent than clinically recognized.

Pathophysiology

Normal swallowing is a complex process involving highly coordinated contraction and relaxation of the masticatory muscles, teeth, tongue, pharynx, and esophagus. This process includes motor and nonmotor components, as well as dopamine and nondopamine-mediated systems. The process can also be divided into oropharyngeal and esophageal phases. At the neuronal level, swallowing is mediated by the nucleus tractus solitarius and substantia reticularis via voluntary and autonomic afferent and efferent neural projections.

While voluntary activity is largely nondopaminergic, bradykinesia and rigidity primarily affect the oropharyngeal phase, suggesting dopamine-mediated extrapyramidal involvement (52–54). Dysfunction of the esophageal phase has been attributed to central damage to the DMN of the vagus and peripheral dopamine depletion. The upper esophageal sphincter has been found to exhibit incomplete relaxation in up to 25% of PD patients (51), possibly due to involvement of the DMN. Lewy bodies have been found in the myenteric plexi of the distal one-third of the esophagus of PD patients, supporting peripheral involvement (55).

The literature is inconsistent regarding the effects of dopamine replacement on dysphagia (54,56,57). Monte et al. (54) demonstrated that any apparent benefit may actually be mediated by intercurrent medication-induced dyskinesia, as dyskinetic patients performed better in oropharyngeal swallowing function than nondyskinetic patients. Generally, swallowing is more coordinated when medications are working (i.e., the "ON" state).

Impact of Subthalamic Nucleus-Deep Brain Stimulation

Dysphagia has been reported as an adverse event in some of the published outcome studies, occurring in approximately 4% to 8% of patients followed (58–60). It is unclear whether the reported worsening of swallowing function is a direct result of STN-DBS or a progression of disease with further involvement of nondopaminergically mediated pathways. Only one study has directly evaluated postoperative dysphagia (61). Bejjani et al. (61) found swallowing function after STN-DBS off medication to be similar to preoperative functioning on medication in 10 patients, consistent with the fact that there is some dopaminergically-mediated component to swallowing. Further studies are needed to assess the true impact of STN-DBS on swallowing function.

Hyperhidrosis and Seborrhea

Epidemiology

Nearly two-thirds of PD patients report sweating abnormalities (8,62,63), with the majority suffering from hyperhidrosis. Seborrheic dermatitis affects more than 50% of PD patients (64). It has been suggested that excessive perspiration and sebum production may worsen as a nonmotor "off" symptom (8,64–66), and hyperhidrosis is particularly exacerbated by accompanying dyskinesias (62). Many PD patients describe these symptoms as a source of significant physical, social, and emotional disability (62).

Pathophysiology

Sweating occurs when the anterior hypothalamus activates the sympathetic sudomotor reflex, causing eccrine sweat production and peripheral vasodilation via postganglionic cholinergic fibers (67). In PD, it is hypothesized that hyperhidrosis arises from preganglionic dysregulation early in the disease process, progressing to postganglionic pathology later (63). Dopaminergic replacement therapies can improve symptoms in early disease (66), though sweating can also be a side effect of dopamine excess. Seborrhea is thought to arise from dopamine depletion that leads to release of melanocyte-stimulating hormone and sebum (68). In addition, bradykinesia and immobility leads to stasis of secreted sebum, yeast growth, and subsequent dermatitis (68). Improved motor function alone may also relieve excessive seborrhea and hyperhidrosis (62,64,66). Similar to hyperhidrosis, there is evidence that dopamine replacement directly mitigates sebum production (64,69).

Impact of Subthalamic Nucleus-Deep Brain Stimulation

Currently, there are no published studies addressing the impact of STN-DBS on hyperhidrosis or seborrhea in PD. There is experimental evidence that STN-DBS may decrease sympathetic skin response (70).

Temperature Dysregulation

Epidemiology

Recent descriptive statistics on temperature dysregulation in PD are lacking. Appenzeller and Goss (1971) described failure of thermoregulation in 18 out of 25 patients, measured by reflex vasodilatation of digits in response to increasing body temperature (71).

Pathophysiology

Temperature dysregulation issues in PD usually manifest as heat intolerance, likely arising from reduced sweating response and impaired peripheral vasodilatation via somatosympathetic reflexes (71). Poorly delineated mechanisms of sympathetic hyperactivity and dysregulated basal ganglionic involvement also lead to the overproduction of heat (18). Involvement of dopaminergic systems within the basal ganglia is also supported by the neuroleptic malignant syndrome (NMS) characterized by hyperthermia and rigidity in the setting of dopamine withdrawal or D2-receptor blockade. Conversely, there is also evidence for lowered nocturnal core body temperature in PD (72).

In addition to causing the discomfort of heat intolerance, thermoregulatory mechanisms may impact motor symptoms in PD. Meigal and Lupandin (73) reviewed the evidence for a "thermoregulation-dependent component" of PD. Analogous to a "cold shivering," tremor may involuntarily activate to overcome misperceived heat loss. Similarly, there is evidence that decreased body temperature activates flexor musculature, which may contribute to stooped posture and festinating gait. Animal models have identified the "efferent tract of shivering" to be the ventromedial and dorsomedial hypothalamus, caudate nucleus, putamen, globus pallidus, substantia nigra, red nucleus, mesencephalic reticular formation, and the lateral portion of reticular formation of pons and medulla (74,75). This shows considerable overlap with the primary pathological damage seen in PD.

Impact of Subthalamic Nucleus-Deep Brain Stimulation

Temperature dysregulation has not been studied directly in STN-DBS. In 2004, Linazasoro et al. (76) described a case of STN-DBS masking "possible" NMS in PD. Hyperthermia, hyperhidrosis, and hypertension were presumed due to NMS from levodopa withdrawal, while lack of rigidity was attributed to a subthalamotomy effect. In this single case, there was an absence of effect on temperature regulation by STN-DBS though conclusions cannot be drawn based on this limited experience.

Urologic Dysfunction

Epidemiology

Urologic dysfunction affects up to 70% of PD patients (77,78). The extent of dysfunction increases with progression of PD (77).

Pathophysiology

Loss of bladder control in PD is multifactorial. Decreased bladder capacity (79), detrusor hyperreflexia (77), motor fluctuations (80), and diminished mobility

(81,82) have been suggested as contributing factors of incontinence. Several animal models support the theory of basal ganglionic control of the bladder (18) and administration of D1-agonists provides improved urinary control in nonhuman primates (83). In humans, levodopa treatment usually worsens detrusor hyperreflexia; this may enhance emptying during the voiding phase, but it may aggravate incontinence during the filling phase (84a). If functional micturition is worsened by diminished mobility, dopamine replacement may provide some relief.

Impact of Subthalamic Nucleus-Deep Brain Stimulation

Cystometrogram studies demonstrate that stimulation of the globus pallidus reduces detrusor hyperreflexia in rats (85); in humans, STN-DBS should provide a similar effect. Two prospective studies have evaluated STN-DBS and urinary function. Finazzi-Agro et al. (86) reported significantly increased bladder capacity and reflex volume in five patients with bilateral STN-DBS; detrusor hyperreflexia showed a trend for improvement. A larger trial by Seif et al. demonstrated significantly increased bladder capacity and reduced voiding desire (i.e., urge) after bilateral STN-DBS in 16 patients (87). These preliminary findings suggest a positive impact of STN-DBS on urinary function.

Sexual Dysfunction

Epidemiology

Sexual dysfunction in PD is a common disorder, affecting men more often than women. Rates of sexual dissatisfaction have been reported as 59% in men and 36% in women (88).

Pathophysiology

Modulation of sexual desire in PD is a complex process involving both dopaminergic and nondopaminergic mechanisms. Considering sexual behavior in two stages (anticipatory and consummatory), two central dopaminergic systems are implicated. The anticipatory stage involves the mesolimbic-mesocortical system with arousal, motivation, and reward, while the consummatory stage requires motor coordination from the nigrostriatal system (88,89). The motor stage is more critical in men for erection and ejaculation. Other nonmotor features of urologic dysfunction, sleep disturbances, mood changes, and diminished cognition may also impact libido. Dopamine replacement with levodopa or dopamine agonists generally improves sexual function, particularly in younger patients (90,91). Hypersexuality has been reported in several patients after initiation of dopaminergic therapy as well (92–95), possibly from additional activation of the D3-receptors of the mesolimbic system. Hypersexuality as a manifestation of an impulse control disorder associated with dopaminergic therapy has become increasingly recognized (92).

Impact of Subthalamic Nucleus-Deep Brain Stimulation

A single published trial reported improved sexual well-being as a primary outcome following STN-DBS (95). Castelli et al. found increased frequency, increased satisfaction, and decreased avoidance of sexual activity in men less than 60. While there was no significant change in sexual functioning for women in this study, depression scores improved; this has been shown to be highly correlated with sexual well-being in other studies (96,97).

Others have reported hypersexuality following STN-DBS as an adverse effect (61,98). Hypersexuality with mania affected five out of 57 reported patients from two case series, though an accurate incidence would require larger studies (61,98). The mechanism for excessive arousal is unknown.

DISORDERS OF SMELL

Epidemiology

Significant olfactory deficits occur in PD, affecting more than 70% of individuals of varying stages of disease (99,100). It has been suggested that seemingly idiopathic hyposmia may represent a preclinical marker of PD, conferring at least a 10% risk of developing the disease among first degree relatives of PD patients (101).

Pathophysiology

Early pathologic changes, including Lewy bodies, have been found in the olfactory bulb and the anterior olfactory nucleus (103). Subsequent neurodegeneration of the olfactory tract correlates with disease duration (104) and olfactory function may worsen with more severe PD (102). Treatment with dopaminergic or cholinergic agents has not demonstrated improvement in olfaction (100,105).

Impact of Subthalamic Nucleus-Deep Brain Stimulation

One published trial evaluated olfaction as a primary outcome of treatment with STN-DBS (106). Hummel et al. demonstrated improvement in mean odor discrimination among nine hyposmic PD patients with bilateral STN-DBS. There was no change in odor threshold measures. The authors propose an indirect effect of DBS on olfaction, perhaps through release of inhibitory cortical-basal ganglionic projections. This is supported by two case reports of subjectively improved olfaction after transcranial electromagnetic stimulation of the entire head, which may also block inhibitory processes (107).

SPEECH DISORDERS

Epidemiology

Speech disorders are common in PD, reported in up to 89% of patients with advanced disease (108,109). More simple disorders of voice (loudness, pitch, rate, breathiness) typically precede complex perturbations of articulation, fluency, and prosody (110,111).

Pathophysiology

Like swallowing function, normal speech production requires the coordination of multiple modalities, as laryngeal, respiratory, and articulatory functions are required to create intelligible speech. Speech dysfunction in PD is complex and probably multifactorial. Basal ganglionic pathology of PD may result in "hypokinetic dysarthria" with hypophonia, monotony, breathiness, and hoarseness (112,113). Discoordinated chest wall and respiratory muscle movements, coupled with reduced airflow across the vocal folds, can also contribute to hypokinetic dysarthria (112). Other factors, such as glottal incompetence (114), poor vocal fold closure (115,116), impaired fold vibration (115), and laryngeal tremor (115) may also contribute to speech disability. In addition, poor articulation with imprecise consonants, stuttering, pallilalia, and impaired prosody has also been described in PD patients, representing more definitively nonmotor symptomatology (109,111). Greater description of the features of hypokinetic dysarthria is beyond the scope of this chapter, and more detailed reviews are available in the literature (112,113,117).

Sensory feedback has also been implicated in the pathophysiology of speech disability. It has been proposed that the basal ganglia assist in deciphering afferent sensory information to help guide coordinated motor movements and impaired speech in PD may arise from damage to this feedback loop (118). A recent study of two PD patients undergoing STN-DBS surgery (prior to stimulation) revealed that neuronal activity as measured by microelectrode activity within the STN directly correlated to vocal tasks, likely related to planning of speech (119). Poststimulation data has not been published. Few positive reports of dopaminergic therapy on speech have been reported either (117,120,121), consistent with the notion that hypokinetic dysarthria may be a nonmotor, nondopaminergic complication of PD. Furthermore, even if dopaminergic agents slightly improve vocalization early, subsequent worsening dyskinesias can exacerbate dysarthria as the disease progresses (122).

Impact of Subthalamic Nucleus-Deep Brain Stimulation

The effect of STN-DBS upon speech has been evaluated in several studies, and the results remain mixed. It has been proposed that simple motor aspects of speech (hypophonia, breathiness) may improve in a similar manner to other motor aspects of the disease, while overall articulation from complex coordination of multiple neuronal circuits are less responsive (123). Several authors have reported improvements in lingual and phonic parameters after STN-DBS, likely the result of motor benefits of lip, tongue, and pharyngeal movements (124–128). Other publications have shown deleterious effects following STN-DBS surgery on speech (129,130). In the largest long-term series of STN-DBS published to date, Krack et al. (129) found that speech continued to decline for five years postsurgery. Speech may be a symptom less amenable to surgical intervention that continues to deteriorate as part of the natural history of disease. There is no clear evidence that there is causality between STN-DBS surgery and worsening speech, but there are the descriptions of worsened dysarthria and hypophonia published as side effects (16). This side effect, particularly at higher levels of stimulation, may arise from diffusion of current from the STN to the corticobulbar fibers controlling laryngeal, pharyngeal, and lingual muscles (123,131) and should improve with adjustment and optimization of stimulation parameters.

SLEEP DISORDERS AND FATIGUE

Epidemiology

Sleep disorders comprise a varied and under-recognized constellation of abnormalities causing significant morbidity in PD. Problems include restless legs syndrome (RLS) and periodic limb movements disorder (PLMD), REM-sleep behavior disorder (RBD), shifting circadian rhythms, and insomnia (132). Resultant excessive daytime sleepiness (EDS) has been recognized in over 50% of PD patients (132). Distinct from sleepiness, fatigue in PD describes exhaustion or loss of energy without the need for more sleep (133). It affects about 50% of patients with PD (134), and it is not related to stage or duration of disease (135).

Pathophysiology

The pathophysiology of sleep disturbances in PD depends upon the particular disturbance. Descriptions of fatigue are so nonspecific that discreet localization within the neuroaxis is not practical.

RLS describes an urge to move the legs while at rest, worse at night, and relieved by movement (136). PLMD describes periodic episodes of repetitive stereotypical movements of the legs associated with sleep disturbance (137). Collectively, these movements may occur from dopaminergic depletion in the nigro-striatal pathway, possibly mediated or exaggerated in the setting of iron deficiency (138).

RBD results in motor activity during the usual atonic REM-stage of sleep, likely arising from disruption of the complex network of dopaminergic, cholinergic, noradrenergic, and serotonergic pathways in the brainstem that are involved in the pathology of PD (139). In early PD, neuronal dropout and Lewy body deposition occurs rostrally through the brainstem. This stepwise involvement of the medullary nucleus reticularis magnocellularis, the pontine locus ceruleus, and the midbrain pedunculopontine nucleus (PPN) and substantia nigra could explain why RBD precedes significant parkinsonism in many patients.

In shifting circadian rhythms (under suprachiasmatic nuclear control), the trend for earlier sleep onset results in earlier morning awakenings (140). This may be exaggerated in the PD patient whose sleep is already disrupted by RLS/PLMD or RBD.

Primary insomnia, as fragmented sleep and increased sleep latency, is more common in PD patients, though a particular pathologic correlate is not known (141). Worsened nighttime motor symptoms (tremor, dystonia, akinesia) can also contribute to disrupted sleep.

EDS may result from any nighttime disruption of sleep, and it typically worsens in the PD patient in conjunction with worsening cognitive impairment; each symptom can exacerbate the other, leading to a vicious cycle (133). "Sleep attacks" are defined by the irresistible urge to sleep not preceded by sleepiness (classically seen in narcolepsy) (132,142). These phenomena are recognized in PD patients, but the risk can be quadrupled in patients taking dopamine agonists (ergot and nonergot) (142,143). A less pronounced risk is seen with levodopa therapy.

Impact of Subthalamic Nucleus-Deep Brain Stimulation

Sleep generally gets better after STN-DBS. Sleep architecture, sleep quality and sleep duration improve, associated with reduced nighttime symptoms of akithisia, dystonia, cramps, and tremor (144–150). Along with reduction in motor symptoms, other hypotheses for sleep improvements relate to secondary benefits of STN-DBS including improved mood and reduction of dopaminergic agents (147). A primary response to STN-DBS is also a possibility, as it has been proposed that inhibition of STN output to the PPN diminishes its influence upon disrupted sleep-wake cycles (147).

In contrast to its beneficial effect upon overall sleep, STN-DBS has demonstrated inconsistent results with regard to RLS, RBD, and EDS. Kedia et al. (151) described the new appearance of RLS in 11 out of 195 patients following STN-DBS. It was proposed that the reduction of dopaminergic agents could have "unmasked" latent symptoms. Conversely, Driver-Dunckley et al. (152) reported six advanced PD patients with improved symptoms after bilateral STN-DBS, even with decreased dopamine equivalent usage. Others have reported no effect (Iranzo, Hjort, Lyons, Monaca). There are no reports of benefit or detriment of STN-DBS on RBD. Most authors report no change in the EDS after STN-DBS (145,146,150), while others reported improvement (153) and worsening (154). Finally, Krack et al. (155) described fatigue and "lack of initiative" in two out of eight STN-DBS patients, attributing it to medication withdrawal postoperatively. Fatigue has not adequately been assessed as an outcome measure in STN-DBS trials.

METABOLIC DISORDERS AND WEIGHT CHANGES

Epidemiology

Weight loss commonly occurs in PD, affecting more than half of patients (156). In one study of 51 PD cases and 49 age- and sex-matched controls, four times as many PD patients reported weight loss of at least 10 pounds versus controls, with a mean weight loss of 7.2 pounds (157).

Pathophysiology

Loss of weight in PD has been attributed to an increase in resting energy expenditure in the form of dyskinesia (158). Diminished food intake may be due to bradykinesia with increased chewing time, gastroparesis with early satiety, and swallowing dysfunction. Depression commonly occurs in PD and may also result in decreased appetite and intake. Finally, dopaminergic medication side effects such as nausea and vomiting also contribute to decreased intake (158,159).

Impact of Subthalamic Nucleus-Deep Brain Stimulation

Weight gain has become a well-recognized consequence of STN-DBS, though whether it is transitory, or permanent is not known. Several studies have specifically evaluated weight gain in STN-DBS, while others have reported it as a side effect. Barichella et al. (160) followed 30 patients (22 male, 8 female) up to 12 months postoperatively and found that all but one of the patients in the study gained weight. Average weight gain in these patients was 9.3 kg. Similarly, Macia et al. (161) found that all of 18 post-STN-DBS patients studied experienced weight gain with an average increase of 9.7 kg within the first three months. Other investigators have reported a high prevalence of weight gain as a side effect in their cohorts (130,154,162–164).

STN-DBS improves rigidity, reduces dyskinesia, and allows the reduction of levodopa requirements—all measures that collectively decrease resting energy expenditure and diminish nausea, leading to increased weight. Weight management with attention to proper diet and exercise need to be part of preoperative counseling.

PAIN AND OTHER SENSORY DISTURBANCES

Epidemiology

Sensory disturbances are an underappreciated manifestation of PD. Up to 75% of PD patients experience pain attributed to their disease (8,166,167). Symptoms may arise secondary to painful dyskinesia, akithesia, and dystonia, but up to 30% of patients experience sensations representing a "primary" sensory syndrome not attributable to these (166). Complaints include burning, aching, itching, or tingling sensations in varied parts of the body (168). It has also been shown that concomitant pain in PD leads to significantly lower health-related quality of life for the patients (169).

Pathophysiology

Pain in PD can be considered as a primary syndrome, representing another nonmotor complication of the disease. Chudler and Dong (170) reviewed a multifactorial model of the basal ganglionic role in primary pain, involving nociception, affect, cognition, and modulation. While the details are beyond the scope of this chapter, there is evidence of inhibitory pallidothalamic and nigrothalamic pathways that modulate pain. In PD, loss of dopaminergic neurons from these pathways may trigger excitatory first-order pain fibers to spontaneously transmit at the level of the dorsal horn. Similarly, neurodegeneration may allow for stimulus hypersensitivity within the basal ganglia. Djaldetti et al. (168) confirmed that PD patients demonstrate decreased threshold for thermal pain correlated with the more affected side. This hypersensitivity did not vary with stage or duration of disease. Further, stimulation of the substantia nigra inhibits nociceptive activity from the intralaminar neurons of the thalamus.

Impact of Subthalamic Nucleus-Deep Brain Stimulation

While pallidothalamic and nigrothalamic connections have been implicated in primary pain, the STN has not been singularly recognized. Furthermore, while intractable pain has been treated by DBS for the past half century, the specific targets have always been the sensory thalamus, internal capsule, or periventricular/ periacqueductal grey areas (171). No prospective studies in STN-DBS have evaluated pain as a primary outcome, though surrogate measures of dystonia and dyskinesia have evaluated secondary pain. The effectiveness of STN-DBS in improving dystonia and dyskinesia is well established (16), though STN-DBS effect on pain as a nonmotor symptom has not specifically been reported.

SUMMARY

While STN-DBS is performed to improve the motor symptoms of PD, knowledge of its effects upon the nonmotor aspects of the disease is valuable for the treating physician. Generally, the patient may expect some persistent improvement in urologic function, sexual satisfaction, olfaction, sleep quality, and secondary pain. Transient changes in heart rate (increased) and blood pressure (increased) are also possible. Postoperative weight gain is well described, and this may represent a positive outcome in patients with excessive weight loss prior to surgery. There are no convincing effects of STN-DBS upon gastrointestinal function, skin changes, temperature dysregulation, and primary sensory syndromes in PD. Persistently worsened swallowing and drooling have been noted in patients after STN-DBS, but it is unclear whether these represent a side effect of the surgery or the natural progression of a treatment-resistent nonmotor symptom of PD. Effects upon speech remain mixed, and careful adjustment of stimulation parameters may relieve worsened dysarthria and hypophonia. With an understanding of potential nonmotor outcomes from surgery, the patient and caregiver can have realistic expectations of the full potential of STN-DBS in treating PD.

REFERENCES

1. Parkinson, J. An Essay on the Shaking Palsy. London: Sherwood, Neely, and Jones; 1817.
2. Hughes AJ, Daniel SE, Kilford L, Lees AJ. Accuracy of clinical diagnosis of idiopathic Parkinson's disease: a clinico-pathological study of 100 cases. J Neurol Neurosurg Psychiatry 1992; 55:181–184.
3. Shulman LM, Taback RL, Bean J, Weiner WJ. Comorbidity of the non-motor symptoms of Parkinson's disease. Mov Disord 2001; 16(3):507–510.
4. Aarsland D, Andersen K, Larsen J, Lolk A, Kragh-Sørensen P. Prevalence and characteristics of dementia in Parkinson disease: an 8-year prospective study. Arch Neurol 2003; 60:387–392.
5. Emre M. Dementia associated with Parkinson's disease. Lancet 2003; 2:229–237.
6. Hobson P, Meara J. Risk and incidence of dementia in a cohort of older subjects with Parkinson's disease in the United Kingdom. Mov Disord 2004; 19:1043–1049.
7. Singer C, Weiner WJ, et al. Autonomic dysfunction in men with PD. Eur Neurol 1992; 32:134–140.
8. Witjas T, Kaphan E, Azulay JP, Blin O, Ceccaldi M, Pouget J, Poncet M, Cherif AA. Nonmotor fluctuations in Parkinson's disease: frequent and disabling. Neurology 2002; 59:408–413.
9. Fahn S, Elton RL, Members of UPDRS Development Committee. Unified Parkinson Disease Rating Scale. In: Fahn S, Marsden CD, Calne DB, eds. Recent Developments in Parkinsons Disease. Florham Park, NJ: Macmillan Health Care Information, 1987:153–164.
10. The Movement Disorder Society Task Force for Rating Scales for Parkinson's Disease. The Unified Parkinson's Disease Rating Scale (UPDRS): status and recommendations. Mov Disord 2003; 18:738–750.
11. Shulman LM, Taback RL, Rabinstein AA, Weiner WJ. Non-recognition of depression and other non-motor symptoms in Parkinson's disease. Parkinsonism and Related Disroders 2002; 8(3):193–197.
12. Goetz C. Letter to the editor: Re: UPDRS: Status and Recommendations. Mov Disord 2004; 19(5):605.
13. Miyasaki JM, Shannon K, Voon V, et al. Quality Standards Subcommittee of the American Academy of Neurology. Practice Parameter: evaluation and treatment of depression, psychosis, and dementia in Parkinson disease (an evidence-based review): report of the Quality Standards Subcommittee of the American Academy of Neurology. Neurology 2006; 66:996–1002.
14. Albin RL, Young AB, Penney JB. The functional anatomy of basal ganglia disorders. Trends Neurosci 1989; 12:366–375.

15. DeLong MR: Primate models of movement disorders of basal ganglia origin. Trends Neurosci 1990; 13:281–285.
16. Kleiner-Fisman G, Herzog J, Fisman D, et al. Subthalamic nucleus deep brain stimulation: summary and meta-analysis of outcome. Mov Disord 2006; S290–S304.
17. Kimura M. Role of basal ganglia in behavioral learning. Neurosci Res 1995; 22:353–358.
18. Pazo JH, Belforte JE. Basal ganglia and functions of the autonomic nervous system. Celular and Molecular Neurobiology 2002; 22(5/6):645–654.
19. Brown LL, Feldman SM. The organization of somatosensory activity in dorsolateral striatum of the rat. Prog Brain Res 1993; 99:237–250.
20. Langston JW. The Parkinson's complex: parkinsonism is just the tip of the iceberg. Ann Neurol 2006; 59(4):591–596.
21. Drapier S, Raoul S, Drapier D, et al. Only physical aspects of quality of life are significantly improved by bilateral subthalamic stimulation in Parkinson's disease. Journal of Neurology 2005; 252(5):583–588.
22. Micieli G, Tosi P, Marcheselli P, Cavallini A. Autonomic dysfunction in Parkinson's disease. Neurological Sciences 2003; 24:S32–S34.
23. Golstein DS, Holmes CS, Dendi R, Bruce SR, Li ST. Orthostatic hypotension from sympathetic denervation in Parkinson's disease. Neurology 2002; 58: 1247–1255.
24. Senard JM, Brefel-Courbon C, Rascol O, Montrastuc JL. Orthostatic hypotension in patients with Parkinson's disease: Pathophysiology and management. Drugs Aging 2001; 18:495–505.
25. Dewey RB. Autonomic dysfunction in Parkinson's disease. Neurol Clin 2004; 22:S127–S139.
26. Micieli G, Martignoni F, Cavalinlini A, Sandrini G, Nappi G. Postprandial and orthostatic hypotension in Parkinson's disease. Neurology 1987; 37:386–393.
27. Orimo S, Oka T, Miura H, Tsuchiya K, Mori F, Wakabayashi K. Sympathetic cardiac denervation in Parkinson's disease and pure autonomic failure but not in multiple system atrophy. J Neurol Neurosurg Psychiatry 2002; 73:776–777.
28. Chaudhuri KR, Ellis C, Love-Jones S, et al. Postprandial hypotension and parkinsonian state in Parkinson's disease. Mov Disord 1997; 12(6):877–884.
29. Lin MT, Yang JJ. Stimulation of the nigrostriatal dopamine system produces hypertension and tachycardia. Am J Physiol 1994; 266:H2489–H2496.
30. Holmberg B, Corneliusson O, Elam M. Bilateral stimulation of nucleus subthalamicus in advanced Parkinson's disease: No effects on, and of, autonomic dysfunction. Mov Disord 2005; 20(8):976–981.
31. Haapaniemi TH, Kallio MA, Korpelainen JT, et al. Levodopa, bromocriptine and selegiline modify cardiovascular responses in Parkinson's disease. J Neurol 2000; 247:868–874.
32. Kujawa K, Leurgans S, Raman R, Blasucci L, Goetz CG. Acute orthostatic hypotension when starting dopamine agonists in Parkinson's disease. Arch Neurol 2000; 57:1461–1463.
33. Linthorst ACE, Van den Buuse M, De Jong W, Versteeg DHG. Electrically stimulated [3H]dopamine and [14C]acetylcholine release from nucleus caudatus slices: differences between spontaneously hypertensive rats and Wistar-Kyoto rats. Brain Res 1990; 509:266–272.

34. Sauleau P, Raoul S, Lallement F, et al. Motor and non motor effects during intraoperative subthalamic stimulation for Parkinson's disease. J Neurol 2005; 252(4):457–464.
35. Kaufmann H, Bhattacharya KF, Voustianiouk A, Gracies JM. Stimulation of the subthalamic nucleus increases heart rate in patients with Parkinson disease. Neurology 2002; 59:1657.
36. Hardoff R, Sula M, Tamir A, et al. Gastric emptying time and gastric motility in patients with Parkinson's disease. Mov Disord 2001; 16(6):1041–1047.
37. Edwards L, Quigley EM, Hofman R, Pfeiffer RF. Gastrointestinal symptoms in Parkinson disease: 18-month follow-up study. Mov Disord 1993; 8:83–86.
38. Magerkurth C, Schnitzer R, Braune S. Symptoms of autonomic failure in Parkinson's disease: prevalence and impact on daily life. Clin Auton Res 2005; 15:76–82.
39. Thomaides T, Karapanayiotides T, Zoukos Y, et al. Gastric emptying after semisolid food in multiple system atrophy and Parkinson disease. J Neurol 2005; 252:1055–1059.
40. Soykan I, Sarosiek I, Shifflett J, Wooten GF, McCallum RW. Effect of chronic oral domperidone therapy on gastrointestinal symptoms and gastric emptying in patients with Parkinson's disease. Mov Disord 1997; 12:952–957.
41. Jost WH. Gastrointestinal motility problems in patients with Parkinson's disease. Effects of antiparkinsonian treatment and guidelines for management. Drugs Aging 1997; 10:249–258.
42. Eadie MJ, Tyrer JH. Alimentary disorder in parkinsonism. Australas Ann Med 1965; 14:13–22.
43. Edwards LL, Quigley EM, Pfeiffer RF. Gastrointestinal dysfunction in Parkinson's disease: frequency and pathophysiology. Neurology 1992; 42:726–732.
43a. Pazo JH, Medina JH, Tumilasci OR. The role of caudate-putamen nucleus in salivary secretion induced by L-DOPA. Neuropharmacology 1982; 21(3):261–265.
44. Proulx M, De Courval FP, Wiseman MA, Panisset M. Salivary production in Parkinson's disease. Mov Disord 2005; 20(2):204–207.
45. Bateson MC, Gibberd FB, Wilson RS. Salivary symptoms in Parkinson disease. Arch Neurol 1973; 29:274–275.
46. Thobois S, Mertens P, Guenot M, et al. Subthalamic nucleus stimulation in Parkinson's disease: clinical evaluation of 18 patients. J Neurol 2002; 249:529–534.
47. Hariz MI, Johansson F, Shamsgovara P, Johansson E, Hariz GM, Fagerlund M. Bilateral subthalamic nucleus stimulation in a parkinsonian patient with preoperative deficits in speech and cognition: persistent improvement in mobility but increased dependency: a case study. Mov Disord 2000; 15(1):136–139.
48. Esselink RA, de Bie RM, de Haan RJ, et al. Unilateral pallidotomy versus bilateral subthalamic nucleus stimulation in PD: a randomized trial. Neurology 2004; 62:201–207.
49. Edwards LL, Pfeiffer RF, Quigley EM, Hofman R, Balluff M. Gastrointestinal symptoms in Parkinson's disease. Mov Disord 1991; 6:151–156.
50. Goetz CG, Lutge W, Tanner CM. Autonomic dysfunction in Parkinson's disease. Neurology 1986; 36:73–75.
51. Ali GN, Wallace KL, Schwartz R, DeCarle DJ, Zagami AS, Cook IJ. Mechanisms of oral-pharyngeal dysphagia in patients with Parkinson's disease. Gastroenterology 1996; 110:383–392.

52. Bushmann M, Dobmeyer SM, Leeker L, Perlmutter JS. Swallowing abnormalities and their response to treatment in Parkinson's disease. Neurology 1989; 39: 1309–1314.
53. Palmer ED. Dysphagia in parkinsonism. JAMA 1974; 229:1349.
54. Monte FS, da Silva-Junior FP, Braga-Neto P, Nobre e Souza MA, Sales de Bruin VM. Swallowing abnormalities and dyskinesia in Parkinson's disease. Mov Disord 2005; 20:457–462.
55. Wakabayashi K, Takahashi H, Takeda S, Ohama E, Ikuta F. Parkinson's disease: the presence of Lewy bodies in Auerbach's and Meissner's plexuses. Acta Neuropathol (Berl) 1988; 76:217–221.
56. Tison F, Wiart L, Guatterie M, et al. Effects of central dopaminergic stimulation by apomorphine on swallowing disorders in Parkinson's disease. Mov Disord 1996; 11:729–732.
57. Hunter PC, Crameri J, Austin S, Woodward MC, Hughes AJ. Response of parkinsonian swallowing dysfunction to dopaminergic stimulation. J Neurol Neurosurg Psychiatry 1997; 63:579–583.
58. Ostergaard K, Sunde N, Dupont E. Effects of bilateral stimulation of the subthalamic nucleus in patients with severe Parkinson's disease and motor fluctuations. Mov Disord 2002; 17:693–700.
59. Valldeoriola F, Pilleri M, Tolosa E, Molinuevo JL, Rumia J, Ferrer E. Bilateral sub-thalamic stimulation monotherapy in advanced Parkinson's disease: long-term follow-up of patients. Mov Disord 2002; 17:125–132.
60. Krause M, Fogel W, Heck A, et al. Deep brain stimulation for the treatment of Parkinson's disease: subthalamic nucleus versus globus pallidus internus. J Neurol Neurosurg Psychiatry 2001; 70:464–470.
61. Bejjani BP, Gervais D, Arnulf I, et al. Axial parkinsonian symptoms can be improved: the role of levodopa and bilateral subthalamic stimulation. J Neurol Neurosurg Psychiatry 2000; 68:595–600.
62. Swinn L, Schrag A, Viswanathan R, Bloem BR, Lees A, Quinn N. Sweating dysfunction in Parkinson's disease. Mov Disord 2003; 18:1459–1463.
63. Mano Y, Nakamuro T, Takayanagi T, Mayer RF. Sweat function in Parkinson's disease. J Neurol 1994; 241:573–576.
64. Fischer M, Gemende I, Marsch WC, Fischer PA. Skin function and skin disorders in Parkinson's disease. J Neural Transm 2001; 108:205–213.
65. Raudino F. Non motor off in Parkinson's disease. Acta Neurol Scand 2001; 104:312–315.
66. Sage JI, Mark MH. Drenching sweats as an off phenomenon in Parkinson's disease: treatment and relation to plasma levodopa profile. Ann Neurol 1995; 37:120–122.
67. Cheshire WP, Freeman R. Disorders of sweating. Semin Neurol 2003; 23:399–406.
68. Mastrolonardo M, Diaferio A, Logroscino G. Seborrheic dermatitis, increased sebum excretion, and Parkinson's disease: a survey of (im)possible links. Med Hypotheses 2003; 60:907–911.
69. Burton JL, Cartlidge M, Shuster S. Effect of -dopa on the seborrhea of Parkinsonism. Br J Dermatol 1973; 88:475–479.
70. Priori A, Cinnante C, Genitrini S, et al. Non-motor effects of deep brain stimulation of the subthalamic nucleus in Parkinson's disease: preliminary physiological results. Neurol Sci 2001; 22:85–86.

71. Appenzeller O, Goss JE. Autonomic deficits in Parkinson's syndrome. Arch Neurol 1971; 24:50–57.
72. Pierangeli G, Provini F, Maltoni P, et al. Nocturnal body core temperature falls in Parkinson's disease but not in Multiple-System Atrophy. Mov Disord 2001; 16:226–232.
73. Meigal A, Lupandin Y. "Thermo-regulation dependent component" in pathophysiology of motor disorders in Parkinson's disease? Pathophysiology 2005; 11:187–196.
74. Amini-Sereshki L. Brainstem control of shivering in the cat. II. Facilitation. Am J Physiol 1977; 232:R198–R202.
75. Morimoto A, Murakami N. [14C]deoxyglucose incorporation into rat brain regions during hypothalamic or peripheral thermal stimulation. Am J Physiol 1985; 248:R84–R92.
76. Linazasoro G, Van Blercom N, Castro A, Dapena MD. Subthalamic deep brain stimulation masking possible malignant syndrome in Parkinson disease. Neurology 2004; 63:589–590.
77. Araki I, Kitahara M, Oida T, Kuno S. Voiding dysfunction and Parkinson's disease: urodynamic abnormalities and urinary symptoms. J Urol 2000; 164(5):1640–1643.
78. Araki I, Kuno S. Assessment of voiding dysfunction in Parkinson's disease by the international prostate symptom score. J Neurol Neurosurg Psychiatry 2000; 68(4):429–433.
79. Gray R, Stern G, Malone-Lee J. Lower urinary tract dysfunction in Parkinson's disease: changes relate to age and not disease. Age Ageing 1995; 24:499–504.
80. Uchiyama T, Sakakibara R, Hattori T, Yamanishi T. Short-term effect of a single levodopa dose on micturition disturbance in Parkinson's disease patients with the wearing-off phenomenon. Mov Disord 2003; 18(5):573–578.
81. Giladi N, Kao R, Fahn S. Freezing phenomenon in patients with parkinsonian syndromes. Mov Disord 1997; 12(3):302–305.
82. Lemack GE, Dewey RB Jr, Roehrborn CG, O'Suilleabhain PE, Zimmern PE. Questionnaire-based assessment of bladder dysfunction in patients with mild to moderate Parkinson's disease. Urology 2000; 56(2):250–254.
83. Yoshimura N, Mizuta E, Yoshida O, Kuno S. Therapeutic effects of dopamine D1/D2 receptor agonists on detrusor hyperreflexia in 1-methyl-4-phenyl-1,2,3,6-tetrahydropyridine-lesioned parkinsonian cynomolgus monkeys. J Pharmacol Exp Ther 1998; 286:228–233.
84. Uchiyama T, Sakakibara R, Hattori T, Yamanishi T. Short-term effect of a single levodopa dose on micturition disturbance in Parkinson's disease patients with the wearing-off phenomenon. Mov Disord 2003; 18(5):573–578.
85. Pazo JH. Caudate-putamen and globus pallidus influences on a visceral reflex. Acta Physiol Lat Am 1976; 26(4):260–266.
86. Finazzi-Agro E, Peppe A, D'Amico A, et al. Effects of subthalamic nucleus stimulation on urodynamic findings in patients with Parkinson's disease. J Urol 2003; 169(4):1388–1391.
87. Seif C, Herzog J, van der Horst C, et al. Effect of subthalamic deep brain stimulation on the function of the urinary bladder. Ann Neurol 2004; 55(1):118–120.
88. Brown RG, Jahanshahi M, Quinn N, Marsden CD. Sexual function in patients with Parkinson's disease and their partners. J Neurol Neurosurg Psychiatry 1990; 53:480–486.

89. Melis MR, Argiolas A. Dopamine and sexual behavior. Neurosci Biobehav Rev 1995; 19:19–38.

90. Pohanka M, Kanovsky P, Bares M, Pulkrabek J, Rektor I. The long-lasting improvement of sexual dysfunction in patients with advanced, fluctuating Parkinson's disease induced by pergolide: evidence from the results of an open, prospective, one-year trial. Parkinsonism Relat Disord 2005; 11:509–512.

91. Kanovsky P, Bares M, Pohanka M, Rektor I. Penile erections and hypersexuality induced by pergolide treatment in advanced, fluctuating Parkinson's disease. J Neurol 2002; 249:112–114.

92. Klos K, Bower J, Josephs K, Matsumoto J, Ahlskog J. Pathological hypersexuality predominantly linked to adjuvant dopamine agonist therapy in Parkinson's disease and multiple system atrophy. Parkinsonism & Related Disorders 2005; 11(6):381–386.

93. Uitti RJ, Tanner CM, Rajput AH, Goetz CG, Klawans HL, Thiessen B. Hypersexuality with antiparkinsonian therapy. Clin Neuropharmacol 1989; 12:375–383.

94. Giovannoni G, O'Sullivan JD, Turner K, Manson AJ, Lees AJ. Hedonistic homeostatic dysregulation in patients with Parkinson's disease on dopamine replacement therapies. J Neurol Neurosurg Psychiatry 2000; 68:423–428.

95. Castelli L, Perozzo P, Genesia ML, et al. Sexual well-being in parkinsonian patients after deep brain stimulation of the subthalamic nucleus. J Neurol Neurosurg Psychiatry 2004; 75:1260–1264.

96. Jacobs H, Vieregge A, Vieregge P. Sexuality in young patients with Parkinson's disease: a population based comparison with healthy controls. J Neurol Neurosurg Psychiatry 2000; 69:550–552.

97. Welsh M, Hung L, Waters CH. Sexuality in women with Parkinson's disease. Mov Disord 1997; 12:923–927.

98. Romito LM, Scerrati M, Contarino MF, et al. Long-term follow up of subthalamic nucleus stimulation in Parkinson's disease. Neurology 2002; 58:1546–1550.

99. Hawkes CH, Shephard BC, Daniel SE. Olfaction disorders in Parkinson's disease. J Neurol Neurosurg Psychiatry 1997; 62:436–446.

100. Doty RL, Stern MB, Pfeiffer C, Gollomp SM, Hurtig HI. Bilateral olfactory dysfunction in early stage treated and untreated idiopathic Parkinson's disease. J Neurol Neurosurg Psychiatry 1992; 55:138–142.

101. Ponsen MM, Stoffers D, Booij J, van Eck-Smit BL, Wolters ECh, Berendse HW. Idiopathic hyposmia as a preclinical sign of Parkinson's disease. Ann Neurol 2004; 56:173–181.

102. Stern MB, Doty RL, Dotti M, et al. Olfactory function in Parkinson's disease subtypes. Neurology 1994; 44:266–268.

103. Braak H, Del Tredici K, Rub U, et al. Staging of brain pathology related to sporadic Parkinson's disease. Neurobiol Aging 2003; 24:197–211.

104. Pearce RKB, Hawkes CH, Daniel SE. The anterior olfactory nucleus in Parkinson's disease. Mov Disord 1995; 10:283–287.

105. Quinn NP, Rossor MN, Marsden CD. Olfactory threshold in Parkinson's disease. J Neurol Neurosurg Psychiatry 1987; 50(1):88–89.

106. Hummel T, Jahnke U, Sommer U, Reichmann H, Muller A. Olfactory function in patients with idiopathic Parkinson's disease: effects of deep brain stimulation in the subthalamic nucleus. J Neural Transm 2005; 112:669–676.

107. Sandyk R. Treatment with AC pulsed electromagnetic fields improves olfactory function in Parkinson's disease. Int J Neurosci 1999; 97:225–233.

108. Hartelius L, Svensson P. Speech and swallowing symptoms associated with Parkinson's disease and multiple sclerosis: a survey. Folia Phoniatr Logop 1994; 46:9–17.

109. Logemann JA, Fisher HB, Boshes B, Blonsky ER. Frequency and cooccurrence of vocal tract dysfunctions in the speech of a large sample of Parkinson patients. J Speech Hear Disord 1978; 43:47–57.

110. Ho AK, Iansek R, Marigliani C, Bradshaw JL, Gates S. Speech impairment in a large sample of patients with Parkinson's disease. Behav Neurol 1998; 11:131–137.

111. Sapir S, Pawlas AA, Ramig LO, et al. Voice and speech abnormalities in Parkinson's disease: relation to severity of motor impairment, duration of disease, medication, depression, gender, and age. Journal of Medical Speech Language Pathology 2001; 9:213–226.

112. Trail M, Fox C, Ramig LO, Sapir S, Howard J, Lai EC. Speech treatment for Parkinson's disease. NeuroRehabilitation 2005; 20:205–221.

113. Schulz GM, Grant MK. Effects of speech therapy and pharmacologic and surgical treatments on voice and speech in Parkinson's disease: a review of the literature. J Commun Disord 2000; 33:59–88.

114. Smith ME, Ramig LO, Dromey C, Perez KS, Samandari R. Intensive voice treatment in Parkinson disease: laryngostroboscopic findings. J Voice 1995; 9:453–459.

115. Perez KS, Ramig LO, Smith ME, Dromey C. The Parkinson larynx: tremor and videostroboscopic findings. J Voice 1996; 10:354–361.

116. Hirose H. Pathophysiology of motor speech disorders (dysarthria). Folia Phoniatr (Basel) 1986; 38:61–88.

117. Pinto S, Ozsancak C, Tripoliti E, Thobois S, Limousin-Dowsey P, Auzou P. Treatments for dysarthria in Parkinson's disease. Lancet Neurol 2004; 3:547–556.

118. Schneider JS, Diamond SG, Markham CH. Deficits in orofacial sensorimotor function in Parkinson's disease. Ann Neurol 1986; 19:275–282.

119. Watson P, Montgomery EB Jr. The relationship of neuronal activity within the sensori-motor region of the subthalamic nucleus to speech. Brain Lang 2006; 97:233–240.

120. Nakano KK, Zubick H, Tyler HR. Speech defects of parkinsonian patients. Effects of levodopa therapy on speech intelligibility. Neurology 1973; 23:865–870.

121. Cahill LM, Murdoch BE, Theodoros DG, Triggs EJ, Charles BG, Yao AA. Effect of oral levodopa treatment on articulatory function in Parkinson's disease: preliminary results. Motor Control 1998; 2:161–172.

122. Marsden CD, Parkes JD. Bromocriptine in parkinsonism. Lancet 1976; 2:419–420.

123. Pinto S, Gentil M, Krack P, et al. Changes induced by levodopa and subthalamic nucleus stimulation on parkinsonian speech. Mov Disord 2005; 20:1507–1515.

124. Rousseaux M, Krystkowiak P, Kozlowski O, Ozsancak C, Blond S, Destee A. Effects of subthalamic nucleus stimulation on parkinsonian dysarthria and speech intelligibility. J Neurol 2004; 251:327–334.

125. Pinto S, Gentil M, Fraix V, Benabid AL, Pollak P. Bilateral subthalamic stimulation effects on oral force control in Parkinson's disease. J Neurol 2003; 250: 179–187.

126. Gentil M, Chauvin P, Pinto S, Pollak P, Benabid AL. Effect of bilateral stimulation of the subthalamic nucleus in parkinsonian voice. Brain and Language 2001; 8: 233–240.

127. Gentil M, Pinto S, Pollack P, Benabid A. Effect of bilateral stimulation of the subthalamic nucleus on parkinsonian dysarthria. Brain and Language 2003; 85(2): 190–196.

128. Hoffman-Ruddy B, Schulz G, Vitek J, Evatt M. A preliminary study of the effects of sub thalamic nucleus (STN) deep brain stimulation (DBS) on voice and speech characteristics in Parkinson's Disease (PD). Clinical Linguistics & Phonetics 2001; 15(1–2):97–101.

129. Krack P, Batir A, Van Blercom N, et al. Five-year follow-up of bilateral stimulation of the subthalamic nucleus in advanced Parkinson's disease. New England Journal of Medicine 2003; 349(20):1925–1934.

130. Romito LM, Scerrati M, Contarino MF, Iacoangeli M, Bentivoglio AR, Albanese A. Bilateral high frequency subthalamic stimulation in Parkinson's disease: long-term neurological follow-up. J Neurosurg Sci 2003; 47:119–128.

131. Krack P, Fraix V, Mendes A, Benabid AL, Pollak P. Postoperative management of subthalamic nucleus stimulation for Parkinson's disease. Mov Disord 2002; 17(suppl 3):S188–S197.

132. Hobson DE, Lang AE, Martin WR, Razmy A, Rivest J, Fleming J. Excessive daytime sleepiness and sudden-onset sleep in Parkinson disease: a survey by the Canadian Movement Disorders Group. JAMA 2002; 287(4):455–463.

133. Adler CH, Thorpy MJ. Sleep issues in Parkinson's disease. Neurology 2005; 64:S12–S20.

134. Friedman JH, Friedman H. Fatigue in Parkinson's disease: a nine-year follow-up. Mov Disord 2001; 16:1120–1122.

135. Abe K, Takanashi M, Yanagihara T. Fatigue in patients with Parkinson's disease. Behav Neurol 2000; 12:103–106.

136. Allen RP, Picchietti D, Hening WA, Trenkwalder C, Wlaters AS, Montplaisir J. Restless legs syndrome: diagnostic criteria, special considerations, and epidemiology. A report from the restless legs syndrome diagnosis and epidemiology workshop at the National Institutes of Health. Sleep Med 2003; 4:101–119.

137. American Sleep Disorder Association (ASDA), Atlas Task Force of the American Sleep Disorders Association. Recording and scoring leg movements, Sleep 16 1993, 748–759.

138. Allen R. Dopamine and iron in the pathophysiology of restless legs syndrome (RLS). Sleep Med 2004; 5(4):385–391.

139. Boeve BF, Silber MH, Ferman TJ. REM sleep behavior disorder in Parkinson's disease and dementia with Lewy bodies. J Geriatr Psychiatry Neurol 2004; 17:146–157.

140. Dagan Y. Circadian rhythm sleep disorders (CRSD). Sleep Med Rev 2002; 6: 45–54.

141. Tandberg E, Larsen JP, Karlsen K. Excessive daytime sleepiness and sleep benefit in Parkinson's disease: a community-based study. Move Disord 1999; 14:922–927.

142. Frucht S, Rogers JD, Greene PE, Gordon MF, Fahn S. Falling asleep at the wheel: motor vehicle mishaps in persons taking pramipexole and ropinirole. Neurology 1999; 52:1908–1910.

143. Arnulf I. Excessive daytime sleepiness in parkinsonism. Sleep Med Rev 2005; 9(3):185–200.

144. Arnulf I, Bejjani BP, Garma L, et al. Improvement of sleep architecture in PD with subthalamic nucleus stimulation. Neurology 2000; 55(11):1732–1734.

145. Hjort N, Ostergaard K, Dupont E. Improvement of sleep quality in patients with advanced Parkinson's disease treated with deep brain stimulation of the subthalamic nucleus. Mov Disord 2004; 19(2):196–199.

146. Iranzo A, Valldeoriola F, Santamaria J, Tolosa E, Rumia J. Sleep symptoms and polysomnographic architecture in advanced Parkinson's disease after chronic bilateral subthalamic stimulation. J Neurol Neurosurg Psychiatry 2002; 72:661–664.

147. Monaca C, Ozsancak C, Jacquesson JM, et al. Effects of bilateral subthalamic stimulation on sleep in Parkinson's disease. J Neurol 2004; 251(2):214–218.

148. Cicolin A, Lopiano L, Zibetti M, et al. Effects of deep brain stimulation of the subthalamic nucleus on sleep architecture in parkinsonian patients. Sleep Med 2004; 5(2):207–210.

149. Antonini A, Landi A, Mariani C, DeNotaris R, Pezzoli G. Deep brain stimulation and its effect on sleep in Parkinson's disease. Sleep Med 2004; 5(2):211–214.

150. Lyons KE, Pahwa R. Effects of bilateral subthalamic nucleus stimulation on sleep, daytime sleepiness, and early morning dystonia in patients with Parkinson disease. J Neurosurg 2006; 104:502–505.

151. Kedia S, Moro E, Tagliati M, Lang AE, Kumar R. Emergence of restless legs syndrome during subthalamic stimulation for Parkinson disease. Neurology 2004; 63(12):2410–2412.

152. Driver-Dunckley E, Evidente VG, Adler CH, et al. Restless legs syndrome in Parkinson's disease patients may improve with subthalamic stimulation. Mov Disord 2006 May 2 [Epub ahead of print].

153. Lopiano L, Rizzone M, Bergamasco B, et al. Daytime sleepiness improvement following bilateral chronic electrical stimulation of the subthalamic nucleus in Parkinson's disease. Eur Neurol 2001; 46(1):49–50.

154. Volkmann J, Allert N, Voges J, et al. Safety and efficacy of pallidal or subthalamic nucleus stimulation in advanced PD. Neurology 2001; 56:548–551.

155. Krack P, Pollak P, Limousin P, Hoffmann D, Xie J, Benazzouz A, Benabid AL. Subthalamic nucleus or internal pallidal stimulation in young onset Parkinson's disease. Brain 1998; 121:451–457.

156. Abbott RA, Cox M, Markus H, Tomkins A. Diet, body size and micronutrient status in Parkinson's disease. Eur J Clin Nutr 1992; 46(12):879–884.

157. Beyer PL, Palarino MY, Michalek D, Busenbark K, Koller WC. Weight change and body composition in patients with Parkinson's disease. J Am Diet Assoc 1995; 95(9):979–983.

158. Markus HS, Cox M, Tomkins AM. Raised resting energy expenditure in Parkinson's disease and its relationship to muscle rigidity. Clin Sci (Lond) 1992; 83(2):199–204.

159. Levi S, Cox M, Lugon M, Hodkinson M, Tomkins A. Increased energy expenditure in Parkinson's disease. BMJ 1990; 301:1256–1257.

160. Barichella M, Marczewska AM, Mariani C, et al. Body weight gain rate in patients with Parkinson's disease and deep brain stimulation. Mov Disord 2003; 18:1337–1340.

161. Macia F, Perlemoine C, Coman I, et al. Parkinson's disease patients with bilateral subthalamic deep brain stimulation gain weight. Mov Disord 2004; 19(2):206–212.

162. Moro E, Scerrati M, Romito LM, Roselli R, Tonali P, Albanese A. Chronic subthalamic nucleus stimulation reduces medication requirements in Parkinson's disease. Neurology 1999; 53:85–90.

163. Tamma F, Rampini P, Egidi M, et al. Deep brain stimulation for Parkinson's disease: the experience of the Policlinico-San Paolo Group in Milan. Neurol Sci 2003; 24(suppl 1):S41–S42.

164. Doshi PK, Chhaya NA, Bhatt MA. Bilateral subthalamic nucleus stimulation for Parkinson's disease. Neurol India 2003; 51:43–48.

165. Goetz CG, Tanner CM, Levy M, Wilson RS, Garron DC. Pain in Parkinson's disease. Mov Disord 1986; 1(1):45–49.

166. Quinn NP, Koller WC, Lang AE, Marsden CD. Painful Parkinson's disease. Lancet 1986; 1(8494):1366–1369.

167. Ford B. Pain in Parkinson's disease. Clin Neurosci 1998; 5:63–72.

168. Djaldetti R, Shifrin A, Rogowski Z, Sprecher E, Melamed E, Yarnitsky D. Quantitative measurement of pain sensation in patients with Parkinson disease. Neurology 2004; 62:2171–2175.

169. Quittenbaum BH, Grahn B. Quality of life and pain in Parkinson's disease: a controlled cross-sectional study. Parkinsonism & Related Disorders 2004; 10(3):129–136.

170. Chudler EH, Dong WK. The role of the basal ganglia in nociception and pain. Pain 1995; 60:3–38.

171. Bittar RG, Kar-Purkayastha I, Owen SL, et al. Deep brain stimulation for pain relief: a meta-analysis. J Clin Neurosci 2005; 12(5):515–519.

15

Neuropsychology of Deep Brain Stimulation in Parkinson's Disease

Paul J. Moberg

Departments of Psychiatry and Neurology, University of Pennsylvania School of Medicine, and Parkinson's Disease Research, Education, and Clinical Center (PADRECC), Philadelphia Veterans Affairs Medical Center, Philadelphia, Pennsylvania, U.S.A.

Kathryn Kniele

Department of Psychiatry and Behavioral Sciences, Medical University of South Carolina, Charleston, South Carolina, U.S.A.

Jacqueline H. Rick

Department of Psychiatry, University of Pennsylvania School of Medicine, and Parkinson's Disease Research, Education, and Clinical Center (PADRECC), Philadelphia Veterans Affairs Medical Center, Philadelphia, Pennsylvania, U.S.A.

INTRODUCTION

A progressive and debilitating neurodegenerative process, Parkinson's disease (PD) is characterized by systemic degeneration of dopaminergic neurons, with selective loss in the brain's basal ganglia—a bundle of neuron fibers consisting of the corpus striatum, subthalamic nucleus (STN), and substantia nigra. Overt PD symptomatology typically emerges after 70% of dopaminergic reduction in the nigrostriatal regions (1). Primary behavioral manifestations of the disorder include resting tremor, bradykinesia, postural instability, and rigidity. As such, PD is regarded primarily as a movement disorder. However, various

247

secondary "nonmotor" disturbances are common in PD, likely due to disruption of noradrenergic and serotonergic neurotransmitter systems, as well as systemic disruption of the dopaminergic system. These nonmotor symptoms include psychiatric and cognitive changes, as well as autonomic, sleep, and sensory disorders. Changes in mood and cognition are common in the advanced stages of PD, though they may antedate the onset of obvious motor symptoms. Psychiatric complications of PD include anxiety, depression, apathy, hypersexuality, and other neuropsychiatric symptoms ranging from vivid dreams to psychosis and delirium. Changes in cognitive functioning are common and may range from none or slight impairment of cognitive abilities to frank dementia.

COURSE OF PARKINSON'S DISEASE-RELATED COGNITIVE IMPAIRMENT

Although the typical course of PD involves onset of motor symptoms followed by progressively worsening cognitive functioning, it is possible for the nonmotor symptoms to emerge first. Indeed, there are various phenotypes of PD progression, with distinct initial symptomatology and progressive course. Cognitive impairment associated with idiopathic PD may take years to develop, or symptoms may manifest early in the course of the disease (2). Similarly unpredictable, cognitive impairments may be stable and of insufficient magnitude to affect daily functioning or they may occur in severe, progressive, and debilitating fashion. Although an historical debate exists regarding whether cognitive deterioration in PD represented a disease-related process or a distinct phenomenon superimposed on the disease process, it is now understood that mental decline is common in PD (3) and represents a behavioral manifestation of disease progression. Despite variability in presentation and severity of cognitive symptomatology in PD, current estimates suggest that up to 80% of PD patients demonstrate measurable cognitive impairment at some point during the disease course (4).

NEUROPSYCHOLOGICAL FUNCTIONING IN PARKINSON'S DISEASE

The most commonly reported neuropsychological finding in PD is impaired executive functioning. Executive functions include the ability to plan, initiate, and monitor behavior, as well as think abstractly, solve problems, and adapt to novel environmental stimuli. The myriad of difficulties in this domain is collectively referred to as dysexecutive syndrome and reflects underlying cortical and subcortical pathophysiology. Compared with groups of healthy controls, clinical samples of patients with PD demonstrate significantly more impaired performance on measures of executive functioning (5). Indeed, mild impairments in executive functioning are often present in the prodromal stage of the disease (6,7) and executive functions appear to be the most susceptible to decline (8).

Visuospatial functions also appear to be affected. Patients may demonstrate difficulty in visual attention (5), constructional praxis, visual and spatial perception (9), and mental rotation (10). One of the earliest signs of altered visuospatial perception may be changes in handwriting, with those affected by PD demonstrating characteristic micrographia (11). Findings of visuospatial impairment in PD are equivocal though, as some studies comparing age- and education-matched healthy controls to patients with PD fail to support the idea of a generalized visuospatial deficit (12). In fact, several researchers hypothesize that the observed visuospatial deficits in PD may be attributable to the executive demand of visuospatial tasks, and thus represent a manifestation of dysexecutive syndrome (13,14).

In addition to executive and visuospatial deficits, impairments in controlled word-list generation (i.e., verbal fluency) (15), attention (16), and working memory (17) are also characteristic of PD. There is evidence of impaired verbal learning and memory, though poor performance on these tasks appears to be related to failure to use efficient strategies for encoding and retrieving information (14). Psychomotor slowing is also commonly observed (5).

DEMENTIA IN PARKINSON'S DISEASE

Dementia in PD is characterized by impaired executive functioning, decreased visuospatial ability, and fluctuating attention—similar to those neuropsychological deficits observed earlier on in the disease course, though of greater severity. Thus, there is a positive predictive value in identifying prodromal neuropsychological impairment in PD (18). Aphasia and agnosia are uncommon in PD-related dementia (PDD) (19). The incidence of dementia in the population of patients with PD is higher, up to six times higher, than among peers without the disease (20). In cross-sectional samples, 10% to 20% of patients with PD meet criteria for dementia (21). In prospective community and clinic-based samples, up to 30% meet criteria for dementia within less than five years (4,22). This number increases dramatically over time. Aarsland et al. (2005) followed 224 patients with PD over eight years and observed that 78.2% of them developed dementia within the eight-year follow-up. In that study, the four-year prevalence of dementia was three times that of the non-PD population sample control group, indicating that PD constitutes a risk factor for dementia (23). A recent review of largely community-based prevalence studies of dementia in PD suggests that 24% to 31% of PD patients meet criteria for dementia, depending on the diagnostic criteria used (24). Although it is unclear whether PDD is related to the age of onset of disease, risk factors for PDD include older age, depression, family history of dementia, hallucinations (4), and severity and subtype of motor symptoms (25,26).

Pathophysiology of Dementia in Parkinson's Disease

PDD appears to be directly related to an interaction between neuronal loss in the substantia nigra of the basal ganglia superimposed on age-related pathological changes (27), particularly in cortical and limbic structures. Neuroanatomical findings suggest that dementia in PD is similar to dementia of the Lewy body type (DLB), and it has been argued that they are part of the same spectrum of disorders (14). Specifically, Aarsland et al. (2003) reported that the presence of hallucinations, a common finding in DLB, predicted dementia in PD, supporting the hypothesis that PDD and DLB are similar spectrum disorders. Furthermore, the presence of limbic or neocortical Lewy body disease was found to be significantly associated with the rate of cognitive decline, again suggesting shared underlying neuropathology in PDD and DLB (28,29).

Many PD patients with dementia also have Alzheimer's disease (AD). However, accurate estimation of the incidence of AD in PD patients is difficult given that progressive deterioration of cognitive abilities is characteristic of PD itself and that accurate diagnosis of AD may only be provided post mortem. Although some AD neuropathological changes such as the presence of neurofibrillary tangles and amyloid neuritic plaques have been observed in individuals with PDD (29), evidence fails to support the hypothesis that PDD and AD are causally related.

Prevalence and Impact of Impaired Cognition and Dementia in Parkinson's Disease

Persons with PD and cognitive disturbance report greater impairments in everyday living and poor quality of life (QOL) (30). QOL in patients with chronic disease includes aspects of physical and emotional health, as well as cognitive functioning. Indeed, neuropsychological functioning ranks as one among five major dimensions relating to patients' reported QOL (31). Furthermore, dementia in PD is a poor prognostic indicator, associated with higher mortality rates (32,33) and increased caregiver burden (34). According to data from the Centers for Disease Control and Prevention, approximately 1% of the United States population over age 65 (estimated to be approximately 2,000,000 based on U.S. Census data) carries a diagnosis of PD. With upwards of one-quarter of those patients suffering from Parkinson's-related cognitive impairment or dementia, and the significant negative impact of PDD on patient and caregiver QOL and patient survival, consideration of cognitive decline in PD is an important aspect when considering treatments for the disease.

TREATMENT FOR PARKINSON'S DISEASE

There are several available treatments for PD, though none are able to completely halt or reverse the disease process. Rather, symptomatic treatment is aimed at maintaining patients' functioning and QOL. Primary treatments include pharmacological and surgical interventions, and the refinement of these techniques over time has had considerable positive impact, with PD patients living longer and experiencing less disability.

PHARMACOLOGICAL MANAGEMENT OF PARKINSON'S DISEASE

The United States Food and Drug Administration (FDA) has approved over a dozen pharmacological agents for the treatment of PD. Levodopa (L-dopa) is the gold standard, first-line treatment for PD. It is often used in combination with dopamine receptor agonist agents such as carbidopa and bromocriptine. Other adjunctive or alternative therapies include anticholinergic agents (e.g., benztropine mesylate), MAO-ß-inhibitors (e.g., selegeline hydrochloride and the recently FDA-approved rasagiline), COMT inhibitors (e.g., entacapone and tolcapone), as well as apomorphine (AMP), a selective dopamine receptor agonist. Although the efficacy of these agents is often measured by improvements in motor functioning, it is clear that they also have some impact on the nonmotor symptoms of PD, including cognition. For example, L-dopa has been shown to improve attention, executive functioning (35), and verbal and visual memory (36,37). Although subcutaneous infusion of apomorphine (APM-csi) improves motor ability in patients with PD (38), the treatment appears to have deleterious effects on visuospatial ability and processing speed (39). Similarly, the use of anticholinergic agents may aggravate existing neuropsychological impairments and may lead to confusion, impaired memory, and sedation in patients. The cognitive effects of these medications is of particular concern as there is tolerance, and patients often must increase dosage of the medication over time to maintain control of symptoms.

Pharmacological Treatment of Cognitive Disturbance and Dementia in Parkinson's Disease

Recently, the Quality Standards Subcommittee of the American Academy of Neurology released a report stating that cholinesterase inhibitors, such as donepezil or rivastigmine, are effective treatments for dementia in PD (40). In June 2006, the FDA approved rivastigmine tartrate (Exelon®), manufactured by Novartis, as the first approved medication for treatment of PDD. As a class, these agents have been found to improve cognitive and functional abilities, as well as reduce behavioral disturbance and psychoses (41). However, it should be noted that improvements in cognition may be modest and these treatments may exacerbate motor symptoms.

SURGICAL INTERVENTIONS IN PARKINSON'S DISEASE

Though often reserved for individuals with the most severe forms of PD or those who fail to respond adequately to pharmacological treatment, surgical interventions have been successful in controlling at least the motor symptoms of the disease. Stereotactic lesioning of the globus pallidus interna (GPi) (i.e., pallidotomy) and surgical removal of the thalamus (i.e., thalatomy) were the surgical treatments of choice in the 1950s and 1960s (42). The negative sequelae of pallidotomy include scotoma in the visual field, injury to the internal capsule, facial paresis, and, rarely, intracerebral hemorrhage. As with thalamotomy, dysarthria, dysphagia, and impaired cognition can be observed after pallidotomy. As such, with the advent of powerful pharmacological agents and more refined surgical techniques, such procedures are currently not the standard of practice.

Subthalamic Deep Brain Stimulation

Advances in surgical techniques along with greater understanding of the pathophysiology of PD have allowed the use of deep brain stimulation (DBS) techniques in treating PD (43). Specifically, deep brain stimulation of the subthalamic nucleus (STN DBS) confers obvious and significant motor benefits (44,45,45a). Approved by the FDA for use in the surgical treatment of PD, STN DBS has become an accessible and acceptable therapeutic option for treatment in patients with advanced disease that is complicated by wearing off motor fluctuations and dyskinesias. Bilateral STN DBS is efficacious in the treatment of motor symptoms (i.e., dyskinesias and fluctuations) in advanced PD (45,45a). Among the most notable improvements are reduced tremor, bradykinesia, rigidity, dystonia, motor fluctuations, and drug-induced dyskinesias as well as improved ability to perform activities of daily living. Its benefits over existing surgical interventions (e.g., pallidotomy, thalatomy) include reversibility, decreased risk of reoperation, and decreased morbidity. However, serious complications including infection, ischaemic stroke, subdural hematoma, and intracerebral hemorrhage can occur (46). Presently, several hundred patients have undergone STN DBS.

Mechanism of Action

The procedure consists of implantation of an electrode either unilaterally or bilaterally into the STN. A wire extends subcutaneously from the site of implantation into the patient's chest wall, where an implantable pulse generator is inserted into a pocket beneath the skin. This allows for manipulation of stimulation parameters to individualize treatment. Though the exact mechanism of action in regulating motor symptoms is unknown, STN DBS may exert its effects by inhibiting neuronal activity in the overactive subthalamic nucleus (47).

Cognitive Effects of Subthalamic Nucleus Deep Brain Stimulation in Parkinson's Disease

STN DBS may offer an attractive alternative to lesioning techniques if it can be established that there is less cognitive morbidity than that associated with ablative procedures (48). In a controlled comparison study of 16 patients with treatment refractory PD, nine patients with STN DBS placement and seven patients undergoing continuous APM-csi, it was observed that the STN DBS group performed significantly worse on verbal fluency at six months and speeded naming at the six-month and one-year follow-ups (38). These changes were independent of pre- or postsurgical depression scores and pre- or postdose of L-dopa and were thus attributed to the direct effects of STN DBS. Conversely, minor improvements in verbal fluency, confrontation naming, mood, and QOL have been reported for STN DBS (43). Neuropsychological changes following STN DBS may be attributable to the electrical stimulation of specific brain structures or inhibition of overactivity in the thalamic region. There may also be direct mechanical damage that occurs in positioning the electrode and its penetration through cortical structures that could affect postsurgical cognitive outcomes (38).

Given that STN DBS techniques for PD are in their relative infancy and equivocal results of observational studies, the true impact of STN DBS on cognition in patients with PD is unclear. Furthermore, a number of methodological issues in studies reporting cognitive changes following DBS call into question the true magnitude of the observed differences (43). Specifically, PD patients with dementia or severe cognitive deficit are often prohibited from undergoing the procedure, thus limiting the possible range of improvement on cognitive functioning tasks postsurgery. In addition, the heterogeneity of postsurgical variables such as error in placement of electrodes, length of elapsed time between pre- and postoperative neuropsychological evaluations, stimulator parameter settings, and postsurgical medication regimen are also factors. The ecological validity of the neuropsychological tests used to measure cognitive performance is questionable at times, and few have examined the impact of the surgery on patients with and without cognitive deficits pre- and post-STN DBS.

The lack of data on such an important outcome variable is disturbing, given that the motor, psychiatric, and cognitive concomitants of PD may lead to social embarrassment, loneliness, and dependence on others for functionality. Of those that have evaluated postsurgical QOL of PD patients, results have been equivocal. Ford (2004) reported failure of DBS to improve functional capacity independent of postsurgical medication use as measured by the Hoehn and Yahr stage (49), whereas others have noted specific improvement across QOL domains (50). For example, Castelli et al. evaluated depression, anxiety, and sexual well-being in 31 patients submitted to STN DBS preoperatively and 9 to 12 months postoperatively. In younger male patients, reported sexual well-being and satisfaction increased pre- to post-DBS placement (51). Depression scores on the Beck Depression Inventory (52) also improved pre- to postoperatively. Considering that depression appears to be the most significant factor impairing QOL in PD patients (53), such improvements may be a considerable benefit of STN-DBS treatment.

Although several reviews suggest that STN DBS does not have a deleterious effect on cognition in PD patients, and may actually improve functioning in some domains, there are insufficient data regarding the magnitude of the effects (positive or negative) of the procedure on cognition in patients with PD. As such, we performed a comprehensive literature review to evaluate the overall impact of STN DBS on neuropsychological functioning in PD.

Impact of Subthalamic Nucleus Deep Brain Stimulation on Cognition

Studies examining the neuropsychological sequelae of STN DBS are presented in Table 1. It is notable that many of these studies consist of a small number of

Table 1 Studies Examining Neuropsychological Sequelae of STN DBS: Domains Assessed and Areas Demonstrated Change

Study (first author)	% male	Mean age at surgery	Mean H & Y (off)	Mean disease duration (yrs)	Unilateral, bilateral, or mixed
Alegret (2001)	46.60%	61.1 (8.3)	4.17 (0.83)	16.1 (8.3)	bilateral
Alegret (2004)		62.86 (8.43)		14.14 (3.44)	bilateral
Biseul (2005)	control = 40%, pre- and post = 60%	control = 59.9 (6.9), pre 59.2 (6.9), post = 61.7 (8.2)		pre = 13.7 (4.5) post = 15 (6.2)	bilateral
Castelli (2006)	58%	60.5 (6.5)		15.1 (5.1)	bilateral
Contarino (2006)	64%	57.5 (7.4)		15.5 (5.6)	bilateral
DeGaspari (2006)	73%	59.8 (7.4)		15.8 (3.6)	bilateral
DeGaspari (2006)		60.5 (6.5)	3	12 (2.45)	
Dujardin (2001)	66%	54.78 (8.15)	4.66 (0.71)	13.11 (2.93)	bilatera
Funkiewiez (2003)	58%	54.6 (7.9)			bilateral
Funkiewiez (2004)	56%	55 (8)		15 (5)	bilateral
Gironell (2003)		pall = 62.7(9.9), STN = 56.6(4.8)	pall = 4.2 (0.7), STN = 4.3 (0.6)	pall = 15.8 (5.7) STN = 12.5 (4.8)	bilateral
Moretti (2003)	67%	68.7 (7.89)	4.01	8.91 (2.34)	bilateral
Patel (2003)	63%	56 (11)	pre = 4.1 (0.3), post = 2.5 (0.2)	10 (3.5)	bilateral
Perozzo (2001)	60%	61.6 (6)	4 (0.4)	15.4 (4.9)	bilateral
Perriol (2006)	62%	median = 59 (45-73)	median = 4	median = 14 (4–25)	bilateral
Saint-Cyr (2000)	55%	67 (8)	4 (1.2)	15 (3)	bilateral
Schupbach (2005)	65%	54.9 (9.1)	5	15.2 (5.3)	bilateral
Smeding (2005)	pall = 36%, STN = 30%	pall = 62.1 (8.1), STN = 59.2 (8.6)	pall = 4, STN = 4	pall = 11, STN = 12	bilateral
Whelan (2003)	80%	63.2 (4.8)	pre = 3.2, post = 2.7	10.8 (4.1)	bilateral
Straits-Troster (2000)	86%	65 (12)		8 (3.8)	unilateral-3R, 4L
Troster (2003)	54%	56.6 (11)		9.5 (4.9)	bilateral
Morrison (2004)	DBS = 76%, CPD = 91%	DBS = 59.9 (7.7), CPD = 62.7 (11.5)	DBS = 3.2 (0.8) CPD = 3.3 (0.6)	DBS = 10.8 (3.4) CPD = 10 (3)	bilateral
Pillon (2000)	STN1 = 56%, STN2 = 67%	STN1 = 55.7 (7.5), STN2 = 53.5 (9.7)		STN1 = 15 (4.9), STN2 = 14.2 (5.5)	bilateral
Halbig (2004)	83%	59.9 (7.7)	2.8 (0.5)	16.2 (5)	bilateral
Limousin (1998)	46%	56 (8)		14 (5)	bilateral
Moro (1999)	14%	57.4		15.4	bilateral
Schneider (2003)	25%	62.1 (6.1)		17 (6.3)	bilateral
Schroeder (2002)	43%	59.14 (12.98)		15.29	bilateral
Witt (2004)	74%	57.4 (5.5)		15.1 (5.5)	bilateral
Jahanshahi (2000)	77%	52.8 (4.9)	4.5	15.1 (4.8)	bilateral
Burchiel (1999)	70%	62.8(12)	4	13.6 (5)	bilateral
Brusa (2001)		53.5 (6.18)		15.16 (6.55)	bilateral

Abbreviations: Att, attention; CPD, clinically similar PD control; Front, frontal/executive functions; GC, global; IQ, intelligence quotient; stimulation Vmem, verbal memory; VS, visuospatial; Lang, language; N/a, not applicable; NVMem, nonverbal memory; STN DBS, subthalamic nucle deep brain.

STN, GPi, or mixed	Surgical vs. On/off	Mean follow-up (months)	Functions assessed	Improvements	Declines
TN	surgical	3	VMem, VS, Front, Lang	Front	VMem, VS, Lang
TN	surgical	6 & 12	VMem, Front, Lang, VS, Mood, GC	N/a	Lang
TN	surgical	implant 7.2 (12.1) mo before	GC, Front, Lang	N/a	N/a
TN	surgical	15 (range 12–20 mo)	IQ, VS, Att, VMem, Front, Lang, Mood	Front, Mood	Lang
TN	surgical	12 & 60 mo	GC, IQ, VMem, VS, Lang, Front	GC	Lang, IQ, VS
TN	surgical	15 (9.2) mo	GC, Front, Mood, Lang, IQ, VMem	N/a	Lang
TN	surgical	12	GC, Mood, IQ, Lang, VMem	N/a	Lang, Mood
TN	surgical	3 mo & 1 yr	VMem, Front, Lang, GC	N/a	Front, VMem
TN	surgical	12 patients @ 3 mo, 14 @ 12, 13 @ 24, 10@ 36, 1 @ 48	Mood, GC, Front	Mood	N/a
TN	surgical	12 & 36	GC, Front, VS, VMem, Att, Lang, Mood	Mood	Lang
TN	surgical	6	VMem, NVMem, Att, VS, Front, Lang	N/a	Lang
TN	surgical	1, 6, & 12	Front, IQ, Lang, Mood, VS, VMem	N/a	Lang, Front
TN	surgical	12	Att, VMem, Front, Lang, IQ	N/a	N/a
TN	surgical	6	VMem, NVMem, IQ, Att, Front	N/a	N/a
TN	surgical	12	GC, Mood	N/a	N/a
TN	surgical	3–6 & 9–12	IQ, Front, Lang, VMem, NVMem, Att, Mood	N/a	Lang, VMem, NVMem
TN	surgical	6, 24, 60	GC, Front, mood	N/a	GC, Front
TN	surgical	baseline, 6, & 12	Front, mood, Att, Lang, IQ, GC	N/a	Front
TN	surgical	3	Lang	N/a	Lang (reaction time)
ixed	surgical	STN = 4.4 (1.3) mo	Mood	N/a	N/a
TN	surgical	3.5 mo	Mood, GC, Att, Front, Lang, VS, Vmem, NVMem	N/a	N/a
TN	both	13.3 (7.8) wk after baseline, 9.7 (7.7) days between conditions	Att, Lang, VS, VMem, Front, Mood	N/a	Lang, VMem (surgical)
ixed	both	3 & 12	GC, Front, Lang, VMem, NVMem Mood	Front (off/on), NVMem, Lang	VMem
TN	on/off		Att, GC, Lang, Front, Mood, NVMem, VMem	NVMem, Att	VMem
TN	on/off	1, 3, 6 & 12	Front, GC	N/a	N/a
TN	on/off	1, 3, 6, 12, and annually thereafter	IQ, VMem, Lang, GC	N/a	N/a
TN	on/off	implant 9.3 (6.9) mo prior to study	Mood, VMem, Front, Lang	N/a	N/a
TN	on/off	5	GC, IQ, VS, Front	N/a	Front
TN	on/off	8.8 (6.6) mo after implantation	Lang, Front, GC, Att	Att	N/a
ixed	on/off		Front, Att, Lang, IQ	Front, Att, Lang	Front
ixed	on/off	10 days, 3, 6 & 12 mo	VMem, Att, Mood	Mood	N/a
ixed	on/off (for both stimulator and l-dopa)	4 different conditions each 1 mo apart	Front, Lang, Mood, Other	N/a	N/a

subjects with variable follow-up times. Indeed, a recent study by Parsons et al. (2006) indicated that in order to detect even the most prominent neuropsychological deficits in patients undergoing STN DBS, a minimum sample size of 48 patients is needed. As such, a majority of these studies are under-powered.

Executive Function

Of the 31 studies reported in Table 1, 25 (81%) included in their assessment of cognitive function some measure of frontal/executive function. The majority of investigators utilized the Stroop Color-Word Task (54) and/or the Trail Making Test (55) as putative measures of frontal system functioning. Of the 16 studies that assessed frontal/executive function before and after DBS surgery, two improvements (12%) and five declines (31%) were reported. For example, Castelli et al. (2006) reported an improvement in the Nelson Modified Card Sorting Test an average of 15 months post-DBS surgery. In addition, Alegret et al. (2001) assessed cognitive function in several domains before surgery and three months post-DBS surgery. Although several of the domains tested showed declines at follow-up, performance on Part B of the Trail Making Test showed indications of improvement postsurgery. Although it could be argued that this improvement simply reflected improvements in basic motor function or practice effects, it is notable that subjects' performance on Part A of the Trail Making Test did not show improvements and the motor demands for both tasks are roughly equivalent.

Alternatively, Dujardin et al. (56) and Moretti et al. (57) reported declines in executive function, as measured by the interference condition from the Stroop, 3, 6, and 12 months post-DBS surgery, respectively. In addition, Smeding et al. (2005) (58) reported an increase in the number of errors on the Stroop and Trail Making tasks post-DBS surgery. Schupbach et al. (59) also reported a decline in frontal system function, although they did not specify which tasks were included in the assessment. Interestingly, these investigators observed a declining trend 6, 24, and 60 months post-STN DBS surgery, with the latter assessment yielding a significantly worse performance from baseline. It would appear then that these frontal deficits are robust and persistent.

Lastly, nine of the reported studies examined frontal lobe function in DBS patients "on" and "off" stimulation. One advantage to this type of analysis is that it allows direct comparisons of the effects of stimulation per se and not the effects of surgery plus stimulation (as is seen in standard "pre–post" surgery designs). In addition, since each patient is serving as their own control in such a within-subjects design, this analysis has greater power. Pillon et al. (2000) (60) reported stimulation improvements in patients' performance on the Trail Making Test and reproduction of graphic series. Jahanshahi et al. (61) also reported improvements on stimulation on the Trail Making and Wisconsin Card Sorting Tests; however, a simultaneous decline was observed on the Visual–Visual Conditional Associative Learning test, a task that requires subjects to learn associations between arbitrary objects. Also, Schroeder et al. (62) reported a decline in the change between the control and interference condition in a Stroop task among subjects on and off DBS. The authors indicated that patients off stimulation demonstrated slower reaction times during the control condition and faster reaction times during the interference condition, suggesting less semantic processing on the part of the patients.

Language and Related Functions

Of the 18 studies that investigated language before and after DBS surgery, 12 (67%) observed a decline and no study reported an improvement in language functions relative to baseline levels. This finding is consistent with other reports that have suggested that language function is the single most vulnerable cognitive domain following STN DBS surgery. The majority of studies reviewed observed declines in verbal fluency post-DBS surgery (38,63,64) including studies of semantic (57,65–68), phonemic (57,65,66,68,69), and syllabic frequency (57). Declines were also noted in other language tasks such as the Boston Naming Test (66), lexical decision-making task (70), and the naming condition of the Stroop (38). These declines in performance on verbal fluency tasks were observed after as few as three months post-DBS surgery (71) and as many as 36 months post-DBS surgery (72). Eight studies assessed language function in postsurgical patients on and off stimulation. With the exception of two studies reporting changes in performance on the word condition of the Stroop, all studies examined failed to observe a significant improvement or decline in verbal fluency in the on-stimulation compared with the off-stimulation condition (60,61). This would suggest, therefore, that the previously mentioned language changes in patients post-DBS surgery compared to baseline may reflect a surgical effect rather than a stimulation effect per se.

Memory and Learning

As seen in Table 1, a variety of memory tests were employed across studies, including tests of both verbal and nonverbal memory. In light of the strong language effects noted previously in patients post-STN DBS, one might expect to see a greater difference in verbal memory performance relative to nonverbal abilities. In fact, 14 of the 18 studies (78%) listed in Table 1 that tested memory performance before and after DBS surgery utilized a verbal memory task. Among them, four (22%) found declines in memory performance. For example, Morrison et al. (2004) tested subjects with the Hopkins Verbal Learning Test and the Randt Memory Test, which includes Digit Span subtests, verbal memory for passages, and picture memory. The authors reported an immediate and delayed composite memory score; the delayed recall score, alone, declined at follow-up testing. Alegret et al. (2001) observed a decline in performance on the Rey Auditory Verbal Learning Test (RAVLT). Also, Pillon et al. (2000) tested subjects 3 and 12 months post-DBS surgery. A decline in free recall on the Grober–Buschke Memory Test at three months, which seemed to recover at the 12-month follow-up assessment, was observed. The authors noted that overall their data support few long lasting cognitive effects of DBS treatment.

Saint-Cyr et al. (2000) (65) observed a decline in performance on the long delay free recall and long delay cued recall portions of the California Verbal Learning Test (CVLT). They also reported a decline in a nonverbal memory test of immediate and delayed recall for a complex figure and several designs (i.e., battery of memory efficiency). The authors described that the pattern of the observed memory deficits reflected an encoding deficit as opposed to impairment in free recall. In contrast, previous studies with PD patients have observed poor performance in free recall tests but near normal performance on recognition. Thus, PD patients are thought to have a retrieval deficit. The nature of the specific component memory processes affected by STN DBS is still relatively unclear, and further studies detailing these component processes are clearly needed.

Eight studies listed in Table 1 explored verbal and/or nonverbal memory in patients on versus off stimulation. Halbig et al. (2004) observed an improvement on stimulation on a weather prediction paradigm in which subjects predict rain or shine outcomes based on cues. Alternatively, Halbig et al. (2004) also observed a decline in performance on the verbal multiple-choice follow-up test to the weather prediction task (73). This surprising result warrants further investigation.

Visuospatial and Visuoperceptual Function

Basic visuospatial and visuoperceptual skills appear to have attracted the least research attention in the STN DBS literature. Of the eight papers that examined visuospatial ability before and after DBS surgery, no study reported improvement postsurgery and only one reported decline at the follow-up assessment. Specifically, Alegret et al. (2001) tested judgments of line orientation among a larger battery of cognitive assessments and found a significant decline in performance three months postsurgery. In light of the limited coverage of these functions in STN DBS research, more detailed study of basic visuoperceptual and spatial skills is needed.

Attention

Eight of the investigations reviewed in Table 1 tested attention specifically and no declines or improvements postsurgery were reported. Additionally, five papers detailed the assessment of attention on and off STN DBS. Jahanshahi et al. (2000) utilized two attentional tasks including the missing digit task, where subjects listen to a series of digits and report the one that is not included, and a paced auditory serial addition test which has subjects listen to a series of digits and report the sum of the current and previous digits. On both of these attentional tasks, performance improved on versus off stimulation. Halbig et al. (73) also observed improvements in a sample of 12 patients on versus off stimulation. They utilized a simple motor reaction time task in which subjects had to respond to a visual stimulus. Finally, Witt et al. (74) report that the only cognitive domain that improved with stimulation was attention as measured by a random number generation task. These data suggest that subtle improvements in attention due to stimulation may be missed in standard pre–post surgical designs.

Mood and Affect

The impact of depression and other emotional dysregulation on cognition is well known and must be factored into any assessment of neuropsychological function in PD patients. As changes in affect and mood are covered in Chapter 16, the impact of DBS on these functions will only be briefly summarized here. Twenty-one studies reviewed in Table 1 assessed mood and four reported an improvement in affect following STN DBS. The most common method for evaluating mood was the Beck Depression Inventory (64,72,75,76). Only one study (67) observed a decline in mood ratings post-DBS surgery.

Global Cognition/IQ

Finally, 29 studies reviewed in Table 1 included an assessment of either overall intellectual function (i.e., IQ) or global cognition [e.g., Mini-Mental State Exam (MMSE)]. Contarino et al. (2006) (69) observed a decline in nonverbal intellectual performance on the Raven's Matrices post-DBS surgery. Performance on the Mattis Dementia Rating Scale was also shown to decline postsurgery (59). The only exception to stability or slight decline was seen in a study by Contarino et al., where an improvement on the MMSE was reported over the follow-up period.

Consideration of GPi DBS on Cognition

Although there has been considerably less research on the effects of GPi DBS on cognition, comparison with the effects seen in STN DBS may prove informative. Although both targets have demonstrated clinical efficacy in the treatment of the cardinal motor signs of PD, STN DBS has gained greater popularity and is now considered the site of choice by most centers performing these procedures. This preference seems to stem predominately from the belief that STN DBS provides greater improvement in reducing the motor manifestations of PD and allows a reduction in dopaminergic medication not permitted with GPi DBS (77). Table 2 lists those studies that have examined GPi stimulation in regard to cognition.

As can be seen, out of eight total studies, only three studies examined GPi stimulation exclusively. Of these three, only one study found a decline in cognitive function following surgery (78). In this study, a decline in language function as measured by a semantic verbal fluency task was observed, as was a decline in global cognition as measured by the Mattis Dementia Rating Scale. In the remaining studies examining a mix of GPi and STN DBS, only one additional study reported a decline in frontal lobe functions (61). Well-designed,

Table 2 Studies Examining Neuropsychological Sequelae of GPi DBS: Domains Assessed and Which Areas Demonstrated Change

Study (first author)	% male	Mean age at surgery	Mean H&Y (off)	Mean disease duration (yrs)	Unilateral, bilateral, or mixed	STN, GPi, or mixed	Surgical vs. On/off	Mean follow-up (mo)	Functions assessed	Improvements	Declines
Fields (1999)	83%	48.2 (11.3)		11.33 (5)	mixed	GPi	surgical	2 mo following 1st surgery (unilateral), & 3 mo following 2nd surgery (bilateral)	GC, Att, Front, Lang, VS, Vmem, NVMem, Mood	Mood	N/a
Troster (1997)	67%	50 (12.9)		10 (4.9)	unilateral-6 of 9 patients = left	GPi	surgical	3	GC, Att, Lang, VMem, NVMem, Mood, Front, VS, IQ	Mood	Lang, GC
Vingerhoets (1999)	75%	55 (9.9)	pre = 2.7 (1), post = 1.6 (1)	9.6 (5.7)	unilateral-13 of 20 = left	GPi	surgical	3	VMem, NVMem, VS, Front	N/a	N/a
Straits-Troster (2000)	67%	50.3 (13)		10.3 (4.9)	unilateral-3R 6L	mixed	surgical	2.6 (0.88) mo	Mood	Mood	N/a

										GC (surgery)	N/a
Pillon (2000)	GPi1 = 75%, GPi2 = 60%	GPi1 = 52.5 (6.5), GPi2 = 12.6 (2.7)		GPi1 = 16.3 (3.4), GPi2 = 12.6 (2.7)	bilateral	mixed	both	3 & 12	GC, Front, Lang, VMem, NVMem Mood		
Jahanshahi (2000)	77%	52.8 (4.9)	4.5	15.1 (4.8)	bilateral	mixed	on/off		Front, Att, Lang, IQ	Front, Att, Lang	Front
Burchiel (1999)	70%	46.5 (11)	4	10.6(2)	bilateral	mixed	on/off	10 days, 3, 6 & 12 mo	VMem, Att, Mood	Mood	N/a
Brusa (2001)		53.5 (6.18)		15.16 (6.55)	bilateral	mixed	on/off (for both stimulator and l-dopa)	4 different conditions each 1 mo apart	Front, Lang, Mood, Other	N/a	N/a

Abbreviations: Att, attention; GC, _; GPi, globus pallidus interna; L-dopa, levodopa; N/a, not applicable; NVMem, nonverbal memory; STN subthalamic nucleus; VMem, verbal memory; VS, visuospatial.

head-to-head clinical trials that evaluate motor, nonmotor, and adverse events of both of these approaches are needed.

It is noteworthy that three out of three (100%) studies found improvements in mood following GPi STN when compared with only 11% (3/27) in the STN DBS literature. Although it is difficult to draw any clear conclusions based on the very small sample of GPi DBS studies, it is interesting that positive changes in mood and affect may be differentially affected in GPi DBS when compared with STN DBS. Indeed, preliminary data from Okun et al. (79) suggested that there may be mood changes associated with both STN and GPi DBS. Notably, optimal placement of electrodes in both STN and GPi seems to result in overall improvement in mood and is associated with a lower incidence of adverse mood effects than stimulation outside the optimal site. Data from this study, however, suggested that slight movement dorsal or ventral to the site of optimal motor performance may be associated with more adverse changes in mood with STN stimulation than with GPi stimulation.

SUMMARY AND CONCLUSIONS

As seen in the preceding text, the effect of DBS on neuropsychological function in PD is complex and appears to be influenced by a number of factors related to the illness itself as well as stimulator placement and parameters. The most consistent findings thus far from the extant literature are that moderate declines in verbal fluency and related functions are most commonly seen following STN DBS. It is notable, however, that there have been very few large prospective longitudinal studies, which have included a comprehensive assessment of neuropsychological functions. As PD is a heterogeneous disorder, some of the variability in neuropsychological outcomes after STN DBS may be attributable to subtle subtype differences in the PD populations under study. Indeed, a recent study by Weintraub et al. (2004) identified three different subtypes of PD based on their performance on a verbal list-learning test (i.e., Hopkins Verbal Learning Test—Revised). In this study, cluster analysis was used to classify patients into three memory subgroups based on performance on free recall, intrusion errors, and recall enhancement with recognition. Results revealed three distinct subgroups: an "unimpaired" group that demonstrated intact free recall and few intrusion errors and "impaired retrieval" and "impaired encoding" subgroups with similar impairment on free recall, but the impaired retrieval group demonstrated greater memory improvement with recognition ($P < 0.001$) and had fewer intrusion errors ($P < 0.001$) than the impaired encoding group. The use of such subtyping strategies may hold promise in examining some of the variability seen in the DBS literature. For example, it is possible that those subjects with an "impaired encoding" memory profile may be at greater risk for disruptions of verbal fluency post-STN DBS surgery. The use of such subtyping strategies may prove useful in identifying those patients at greater risk for neurocognitive dysfunction following STN DBS surgery.

A recent quantitative review of the cognitive sequelae of STN DBS generally supports the findings in the current review. Using a random-effects meta-analytic model, Parsons et al. (80) examined the extant literature concerning the effects of STN DBS on cognition. Moderator variables such as confirmation of target by microelectrode recording, verification of electrode placement via radiographic methods, simulation parameters, assessment timepoints, neuropsychological measures, and medication status were also examined. Out of 40 eligible studies, 28 cohort studies (a sample size of 612 patients) were available for meta-analytic review. Results of the meta-analysis revealed small but significant declines in executive functions and verbal learning and memory following STN DBS surgery (Cohens's *d* of 0.08 and 0.21, respectively). Although these findings indicated *statistically significant* declines in these domains following STN DBS, it is noteworthy that the magnitude of these decrements would not be considered to represent *clinically meaningful* declines in function. Consistent with prior findings in the literature and the current review, larger declines in both semantic (Cohen's *d* = 0.73) and phonemic verbal fluency (0.51) were evident across studies. Notably, changes in verbal fluency were not related to patient age, duration of illness, stimulation parameters, or changes in dopaminergic therapy dose after surgery. Despite the noted changes, the results of this detailed meta-analytic study suggest that STN DBS, at least for selected patients, is generally safe from a neuropsychological vantage point. Regardless, the presence of any negative changes in neurocognitive function postsurgery reinforces the need for pre- and postoperative neuropsychological assessment for STN DBS candidates. On the basis of the literature reviewed, emphasis in these assessments on executive functions, verbal learning and memory, and verbal fluency seem prudent and empirically supported. In addition, the effects of GPi DBS on cognition are relatively unexplored at this time, and possible differential neuropsychological effects of this approach when compared with STN DBS have not been tested. Given the different subcortical circuits involved in these DBS approaches, further investigation may help tease apart differences in outcomes and efficacy of these procedures. Lastly, well-controlled, randomized clinical trials will be very important in providing a "gold standard" by which to judge possible changes in neuropsychological function following STN DBS.

REFERENCES

1. Youdim MBH, Riederer P. Understanding Parkinson's disease. Scientific American 1997; 276:52–59.
2. Lees A, Smith E. Cognitive deficits in the early stages of Parksinon's disease. Brain 1983; 106:257–270.
3. Stocchi F, Brusa L. Cognition and emotion in different stages and subtypes of Parkinson's disease. J Neurol 2000; 247:114–121.
4. Aarsland D, Anderson K, Larsen J, Lolk A, Kragh-Sorensen P. Prevalence and characteristics of dementia in Parkinson's disease: an 8-year prospective study. Arch Neurol 2003; 60:387–392.

5. Muslimovic D, Post B, Speelman JD, Schmand B. Cognitive profile of patients with newly diagnosed Parkinson's disease. Neurology 2005; 65:1239–1245.

6. Dubois B, Pillon B. Cognitive deficits in Parkinson's disease. J Neurol 1997; 244: 2–8.

7. Levin BE, Katzen HL. Early cognitive changes and nondementing behavioral abnormalities in Parkinson's disease. Adv Neurol 2005; 96:84–94.

8. Azuma T, Cruz RF, Bayles KA, Tomoeda CK, Montgomery EB, Jr. A longitudinal study of neuropsychological changes in individuals with Parkinson's disease. Int J Geriatr Psych 2003; 18:1115–1120.

9. Uc EY, Rizzo M, Anderson SW, Qian S, Rodnitzky RL, Dawson JD. Visual dysfunction in Parkinson's disease without dementia. Neurology 2005; 65:1907–1913.

10. Crucian GP, Barrett AM, Burk DW, et al. Mental object rotation in Parkinson's disease. J Int Neuropsychol Soc 2005; 9:1078–1087.

11. Becker G, Muller A, Braune S, et al. Early diagnosis of Parkinson's disease. J Neurol 2002; 249:40–48.

12. Brown RG, Marsden CC. Visuospatial function in Parkinson's Disease. Brain 1986; 109:987–1002.

13. Bondi MW, Kaszniak AW, Bayles KA, Vance KT. Contribution of frontal system dysfunction to memory and perceptual abilities in Parkinson's disease. Neuropsychology 1993; 7:89–102.

14. Bosboom JLW, Stoffers D, Wolters EC. Cognitive dysfunction and dementia in Parkinson's disease. J Neural Trans 2004; 111:1303–1315.

15. Peran P, Rascol O, Demonet JF, et al. Deficit of verb generation in nondemented patients with Parkinson's disease. Mov Disord 2003; 18:150–156.

16. Ballard CG, Aarsland D, McKeith I, et al. Fluctuations in attention: PD dementia versus DLB with parkinsonism. Neurology 2002; 59:1714–1720.

17. Owen AM, Iddon JL, Hodges JR, Summers BA, Robbins TW. Spatial and non-spatial working memory at different stages of Parkinson's disease. Neuropsychologia 1997; 35:519–532.

18. Woods SP, Troster AI. Prodromal frontal/executive dysfunction predicts incident dementia in Parkinson's disease. J Int Neuropsychol Soc 2003; 9:17–24.

19. Huber SJ, Shuttleworth EC, Friedenberg DL. Neuropsychological differences between the dementias of Alzheimer's and Parkinson's diseases. Arch Neurol 1989; 46: 1287–1291.

20. Aarsland D, Anderson K, Larsen JP, Lolk A, Nielsen H, Kragh-Sorensen P. Risk of dementia in Parkinson's disease: A community-based, prospective study. Neurology 2001; 56:730–736.

21. Emre M. Dementia associated with Parkinson's disease. Lancet 2003; 2:299–237.

22. Mayeux R, Chen J, Mirabello E, et al. An estimate of the incidence of dementia in idiopathic Parkinson's disease. Neurology 1990; 40:1513–1517.

23. Emre M. Dementia in Parkinson's disease: Cause and treatment. Curr Op Neurol 2004; 17:399–404.

24. Aarsland D, Zaccai J, Brayne C. A systemic review of prevalence studies of dementia in Parkinson's disease. Mov Disord 2005b; 20:1255–1263.

25. Burn DJ, Rowan EN, Allan LM, Molloy S, O'Brien JT, Mckeith IG. Motor subtype and cognitive decline in Parkinson's disease, Parkinson's disease with dementia, and dementia with Lewy bodies. J Neurol Neurosurg Psychiatry 2006; 77:585–589.

26. Marder K, Tang MX, Cote L, Stern Y, Mayeux R. The frequency and associated risk factors for dementia in patients with Parkinson's disease. Arch Neurol 1995; 52: 695–701.

27. Levy G, Schupf N, Tang MX, et al. Combined effect of age and severity on the risk of dementia in Parkinson's disease. Annal Neurol 2002; 51:722–729.

28. Aarsland D, Perry R, Brown A, Larsen JP, Ballard C. Neuropathology of dementia in Parkinson's disease: A prospective, community-based study. Annal Neurol 2005a; 58:773–776.

29. Bertrand E, Lechowicz W, Szpak GM, Lewandowska E, Dymecki J, Wierzba-Bobro-wicz T. Limbic neuropathology in idiopathic Parkinson's disease with concomitant dementia. Folia Neuropathologica 2004; 42:141–150.

30. Weintraub D, Moberg PJ, Duda JE, Katz IR, Stern MB. Effect of psychiatric and other nonmotor symptoms on disability in Parkinson's disease. J Am Geriatr Soc 2004; 52:784–788.

31. Jenkins C, Jono R, Stanton B, Stroup-Benham C. The measurement of health-related quality of life: major dimensions identified by factor analysis. Soc Sci Med 1990; 31:925–931.

32. de Lau LML, Schipper C, Maarten A, Hofman A, Koudstall PJ, Breteler MMB. Prognosis of Parkinson disease: Risk of dementia and mortality: The Rotterdam Study. Arch Neurol 2005; 62:1265–1269.

33. Levy G, Tang MX, Louis ED, et al. The association of incident dementia with mortality in PD. Neurology 2003; 59:1708–1713.

34. Schrag A. Psychiatric aspects of Parkinson's disease: An update. J Neurol 2004; 251:795–804.

35. Lange K, Paul G, Naumann M, Gsell W. Dopaminergic effects on cognitive perform-ance in patients with Parkinson's Disease. J Neural Trans 1995; 46(suppl):423–432.

36. Gasparini M, Fabrizio E, Bonifati V, Meco G. Cognitive improvement during Tolcapone treatment in Parkinson's disease. J Neural Trans 1997; 104:887–894.

37. Kulisevsky J, Garcia-Sanchez C, Berthier M, Barbanoj M, Pascual-Sedano B. Chronic effects of dopaminergic replacement on cognitive function in Parkinson's disease: a two-year follow-up study of previously untreated patients. Mov Disord 2000; 15:613–626.

38. Alegret M, Vallderoriola F, Marti M, et al. Comparative cognitive effects of bilateral subthalamic stimulation and subcutaneous continuous infusion of apomorphine in Parkinson's disease. Mov Disord 2004; 19:1463–1469.

39. Ruzicka E, Roth J, Spackova N, Mecir P, Jech R. Apomorphine induced cognitive changes in Parkinson's disease. J Neurol Neurosurg Psychiatry 1994; 57:998–1001.

40. Miyasaki J, Shannon K, Voon V, et al. Practice parameter: evaluation and treatment of depression, psychosis, and dementia in Parkinson disease (an evidence-based review): report of the Quality Standards Subcommittee of the American Academy of Neurology. Neurology 2006; 66:996–1002.

41. Bullock R. The clinical benefits of rivastigmine may reflect its dual inhibitory mode of action: an hypothesis. Int J Clin Prac 2002; 56:206–214.

42. Olanow C, Marsden C, Lang A, Goetz C. The role of surgery in Parkinson's disease. Neurology 1994; 44:S17–S20.

43. Woods SP, Fields JA, Troster AI. Neuropsychological sequelae of subthalamic nucleus deep brain stimulation in Parkinson's disease: a critical review. Neuropsychol Rev 2002; 12:111–126.

44. Chang V, Chou K. Deep brain stimulation for Parkinson's disease: patient selection and motor outcomes. Medicine & Health 2006; 89:142–144.
45. Krack P, Batir A, Van Blercom N, et al. Five-year follow-up of bilateral stimulation of the subthalamic nucleus in advanced Parkinson's disease. New Engl J Med 2003; 349:1925–1934.
45a. Kleiner-Fisman G, Herzog J, Fisman DN, et al. Subthalamic nucleus deep brain stimulation: summary and meta-analysis of outcomes. Mov Disord 2006; 21(suppl 14):S290–S304.
46. Ford B. Pallidotomy for generalized dystonia. Adv Neurol 2004; 94:287–299.
47. Ceballos-Baumann A, Boecker H, Bartenstein P, et al. A positron emission tomographic study of subthalamic nucleus stimulation in Parkinson disease: enhanced movement-related activity of motor-association cortex and decreased motor cortex resting activity. Arch Neurol 1999; 56:997–1003.
48. Van Horn G, Schiess M, Soukup V. Subthalamic deep brain stimulation: neurobehavioral concerns. Arch Neurol 2001; 58:1205–1206.
49. Hoehn M, Yahr M. Parkinsonism: onset, progression and mortality. Neurology 1967; 17:427–442.
50. Fraix V, Houeto J, Lagrange C, et al. Clinical and economic results of bilateral subthalamic nucleus stimulation in Parkinson's disease. J Neurol Neurosurg Psychiatry 2006; 77:443–449.
51. Castelli L, Perozzo P, Genesia M, et al. Sexual well being in parkinsonian patients after deep brain stimulation of the subthalamic nucleus. J Neurol Neurosurg Psychiatry 2004; 75:1260–1264.
52. Beck A, Ward C, Mendelssohn M, Erbaugh J. An inventory for measuring depression. Arch Gen Psych 1961; 4:561–571.
53. Behari M, Srivastava A, Pandey R. Quality of life in patients with Parkinson's disease. Parkinsonsim Relat Disord 2005; 11:221–226.
54. Stroop J. Studies of interference in serial verbal reactions. J Exp Psychol 1935; 18:643–662.
55. Reitan R. Validity of the trail making test as an indication of organic brain damage. Percep Motor Skill 1958; 8:271–276.
56. Dujardin K, Defebvre L, Krystkowiak P, Blond S, Destee A. Influence of chronic bilateral stimulation of the subthalamic nucleus on cognitive function in Parkinson's disease. J Neurol 2001; 248:603–611.
57. Moretti R, Torre P, Antonello RM, et al. Neuropsychological changes after subthalamic nucleus stimulation: a 12 month follow–up in nine patients with Parkinson's disease. Parkinsonism Relat Disord 2003; 10:73–79.
58. Smeding HMM, Esselink RAJ, Schmand B, et al. Unilateral pallidotomy versus bilateral subthalamic nucleus stimulation in PD: a comparison of neuropsychological effects. J Neurol 2005; 252:176–182.
59. Schupbach WMM, Chastan N, Welter ML, et al. Stimulation of the subthalamic nucleus in Parkinson's disease: a 5 year follow up. J Neurol Neurosurg Psychiatry 2005; 76:1640–1644.
60. Pillon B, Ardouin C, Damier P, et al. Neuropsychological changes between "off" and "on" STN or GPi stimulation in Parkinson's disease. Neurology 2000; 55:411–418.
61. Jahanshahi M, Ardouin CMA, Brown RG, et al. The impact of deep brain stimulation on executive function in Parkinson's disease. Brain 2000; 123:1142–1154.

62. Schroeder U, Kuehler A, Haslinger B, et al. Subthalamic nucleus stimulation affects striato-anterior cingulate cortex circuit in a response conflict task: a PET study. Brain 2002; 125:1995–2004.

63. Gironell A, Kulisevsky J, Rami L, Fortuny N, Garcia-Sanchez C, Pascual-Sedano B. Effects of pallidotomy and bilateral subthalamic stimulation on cognitive function in Parkinson disease. J Neurol 2003; 250:917–923.

64. Castelli L, Perozzo P, Zibetti M, et al. Chronic deep brain stimulation of the subthalamic nucleus for Parkinson's disease: effects on cognition, mood, anxiety, and personality traits. Euro Neurol 2006; 55:136–144.

65. Saint-Cyr JA, Trepanier LL, Kumar R, Lozano AM, Lang AE. Neuropsychological consequences of chronic bilateral stimulation of the subthalamic nucleus in Parkinson's disease. Brain 2000; 123:2091–2108.

66. Morrison CE, Borod JC, Perrine K, et al. Neuropsychological functioning following bilateral subthalamic nucleus stimulation in Parkinson's disease. Archives of Clinical Neuropsychology 2004; 19:165–181.

67. De Gaspari D, Siri C, Di Gioia M, et al. Clinical correlates and cognitive underpinnings of verbal fluency impairment after chronic subthalamic stimulation in Parkinson's disease. Parkinsonism Relat Disord 2006; 12:289–295.

68. De Gaspari D, Siri C, Landi A, et al. Clinical and neuropsychological follow up at 12 months in patients with complicated Parkinson's disease treated with subcutaneous apomorphine infusion or deep brain stimulation of the subthalamic nucleus. J Neurol Neurosurg Psychiatry 2006; 77:450–453.

69. Contarino MF, Daniele A, Sibilia AH, et al. Cognitive outcome five years after bilateral chronic stimulation of subthalamic nucleus in patients with Parkinson's disease. J Neurol Neurosurg Psychiatry 2006.

70. Whelan BM, Murdoch BE, Theodoros DG, Hall B, Silburn P. Defining a role for the subthalamic nucleus within operative theoretical models of subcortical participation in language. J Neurol Neurosurg Psychiatry 2003; 74:1543–1550.

71. Alegret M, Junque C, Vallderoriola F, et al. Effects of bilateral subthalamic stimulation on cognitive function in Parkinson disease. Arch Neurol 2001; 58: 1223–1227.

72. Funkiewiez A, Ardouin C, Caputo E, et al. Long term effects of bilateral subthalamic nucleus stimulation on cognitive function, mood, and behaviour in Parkinson's disease. J Neurol Neurosurg Psychiatry 2004; 75:834–839.

73. Halbig TD, Gruber D, Kopp UA, et al. Subthalamic stimulation differentially modulates declarative and nondeclarative memory. NeuroReport 2004; 15:539–543.

74. Witt K, Pulkowski U, Herzog J, et al. Deep brain stimulation of the subthalamic nucleus improves cognitive flexibility but impairs response inhibition in Parkinson disease. Arch Neurol 2004; 61:697–700.

75. Burchiel KJ, Anderson VC, Favre J, Hammerstad JP. Comparison of pallidal and subthalamic nucleus deep brain stimulation for advanced Parkinson's disease: results of a randomized, blinded pilot study. Neurosurgery 1999; 45:1375–1384.

76. Funkiewiez A, Ardouin C, Krack P, et al. Acute psychotropic effects of bilateral subthalamic nucleus stimulation and levodopa in Parkinson's disease. Mov Disord 2003; 18:524–530.

77. Vitek J. Deep brain stimulation for Parkinson's disease. A critical re-evaluation of STN versus GPi DBS. Stereotact Funct Neurosurg 2002; 78:119–131.

78. Troster AI, Fields JA, Wilkinson SB, et al. Unilateral pallidal stimulation for Parkinson's disease: neurobehavioral functioning before and 3 months after electrode implantation. Am Acad of Neurol 1997; 49:1078–1083.
79. Okun M, Green J, Saben R, Gross R, Foote K, Vitek J. Mood changes with deep brain stimulation of STN and GPi: results of a pilot study. J Neurol Neurosurg Psychiatry 2003; 74:1584–1586.
80. Parsons T, Rogers S, Braaten A, Woods S, Troster A. Cognitive sequalae of subthalamic nucleus deep brain stimulation in Parkinson's disease: a meta-analysis. Lancet Neurol 2006; 5:578–588.

16

Neuropsychiatric Complications and Deep Brain Stimulation in Parkinson's Disease

Daniel Weintraub

*Departments of Neurology and Psychiatry, University of Pennsylvania,
Parkinson's Disease Research, Education, and Clinical Center (PADRECC), and
Mental Illness Research, Education, and Clinical Center (MIRECC), Philadelphia
Veterans Affairs Medical Center, Philadelphia, Pennsylvania, U.S.A.*

Johannes C. Rothlind

*Department of Psychiatry, University of California at San Francisco and
Parkinson's Disease Research, Education, and Clinical Center (PADRECC),
San Francisco Veterans Affairs Medical Center, San Francisco, California, U.S.A.*

INTRODUCTION

Parkinson's disease (PD) is a neurologic syndrome defined by a triad of motor symptoms. However, the frequent co-occurrence of cognitive, affective, and other neurobehavioral disturbance suggests a neuropsychiatric condition with highly varied symptoms. Depression and anxiety disorders, cognitive impairment, and psychosis have long been recognized in some individuals diagnosed with PD (1). Other common, but less well studied, psychiatric manifestations include apathy (2), impulse control disorders (ICDs) (a.k.a., hedonistic homeostatic dysregulation, dopamine dysregulation syndrome, or compulsive behavior) (3), disorders of sleep and wakefulness (4), and pseudobulbar affect.

These neuropsychiatric complications in PD are associated with excess disability, worse quality of life, poorer outcomes, and caregiver distress (1).

Yet, in spite of this and their frequent occurrence, there is incomplete understanding of the epidemiology, phenomenology, risk factors, neuropathophysiology, and optimal treatment strategies for these disorders. Neuropsychiatric complications are typically multimorbid, and there is great intra- and inter-individual variability in presentation. Not surprisingly, there is evidence that psychiatric disorders in PD are under-recognized and under-treated (5). Interestingly, there is evidence that dopaminergic medications may both contribute to the development of some psychiatric symptoms and yet be a form of treatment for others (e.g., dopamine agonists may induce psychosis, but have antidepressant properties).

Deep brain stimulation (DBS) has become an increasingly common form of nonablative surgical treatment for PD. Brain targets most commonly include the subthalamic nucleus (STN) and the globus pallidus interna (GPi). The impact of DBS on psychiatric symptoms and cognition appears varied, with research reporting both improvement and worsening in mental status and psychiatric morbidity post-DBS. This chapter provides an overview of the literature concerning the potential impact of DBS on neuropsychiatric symptoms in PD, and focuses primarily on DBS treatment of the STN, and to a lesser extent on GPi. Common factors may mediate mood, behavior, and cognitive changes during DBS treatment for PD. Because neurocognitive changes are reviewed in detail in the chapter by Moberg (Chapter 15), this chapter will focus on noncognitive psychiatric features noted in DBS patients.

THE NEURAL SUBSTRATE OF DEEP BRAIN STIMULATION AND NEUROPSYCHIATRIC DISORDERS

The motor effects of DBS in PD in part involve inhibition of hyperactive neurons in either the STN or GPi by high-frequency stimulation, with subsequent modulation of the neural circuits connecting the cortex, striatum, and thalamus, also known as the cortico-striatal-thalamo-cortical loops (6). However, some of these loops also subserve cognitive and emotional functioning through connections to the frontal cortex and the limbic system (7). Positron emission tomography and functional magnetic resonance imaging studies during STN DBS have found changes in frontal lobe and limbic system neuronal activity (8–10). Thus, both the mood and cognitive changes that have been associated with STN DBS may in part be a result of alterations in this complex neural circuitry.

In addition, the STN is known to have motor and limbic components, and the total STN area is so small that it is difficult to differentially stimulate its subregions (11). Direct stimulation of structures surrounding the STN (e.g., substantia nigra and GPi) may also result in changes in neuronal function or neurotransmitter systems implicated in psychiatric disorders. For example, there is excitatory glutaminergic outflow from the STN, and the rest of the basal ganglia is innervated by numerous neurotransmitters, including dopamine, serotonin, acetylcholine, excitatory amino acids, GABA, nitric oxide, and adenosine (12). Stimulation of limbic regions within and adjacent to the STN may help explain the psychiatric effects of STN DBS (13,14). Finally, the actual surgical procedure to stereotactically place the electrodes in the STN involves passing the electrodes through the frontal lobes, most commonly bilaterally. It is not known to what extent this procedure can temporarily or permanently affect the neurons of the prefrontal cortex or their associated white matter tracts. However, in general, damage to these regions can result in a frontal lobe syndrome, marked by changes in cognition and behavior.

NEUROPSYCHIATRIC SYMPTOMS IN PATIENTS TREATED WITH DEEP BRAIN STIMULATION

Depression

In a recent comprehensive review (15) of the effect of STN DBS on mood, the authors reported the results of 14 cohort studies and nine case reports or series. Looking at group changes in depression rating scales following DBS, the average score was improved or unchanged in all studies compared to presurgical ratings. Examining changes in depression scores at an individual level, anti-depressant effects (i.e., decrease in score >1 standard deviation of the group mean) were reported in 16.7% to 76.0% of patients and depressant effects (i.e., increase in score >1 standard deviation of the group mean) in 2.0% to 33.3% of patients. Most of the aforementioned studies examined the chronic effects of STN DBS on mood, but there also case reports of acute changes in mood with stimulation (11,13,16). In the only study in the review which included a PD control group not receiving DBS, there were no changes in depression scores from baseline to follow-up in either group (17). A more recent study of 33 nondepressed patients undergoing DBS also found overall improvement in mood postsurgery (18).

However, examining group-average changes in depression rating scale scores is not the same as looking at individual outcomes (19). At an individual level, there have been reports of worsening or de novo depression post-DBS surgery (20,21). Even in studies reporting an overall improvement in mood, it has been reported that between 4% to 17% of patients may experience new or worsening depression in a period ranging from three months to three years postsurgery (15). Most concerning have been case reports of suicide ideation, or completed or attempted suicide after DBS therapy (11,21–24). In one completed suicide case (22), it had not been noted at the time of surgery that the patient had a previous history of severe depression and that the patient's father had committed suicide. This case highlights the importance of obtaining a thorough psychiatric history as part of the pre-DBS evaluation.

There have been attempts to examine predictors or correlates of mood deterioration post-DBS, but results have been inconsistent, save the impact of a history of depression (see subsequently). Arguing against a consistent relation-ship between motor and mood outcomes is the fact that many cases of new-onset or worsening depression have occurred in patients who had improved motor function (24–26), suggesting that other factors [e.g., significant decreases in dopaminergic therapy, the effects of stimulation itself, unrealistic expectations about the degree of improvement postsurgery, or even adverse psychological adjustment to significant improvement in disability (20,26,27)] contribute to the presence of depressive symptoms post-DBS. Although levodopa is reported to have a general mood elevating effect if not antidepressant properties, no study has shown that worsening of mood post-DBS is clearly associated with a decrease in levodopa dosage or other dopaminergic therapy (24).

There are important limitations in the existing research examining the impact of DBS on depression symptoms in PD patients. First, virtually all the research has been uncontrolled, making it impossible to isolate DBS effects. For instance, one study (28) found that mood symptoms were improved post-DBS regardless of whether the stimulator was on or off, suggesting that factors other than the stimulation state are contributing to changes in mood. Secondly, the primary outcome measure for all studies was change in motor symptoms, and the changes in mood state were evaluated as a secondary measure. Thirdly, in all studies there were decreases in dopaminergic medication post-DBS, and this in itself may have impacted on mood symptoms.

Anxiety

Anxiety is frequently comorbid with depression in PD, and anecdotally is often a more disabling symptom. It commonly presents in this population as either generalized anxiety symptoms or discrete anxiety attacks. In a review of 24 cases, clinically significant anxiety was present in about 75% both pre and postoperatively, but the anxiety worsened in the majority of the cases post-DBS surgery in spite of overall motor improvement (22). In addition, two of four patients with agoraphobia (i.e., fear of public places) reported a worsening of these symptoms. Generalized anxiety was frequently associated with a fear of sudden failure of the stimulator, whereas agoraphobia was related to fears of having freezing episodes in public. However, other recent case series found that on average anxiety either improved (18,28) or was unchanged (29) postoperatively, and improvement was retained over a one-year period.

Obsessive-compulsive disorder (OCD) is another type of anxiety disorder that may occur in PD at an increased frequency compared with the general population. There are two case reports of patients with both PD and severe OCD who experienced a dramatic decrease in OCD symptomatology post-DBS surgery (30).

Mania

The aforementioned review (15) of the effect of STN DBS on mood in PD also identified two cohort studies and six individual cases or case series reporting on (hypo)manic states, as defined by states of "laughter," an increase in mania scale scores, or meeting DSM-IV (31) criteria for a manic episode, and there have been additional case reports of (hypo)mania (14,25,32). The two cohort studies reported that transient or permanent (hypo)mania occurred in 4% to 20% of patients (32–35). In one small case series, the manic episodes occurred in all patients within 48 hours of surgery and turning on the stimulators (35). In contrast to depression, most of the cases of mania have been reported to be transient (28), either resolving with psychiatric treatment (25) or changes in DBS electrode contacts (35) or reduction in stimulation amplitude (i.e., decreasing voltage or pulse width) (14).

Psychosis

Psychosis as a complication of STN DBS has been reported, but not commonly. In a recent long-term follow-up of a cohort of STN DBS patients, transient hallucinations (16%) and psychosis (11%) were commonly reported postsurgery, but no information was provided on whether these patients had experienced psychosis preoperatively or on the length of time that lapsed between the surgery and the onset of psychosis (23). None of the patients in this study developed permanent psychosis over a five-year period. In another case series, three patients (6% of sample) developed transient de novo psychosis in the perioperative period, two of which resolved spontaneously and the other with antipsychotic and mood stabilizer treatment (32).

Other Neurobehavioral Changes

Transient confusional states, most likely related to the surgical procedure, have been reported to occur in up to 15% of patients immediately postsurgery (32). Behavioral disorders suggestive of a frontal lobe syndrome have also been reported post-DBS. Damage to the frontal lobes, in this case secondary to surgery-related microtrauma, can result in a syndrome characterized by executive impairment and one or more behavioral changes, including depression, disinhibition (emotional, social, and behavioral), emotional lability, and apathy/abulia, the latter defined as amotivation that manifests itself as a decrease in goal-directed behavior, cognition, and emotion (36–39). In one case series (40), patients on average had an increase in frontal symptomatology 9 to 12 months postoperatively, as scored by their caregivers using the Frontal Lobe Personality Scale (FLOPS) (41). Examining FLOPS subscales, there was significant worsening on the executive dysfunction index and a trend for worsening on the apathy index, but no worsening on the disinhibition index. Specific behavioral changes included perseveration, impulsivity, worse social judgement, emotional lability, and lack of awareness of deficits. Additionally, three patients, all elderly, were reported by their caregivers to have developed frontal behavioral dyscontrol without insight postoperatively. In this case series, the greatest cognitive decline postsurgery was noted in executive abilities, suggesting that the aforementioned behaviors are mediated by damage to the prefrontal cortex.

Perhaps related to the frontal lobe syndrome, another case series reported emotional hyper-reactivity (i.e., affective lability or possibly pseudobulbar affect) in the majority of patients post-DBS surgery (22). Apathy, defined as a loss of interest or motivation, can occur in the context of depression but is also thought to be a distinct psychiatric syndrome in neurodegenerative diseases, including PD (2). It is often associated with damage to the frontal lobes and executive impairment, so it is not surprising that there have been case reports of apathy without depression post-DBS surgery (22,33,42). On the other hand, there have also been reports of improvements in initiative and motivation postoperatively (22).

Finally, there is an increasing awareness of the occurrence of ICDs, such as compulsive gambling and sexual behavior, in PD (3). Although most ICD cases are thought to be associated with the use of dopamine agonists, there have been case reports of both de novo ICD behavior (22) and improvement in ICD-like behaviors post-DBS surgery (43).

ASCERTAINING SPECIFICITY OF DEEP BRAIN STIMULATION EFFECTS

In an attempt to isolate the impact of DBS on psychiatric state, studies have been designed to control for the effects that dopaminergic medication and motor symptoms may have in this regard. In two studies, nondepressed PD patients were evaluated both *on* and *off* PD medications and *on* and *off* DBS (2×2 design), and both levodopa and DBS were found to have distinct, positive effects on feelings of dysphoria, well being, motivation, fatigue, and anxiety (44,45). In another study, no association was found between improvement in motor and mood symptoms, suggesting that any mood benefits derived from STN DBS are independent of its motor effects (40).

Regarding apathy, DBS patients that were *off* medication were found on average to report a decrease in severity of apathy *on* DBS compared with *off* DBS (46). The improvement in apathy was similar to that reported by a matche group on non-DBS patients when tested in the *on* levodopa state compared with *off* levodopa.

ROLE OF PSYCHIATRIC HISTORY

Depression occurs commonly in both the general population and in PD. Thus, it is expected that many patients who undergo DBS will have a history of depression. Four studies (11,22,33,47) have examined the impact of psychiatric history on mood state post-DBS, and three of them (11,22,33) found a significant positive correlation between a history of depression and a depressant effect of STN DBS. As most DBS studies have attempted to exclude patients with significant active depression, it may be that the positive effects of DBS on mood are more likely to occur in nondepressed or mildly depressed patients.

Even though it has been recommended that the presence of clinically significant depression or anxiety at the time of the presurgical evaluation should be exclusion criteria for proceeding with surgery (48,49), retrospective reviews have
documented that thorough psychiatric evaluations and histories are often not obtained
before surgery (22). In a recent prospective study, 40 consecutive PD patients presenting for DBS were thoroughly evaluated for current and lifetime psychiatric history
(50). Lifetime prevalence rates were 60% for depression, 40% for anxiety, 35% for
psychosis, and 10% for medication-induced mania. Of this sample, 23% required psychiatric treatment for current symptoms prior to being considered eligible for DBS.
These results highlight the importance not only of psychiatric evaluation, but also
psychiatric treatment when indicated, before proceeding with DBS surgery.

EFFECTS OF DBS LEAD LOCATION AND STIMULATION PARAMETERS

There is also preliminary evidence that the location of the DBS leads may impact
on mood outcomes. In a dramatic case report (16), a woman experienced severe,
acute, transient depressive symptoms when high-frequency stimulation was
applied to the left substantia nigra instead of the STN. There are other case
reports of changes in mood based on the DBS parameters (11), and one hypothesis
is that use of electrode placements slightly dorsal or ventral to the site for optimal
motor performance may adversely impact mood (13). Although no study found any
clear predictor or clinical correlates of mania post-DBS, in one case series of three
patients, the manic episodes were triggered by stimulation at the lowest (i.e., the
most ventral) of the quadripolar bilateral STN electrodes (35). These episodes
gradually resolved with a change to higher (i.e., more dorsal) electrode contacts.

SUBTHALAMIC NUCLEUS VS. GLOBUS PALLIDUM
INTERNA DEEP BRAIN STIMULATION

The STN has become the preferred target for DBS, in part because it provides
excitatory innervation to a variety of neuronal targets in addition to the GPi
(51) and has been reported to allow a greater reduction in dopaminergic
therapy (13). However, these effects of STN compared with GPi DBS could
have implications for psychiatric outcomes. Although there have been no
published controlled comparative studies of STN and GPi DBS, it has been
suggested that there may be fewer psychiatric complications with GPi DBS
(13,19,27,52,53). However, these conclusions are based on extremely limited
and uncontrolled data, so it appears premature to recommend a particular site
for DBS on the basis of differential psychiatric outcomes.

ACUTE VS. CHRONIC EFFECTS

The length of the time period between DBS surgery and the psychiatric assessments for the different case series and cohort studies has varied widely, from

several weeks up to five years. Some experts believe that in the short-term there tends to be an improvement in depression, occasional induction of euphoria or mania, and cases of disinhibited behavior, while the long-term course has been associated with an increase in apathy and depressive symptoms (44). However, such conclusions were based on the comparison of multiple, uncontrolled studies with widely differing methodologies, making it impossible to differentiate time effects related to DBS from numerous other possible confounding variables, including transient effects related to the acute postsurgical period, changes in dopaminergic therapy over time, and the natural progression of the disease. In addition, there are case series that have reported significant worsening in mood in a subset of DBS patients within weeks of surgery (24).

In two recent uncontrolled studies that followed DBS patients, described as free of major psychiatric pathology presurgically, over a five-year period there was no overall change on a depression rating scale (23,33). In one of the studies (23), the authors characterized adverse events as either transient or permanent. Transient psychiatric effects over this extended period included depression (22%), suicide attempts (11%), hallucinations or psychosis (27%), apathy (11%), disinhibition or emotional lability (14%), and aggressive behavior (8%). Permanent effects included disinhibition or emotional lability (22%), depression (22%), and apathy (11%).

ASSESSMENT AND TREATMENT STRATEGIES

Presurgical Evaluation and Treatment

The assessment of psychiatric symptoms in the context of DBS surgery can be complicated by several factors. First, PD patients being evaluated for psychological well-being pre-DBS surgery have a vested interest in minimizing any psychiatric or cognitive symptoms, as they may fear being deemed a poor surgical candidate if they endorse symptoms. Greater fluctuations in emotional states that occur in association with fluctuating motor disability or other factors (54) may complicate self-ratings, especially when the scale utilized focuses on longer time-frame, whereas state measures may provide information that also fails to reflect a more general level of adjustment. Cognitive deficits and deficits in self-appraisal can also further complicate accurate evaluation in some cases. It may be advisable to supplement patient self-report with other sources of information as part of the assessment process.

There are numerous psychiatric rating instruments that are used in PD to screen for psychiatric symptoms, although a full discussion of them is beyond the scope of this chapter. Examples include the 15-item Geriatric Depression Scale (GDS-15) (55), the Spielberger State Anxiety Inventory (56), and the Parkinson's Psychosis Rating Scale (57). The Neuropsychiatric Inventory (NPI) (58), which is one instrument covering most of the possible psychiatric complications that occur in PD, and includes a version that informants can complete by themselves. More detailed personality assessment may be warranted in some cases. If the presence of a psychiatric disorder remains unclear (i.e., difficult differential diagnosis, conflicting information), complex (e.g., comorbid psychiatric disorders), or severe, it is best to refer the patient to a psychiatrist for evaluation and treatment.

Another important aspect of the presurgical evaluation is to make sure that patients have realistic expectations about the outcome of surgery. This should include a frank discussion about inter-individual variability in outcomes and the fact that the DBS does not halt the progression of PD, which will help patients in performing their own risk:benefit analysis before proceeding with surgery.

If there is evidence for a psychiatric disorder that requires treatment due to its severity, impact on function, or effect on quality of life, many movement disorders specialists are comfortable initiating treatment [e.g., starting a selective serotonin reuptake inhibitor (SSRI) for depression or anxiety, or quetiapine for hallucinations]. If a patient is depressed or anxious and prefers nonpharamacological treatment, it is appropriate to make a referral to a psychologist or other licensed therapist for a course of psychotherapy (e.g., cognitive behavioral therapy). In the event that a psychiatric disorder is worsening or not responding to initial treatment, or if the surgery may need to be delayed due to the symptoms, then it is best to refer the patient for a psychiatric evaluation.

Postsurgical Evaluation and Treatment

There is no controlled research on how best to address neuropsychiatric complications that arise or worsen in the context of STN DBS. The main options are to make parameter adjustments to (or temporarily discontinue) the DBS, to increase or add dopaminergic therapy, to initiate other pharmacotherapy and/or psychotherapy, or to have a period of watchful waiting for mild symptoms that may resolve spontaneously (59).

There are cases where episodes of depression (16,26) or mania (35) occurred only with stimulation of particular contacts, and stimulation of other contacts in the STN improved parkinsonism without altering mood. For patients who have had a substantial decrease in dopaminergic therapy post-DBS surgery, there are case reports of improvement in depressed mood with an increase in the total levodopa equivalent daily dose (20).

Regarding the use of psychiatric medications, there are case reports of depression that have responded to treatment with a SSRI or possibly other antidepressants (11,26,59,60), but severe cases, at times accompanied by suicide ideation or attempts, may necessitate psychiatric hospitalization (26,59).

In general, treatment strategies for anxiety are similar to those for depression (i.e., use of SSRIs), although low-dose benzodiazepine use may be necessary and helpful. However, this class of medication must be used cautiously in PD, as benzodiazepines can lead to sedation, worsening cognition, and gait impairment.

Regarding mania and frontal lobe syndrome, while alterations (or even temporary discontinuation) of DBS may be helpful, it is generally contra-indicated to increase dopaminergic therapy in the context of such disorders. Anecdotally, mood stabilizers (i.e., anticonvulsants) can help with such symptoms (32), and atypical antipsychotic use may be necessary in some cases (25), although even atypical antipsychotics must be used cautiously in patients with advanced PD due to their propensity to worsen parkinsonism. Finally, stimulants are commonly used in the treatment of apathy, though it is not clear if they are helpful in this context.

USE OF DEEP BRAIN STIMULATION IN NON-PARKINSON'S DISEASE PSYCHIATRIC PATIENTS

The DBS is also being explored as a treatment for psychiatric disorders, including depression and OCD, in the general population. In a small case series, it was shown that four of six patients with long-standing treatment-resistant depression had a striking and sustained response to DBS of the subgenual cingulate region (Brodmann area 25) (61). Clinical improvement was associated with a marked reduction in local cerebral blood flow and as well as changes in downstream limbic and cortical sites. Additionally, there also are several small case series reporting improvement in most OCD patients treated with DBS of the anterior limbs of the internal capsules (62,63). No reports were found of the use of STN DBS for the treatment of psychiatric disorders.

CONCLUSION

A review of available studies suggest that on average PD patients experience an improvement in mood post-DBS surgery, although a subset of patients experience an increase in depression severity. Because patients with significant depression may be more commonly excluded from consideration for DBS, it is possible that the generally positive effects of DBS on mood do not generalize to patients with more significant depressive symptoms preoperatively. Regarding management, it may make sense to alter DBS parameters in patients who experience an increase in depression post-DBS before employing other treatment strategies, such as reinstituting higher doses of dopaminergic therapy or initiating antidepressant therapy or psychotherapy.

The impact of DBS on other psychiatric symptoms is less clear. There have been reports of anxiety, psychosis, mania, and behavioral disorders (i.e., frontal lobe syndrome), often transient, after DBS surgery, and while alterations to the DBS parameters may be helpful, it is generally contra-indicated to increase dopa-minergic therapy in such cases. Anecdotally, benzodiazepines, mood stabilizers (i.e., anticonvulsants), and atypical antipsychotics may help in the management of these disorders.

Since patients with current or lifetime psychiatric disorders appear to be at higher risk of adverse outcomes postoperatively, conducting both a thorough preoperative psychiatric evaluation and regular postsurgical psychiatric monitoring is of the utmost importance. It does not appear warranted to exclude a patient from undergoing DBS surgery solely on the basis of a lifetime history of psychiatric disorder, but the presence of significant *current* psychiatric symptoms may warrant at least a delay in the surgery until psychiatric treatment or other measures can be instituted to help improve the patient's mental state. However, it is also important to note that certain psychiatric symptoms may improve post-DBS surgery with a reduction in dopamine-replacement therapy.

Controlled research is needed to better understand both the acute and chronic effects of STN DBS on the psychiatric status of PD patients. One ongoing study ("A Comparison of Best Medical Therapy and Deep Brain Stimulation of Subthalamic Nucleus and Globus Pallidus for the Treatment of Parkinson's Disease," cosponsored by the Department of Veterans Affairs and NINDS) that will help address this issue initially involves randomization to either best medical therapy or DBS for a six-month period, with patients receiving DBS being randomized to either STN or GPi DBS. This type of randomized, controlled study design will provide additional data on the specific subacute and chronic effects of STN DBS on patients' psychiatric state, and will also allow comparison between different types of DBS. Additionally, further controlled study of post-DBS patients in *on–off* drug and stimulation states will allow greater understanding of the acute effects of DBS under different conditions and parameters.

ACKNOWLEDGMENT

Supported by a grant from the National Institute of Mental Health (#067894).

REFERENCES

1. Weintraub D, Stern MB. Psychiatric complications in Parkinson's disease. Am J Geriatr Psychiatry 2005; 13:844–851.
2. Starkstein SE, Mayberg HS, Preziosi TJ, et al. Reliability, validity, and clinical correlates of apathy in Parkinson's disease. J Neuropsychiatry Clin Neurosci 1992; 4:134–139.
3. Dodd ML, Klos KJ, Bower JH, et al. Pathological gambling caused by drugs used to treat Parkinson disease. Arch Neurol 2005; 62:1–5.
4. Aarsland D, Larsen JP, Lim NG, et al. Range of neuropsychiatric disturbances in patients with Parkinson's disease. J Neurol Neurosurg Psychiatry 1999; 67:492–496.
5. Weintraub D, Moberg PJ, Duda JE, et al. Recognition and treatment of depression in Parkinson's disease. J Geriatr Psychiatr Neurol 2003; 16:178–183.

6. Dostrovsky JO, Lozano AM. Mechanisms of deep brain stimulation. Mov Disord 2002; 17:S63–S68.

7. Alexander GE, Delong MR, Strick PL. Parallel organization of functionally segregated circuits linking basal ganglia and cortex. Annu Rev Neurosci 1986; 9:357–381.

8. Schroeder U, Kuehler A, Lang KW, et al. Subthalamic nucleus stimulation affects a frontotemporal network: a PET study. Ann Neurol 2003; 54:445–450.

9. Sestini S, di Luzio AS, Ammannati F, et al. Changes in regional cerebral blood flow caused by deep-brain stimulation of the subthalamic nucleus in Parkinson's disease. J Nucl Med 2002; 43:725–732.

10. Stefurak T, Mikulis D, Mayberg H, et al. Deep brain stimulation for Parkinson's disease dissociates mood and motor circuits: a functional MRI case study. Mov Disord 2003; 18:1508–1541.

11. Doshi PK, Chhaya N, Bhatt MH. Depression leading to attempted suicide after bilateral subthalamic nucleus stimulation for Parkinson's disease. Mov Disord 2002; 17:1084–1100.

12. Ring HA, Serra-Mestres J. Neuropsychiatry of the basal ganglia. J Neurol Neurosurg Psychiatry 2002; 72:12–21.

13. Okun MS, Green J, Saben R, Gross R, Foote KD, Vitek JL. Mood changes with deep brain stimulation of STN and GPi: results of a pilot study. J Neurol Neurosurg Psychiatry 2003; 74:1584–1586.

14. Krack P, Kumar R, Ardouin C, Dowsey PL, McVicker JM, Benabid A-L, et al. Mirthful laughter induced by subthalamic nucleus stimulation. Mov Disord 2001; 16:867–875.

15. Takeshita S, Kurisu K, Trop L, Arita K, Akimitsu T, Verhoeff NPLG. Effect of subthalamic stimulation on mood state in Parkinson's disease: evaluation of previous facts and problems. Neurosurg Rev 2005; 28:179–186.

16. Bejjani BP, Damier P, Arnulf I, et al. Transient acute depression induced by high-frequency deep-brain stimulation. N Engl J Med 1999; 340:1476–1480.

17. Morrison CE, Borod JC, Perrine K, Beric A, Brin MF, Rezai A, et al. Neuropsychological functioning following bilateral subthalamic nucleus stimulation in Parkinson's disease. Arch Clin Neuropsychol 2004; 19:165–181.

18. Kalteis K, Standhardt H, Kryspin-Exner I, Brücke T, Volc D, Alesch F. Influence of bilateral Stn-stimulation on psychiatric symptoms and psychosocial functioning in patients with Parkinson's disease. J Neural Transm 2006; 10:1007/s00702-005-0399-9.

19. Burn DJ, Tröster AI. Neuropsychiatric complications of medical and surgical therapies for Parkinson's disease. J Geriatr Psychiatry Neurol 2004; 17:172–180.

20. Volkmann J, Albert N, Voges J, Weiss PH, Freund H-J, Sturm V. Safety and efficacy of pallidal or subthalamic nucleus stimluation in advanced PD. Neurology 2001; 56:548–551.

21. Bejjani B-P, Dormont B, Pidoux B, Yelnik J, Damier P, Arnulf I, et al. Bilateral subthalamic stimulation for Parkinson's disease by using three-dimensional stereotactic magnetic resonance imaging and electrophysiological guidance. J Neurosurg 2000; 92:615–625.

22. Houeto JL, Mesnage V, Mallet L, et al. Behavioral disorders, Parkinson's disease and subthalamic stimulation. J Neurol Neurosurg Psychiatry 2002; 72:701–707.

23. Schüpbach WMM, Chastan N, Welter ML, Houeto JL, Mesnage V, Bonnet AM, et al. Stimulation of the subthalamic nucleus in Parkinson's disease: a 5 year follow up. J Neurol Neurosurg Psychiatry 2005; 76:1640–1644.

24. Berney A, Vingerhoets F, Perrin A, et al. Effect on mood of subthalamic DBS for Parkinson's disease: a consecutive series of 24 patients. Neurology 2002; 59:1427–1429.
25. Piasecki SD, Jefferson JW. Psychiatric complications of deep brain stimulation for Parkinson's disease. J Clin Psychiatry 2004; 65:845–849.
26. Houeto JL, Damier P, Bejjani BP, Staedler C, Bonnet AM, Arnulf I, et al. Subthalamic stimulation in Parkinson disease: a multidisciplinary approach. Arch Neurol 2000; 57:461–465.
27. Trépanier LL, Kumar R, Lozano AM, Lang AE, Saint-Cyr JA. Neuropsychological outcome of GPi pallidotomy and GPi or STN deep brain stimulation in Parkinson's disease. Brain Cogn 2000; 42:324–347.
28. Daniele A, Albanese A, Contarino MF, Zinzi P, Barbier A, Gasparini F, et al. Cognitive and behavioural effects of chronic stimulation of the subthalamic nucleus in patients with Parkinson's disease. J Neurol Neurosurg Psychiatry 2003; 74: 175–182.
29. Castelli L, Perozzo P, Genesia ML, Torre E, Pesare M, Cinquepalmi A, et al. Sexual well being in parkinsonian patients after deep brain stimulation of the subthalamic nucleus. J Neurol Neurosurg Psychiatry 2004; 75:1260–1264.
30. Mallet L, Mesnage V, Houeto JL, Pelissolo A, Yelnik J, Behar C, et al. Compulsions, Parkinson's disease, and stimulation. Lancet 2002; 360:1302–1304.
31. American Psychiatric Association: Diagnostic and Statistical Manual of Mental Disorders, Fourth Edition, Text Revision. Washington, DC: American Psychiatric Association, 2000.
32. Herzog J, Volkmann J, Krack P, Kopper F, Potter M, Lorenz D, et al. Two-year follow-up of subthalamic deep brain stimulation in Parkinson's disease. Mov Disord 2003; 18:1332–1337.
33. Krack P, Batir A, Van Blercom N, Chabardes S, Fraiz V, Aldouin C, et al. Five-year follow-up of bilateral stimulation of the subthalamic nucleus in advanced Parkinson's disease. N Engl J Med 2003; 13:1925–1934.
34. Romito LM, Scerrati M, Contarino MF, et al. Long-term follow up of subthalamic nucleus stimulation in Parkinson's disease. Neurology 2002; 58:1546–1550.
35. Kulisevsky J, Berthier ML, Gironell A, Pascual-Sedano B, Molet J, Pares P. Mania following deep brain stimulation for Parkinson's disease. Neurology 2002; 59:1421–1424.
36. Fuster JM. Frontal Lobe Syndromes. In: Fogel BS, Schiffer RB, Rao SM, eds. Neuropsychiatry. Baltimore: Williams & Wilkins, 1996:407–413.
37. Isella V, Melzi P, Grimaldi M, et al. Clinical, neuropsychological, and morphometric correlates of apathy in Parkinson's disease. Mov Disord 2002; 17:366–371.
38. Pluck GC, Brown RG. Apathy in Parkinson's disease. J Neurol Neurosurg Psychiatry 2002; 73:636–642.
39. Starkstein SE, Mayberg HS, Preziosi TJ, Andrezejewski P, Leiguarda R, Robinson RG. Reliability, validity, and clinical correlates of apathy in Parkinson's disease. J Neuropsychiatry Clin Neurosci 1992; 4:134–139.
40. Saint-Cyr JA, Trépanier LL, Kumar R, et al. Neuropsychological consequences of chronic bilateral stimulation of the subthalamic nucleus in Parkinson's disease. Brain 2000; 123:2091–2108.
41. Grace J, Stout JC, Malloy PF. Assessing frontal lobe behavioral syndromes with the Frontal Lobe Personality Scale. Assessment 1999; 6:269–284.

42. Bejjani B-P, Dormont B, Pidoux B, Yelnik J, Damier P, Arnulf I, et al. Bilateral sub-thalamic stimulation for Parkinson's disease by using three-dimensional stereotactic magnetic resonance imaging and electrophysiological guidance. J Neurosurg 2000; 92:615–625.

43. Witjas T, Baunez C, Henfy JM, Delfini M, Regis J, Cherif AA, et al. Addiction in Parkinson's disease: impact of subthalamic nucleus deep brain stimulation. Mov Disord 2005; 20:1052–1055.

44. Funkiewiez A, Ardouin C, Krack P, Fraix V, Van Blercom N, Xie J, et al. Acute psychotropic effects of bilateral subthalamic nucleus stimulation and levodopa in Parkinson's disease. Mov Disord 2003; 18:524–530.

45. Schneider F, Habel U, Volkmann J, Regel S, Kornischka J, Sturm V, et al. Deep brain stimulation of the subthalamic nucleus enhances emotional processing in Parkinson's disease. Arch Gen Psychiatry 2003; 60:296–302.

46. Czernecki V, Pillon B, Houeto JL, Welter ML, Mesnage V, Agid Y, et al. Does bilateral stimulation of the subthalamic nucleus aggravate apathy in Parkinson's disease? J Neurol Neurosurg Psychiatry 2005; 76:775–779.

47. Berney A, Vingerhoets F, Perrin A, et al. Effect on mood of subthalamic DBS for Parkinson's disease: A consecutive series of 24 patients [comment]. Neurology 2002; 59:1427–1429.

48. Lopiano L, Rizzone M, Bergamasco B, Tavella A, Torre E, Perozzo P, et al. Deep brain stimulation of the subthalamic nucleus in PD: an analysis of the exclusion causes. J Neurol Sci 2002; 195:167–170.

49. Lang AE, Widner H. Deep brain stimulation for Parkinson's disease: patient selection and evaluation. Mov Disord 2002; 3(suppl 3):S94–S101.

50. Voon V, Saint-Cyr J, Lozano AM, Moro E, Poon YY, Lang, AE. Psychiatric symptoms in patients with Parkinson disease presenting for deep brain stimulation surgery. J Neurosurg 2005; 103:246–251.

51. Olanow CW, Watts RL, Koller WC. An algorithm (decision tree) for the management of Parkinson's disease (2001): treatment guidelines. Neurology 2001; 56(suppl 5): S1–S88.

52. Vitek JL. Deep brain stimulation for Parkinson's disease: a critical re-evaluation of STN versus GPi DBS. Stereotact Funct Neurosurg 2002; 78:119–131.

53. Rodriguez-Oroz MC, Obeso JA, Lang AE, Houeto JL, Pollak P, Rehncrona S, et al. Bilateral deep brain stimulation in Parkinson's disease: a multicentre study with 4 years follow-up. Brain 2005; 128:2240–2249.

54. Richard IH, Frank S, McDermott MP, Wang H, Justus AW, Ladonna KA, et al. The ups and downs of Parkinson disease: a prospective study of mood and anxiety fluctuations. Cognitive and Behavioral Neurology 2004; 17:201–207.

55. Sheikh JI, Yesavage JA. Geriatric Depression Scale (GDS): recent evidence and development of a shorter version. Clin Gerontol 1986; (5):165–173.

56. Spielberger CD, Gorsuch RL, Lushene P, et al. Manual for the State-Trait Anxiety Inventory (Form Y). Palo Alto, CA, USA: Consulting Psychologists Press, Inc., 1983.

57. Friedberg G, Zoldan J, Weizman A, et al. Parkinson Psychosis Rating Scale: a practical instrument for grading psychosis in Parkinson's disease. Clin Neuropharmacol 1998; 21:280–284.

58. Cummings JL, Mega M, Gray K, et al. The Neuropsychiatric Inventory: comprehensive assessment of psychopathology in dementia. Neurology 1994; 44:2308–2314.

59. Thobois S, Mertens P, Guenot M, Hermier M, Mollion H, Bouvard M, et al. Subthalamic nucleus stimulation in Parkinson's disease: clinical evaluation of 18 patients. J Neurol 2002; 249:529–534.
60. Ardouin C, Pillon B, Peiffer E, Bejjani P, Limousin P, Damier P, et al. Bilateral subthalamic or pallidal stimulation for Parkinson's disease affects neither memory nor executive functions: a consecutive series of 62 patients. Ann Neurol 1999; 46:217–223.
61. Mayberg HS, Lozano AM, Voon V, McNeely HE, Seminowicz D, Hamani C, et al. Deep brain stimulation for treatment-resistant depression. Neuron 2005; 45:651–660.
62. Nuttin B, Cosyns P, Demeulemeester H, Gybels J, Meyerson B. Electrical stimulation in anterior limbs of internal capsules in patients with obsessive-compulsive disorders [letter]. Lancet 1999; 354:1526.
63. Nuttin BJ, Gabriëls LA, Cosyns PR, Meyerson B, Andreewitch S, Sunaert S, et al. Long-term electrical capsular stimulation in patients with obsessive-compulsive disorder. Neurosurgery 2003; 52:1263–1274.

17

Quality-of-Life Outcomes Following Stereotactic Surgery for Parkinson's Disease

Andrew Siderowf

Department of Neurology, University of Pennsylvania School of Medicine, Philadelphia, Pennsylvania, U.S.A.

INTRODUCTION

Surgical therapies for Parkinson's disease (PD), notably bilateral stimulation of the subthalamic nuclei (STN), substantially reduce many of the disabling features of advanced PD (1–5). Improvements following surgery for PD include amelioration of motor symptoms in the medication "off" condition, reduction in drug-induced dyskinesias, and decreased requirement for dopaminergic medications for patients having STN stimulation (6). The benefits of surgery on motor function appear to be maintained over prolonged periods of follow-up (7–9).

Since surgery for PD is performed primarily to alleviate symptoms of PD, health-related quality-of-life (HRQL) measures are arguably the most relevant outcomes by which to judge the impact of these procedures. A growing body of literature has addressed the impact of surgery on HRQL. This chapter will review concepts related to patient-reported outcome measures including quality of life (QOL) and HRQL, what factors determine HRQL in PD, and results of studies that have assessed the effects of stereotactic surgery including pallidotomy and deep brain stimulation (DBS) on HRQL.

ASSESSMENT OF QUALITY OF LIFE

QOL and HRQL belong to a family of patient-oriented outcome measures. Patient-oriented outcomes may be distinguished from physiological measures (such as finger-tapping speed or blood pressure) in that they are obtained by patient interview or questionnaire and are more likely to reflect the patient's global impression of their health or well-being (10). These measures include measures of impairment, disability, HRQL, and QOL. In the past, some confusion has existed regarding the meaning of the terms HRQL and QOL and their relationship to each other.

Impairment and Disability

The constructs of impairment, disability, and handicap have been defined by the World Health Organization (11). Impairment is any loss of psychological, physiological, or anatomical function and can be considered equivalent to the symptoms of a disorder. Impairment represents a deviation from normal biomedical function. By contrast, disability is a lack of ability to perform activities of daily living (ADLs), which results from impairment. Of these three concepts, disability is most relevant to HRQL since many measures of HRQL incorporate items related to ability to perform normal daily activities.

Health-Related Quality of Life

HRQL has been defined as "the capacity to perform the usual daily activies for a person's age and major social role" (12). This definition emphasizes the close relationship between functional status and HRQL. HRQL differs from disability principally in this relationship between impairment and role function. A measure of disability would assess a subjects inability to perform a routine task (Can the subject walk 100 yards?), whereas a HRQL instrument would assess this impairment in the context of a specific role (Can the subject walk well enough to perform typical employment activities?). HRQL scales are generally multidimensional, reflecting the desire to capture the effect of impairment on a range of possible roles (social, work, basic ADL function). Although HRQL measures may capture the subjective experience of disability to some extent, they are less subjectively oriented than QOL measures. The vast majority of "QOL" measures used to assess outcomes after surgery for PD are HRQL scales.

Quality of Life

QOL reflects a person's satisfaction with life and may be affected by health status, but also by nonhealth inputs including cultural values, personality traits, economic status, and social relationships (13). Because QOL is less determined by functional status than HRQL, QOL may improve or worsen without any change in health. For example, an amputee may initially experience a decrement in QOL due to loss of ability to take part in hobbies. However, this person's QOL may subsequently improve without any change in functional status, as he/she takes up other hobbies that are unaffected by their disability. QOL may be the most conceptually valid patient-oriented outcomes. However, QOL is subject to considerable measurement challenges, including subjectivity and variability between individual patients in what constitutes QOL, which prevents it from being a widely used outcome measure for medical interventions.

Generic Vs. Disease Specific HRQL Instruments

A large number of HRQL instruments can be used to measure the impact of medical interventions. One major point of distinction for these instruments is whether they are generic or disease-specific. Generic instruments are intended to compare HRQL across diseases and also to compare diseased populations to healthy populations. As a result, generic instruments are sensitive across a range of functional status from no limitations to severe disability. There are many generic HRQL instruments including the Medical Outcomes Study SF-36 (14), the sickness impact profile (SIP) (15), and the Nottingham Health Profile (16). Disease-specific instruments focus on the types of disability and impairments that are found in a specific disorder such as PD. Disease-specific instruments may be more sensitive to small differences in function or improvement due to treatment than generic instruments. Examples of PD-specific HRQL scales are shown in Table 1. At least five different disease-specific HRQL scales have been developed for PD. One of these scales, the quality of life satisfaction-deep brain stimulation (QLS-DBS) was developed specifically for assessment of DBS patients.

Parkinson's Disease Questionnaire-39

The Parkinson's disease Questionnaire (PDQ-39) is a 39 item instrument that has been widely used in population-based and interventional studies (17). The 39 items encompass the following domains: mobility, activities of daily living, emotional well-being, stigma, social support, cognition, communication, and bodily discomfort. For each domain, a score ranging from 0 to 100 is calculated. Higher scores on the PDQ-39 indicate worse HRQL. A summary score from 0 to 100 can also be calculated for the PDQ-39. This summary index is the arithmetic mean of the scores for the individual domains.

Parkinson's Disease Quality of Life

The Parkinson's disease quality of life (PDQL) scale has 37 items that comprise four subscales (18). The subscales include parkinsonian symptoms, systemic symptoms, social function, and emotional function. Higher scores on the PDQL represent better HRQL. The PDQL has been shown to have excellent internal consistency reliability and construct validity.

Table 1 Disease-Specific Health-Related Quality-of-Life Scales for Parkinson's Disease

Scale	Number of items	Number of domains and domain names	Completion time (approximate)
PDQ-39 (17)	39	8: Mobility, activities of daily living, emotional well-being, stigma, social support, cognition, communication, and bodily discomfort.	20–30 min
PDQUALIF (21)	33	7: Social/role function, self-image/ sexuality, sleep, outlook, physical function, independence, and urinary function.	20–30 min
PDQL (18)	37	4: Parkinson's symptoms, systemic symptoms, emotional function, and social function.	15–20 min
PIMS (19)	10	10: Self (positive), self (negative), family relationships, community relationships, safety, leisure, travel, work, financial security, and sexuality.	10–15 min
QLS-DBS (24)	17	Movement disorders 10: controllability of movement, hand dexterity, articulation/speech fluency, ability to swallow, absence of false body sensations, bladder/bowel function, sexual function, sleep, mentation, functional independence, and inconspicuousness of illness. DBS 5: reliability of the stimulator, inconspicuousness of the simulator, independent handling of the stimulator, availability of medical care, and absence of bodily symptoms.	10–40 min

Abbreviations: DBS, deep brain stimulation; PDQ, Parkinson's disease questionnaire; PDQL, Parkinson's disease quality of life; PDQUALIF, Parkinson's disease quality-of-life scale; PIMS, Parkinson's impact scale; QLS-DBS, quality of life satisfaction-deep brain stimulation.

Parkinson's Impact Scale

The Parkinson's impact scale (PIMS) has 10 items that rate self, family relationships, community relationships, safety, leisure, travel, work, financial security, and sexuality on a scale from zero (no problem) to four (severe problem) (19,20). For fluctuating patients, HRQL is rated in the best and worst functional levels. The PIMS was evaluated in a mail survey conducted across Canada. The scale was found to have high test–retest reliability, and construct validity was demonstrated by consistently higher scores in the "off" medication state than in the "on" medication state.

Parkinson's Disease Quality-of-Life Scale

The Parkinson's disease quality-of-life scale (PDQUALIF) consists of 32 items with an additional item that query whether the subjects' symptoms have changed in the past six months (21). The PDQUALIF has seven domains: social/role function, self-image/sexuality, sleep, outlook, physical function, independence, and urinary function that were established in open-ended qualitative interviews with PD patients and their spouses or significant others. The PDQUALIF has been shown to correlate with generic measures of HRQL, to change over time with increasing disease burden (22), and to be responsive to antiparkinsonian interventions (23).

Quality of Life Satisfaction-Deep Brain Stimulation

The QLS-DBS is the only HRQL instrument developed specifically to evaluate the impact of surgery for PD (24). It is based on the generic QLS questionnaire with two modules added specifically to address DBS. The QLS questionnaires first ask the respondent to rate the importance of various aspects of life, and then to report how satisfied they are with each aspect. The final score is a weighted average based on the levels of importance reported in the first part of the rating task. For the DBS-specific questionnaire, two modules are added to the core questionnaire. One module covers domains of function that may be affected by movement disorders. The second module contains items related to the neuro-stimulator (reliability, comfort, etc.) The QLS-DBS was tested in a mailed survey of 113 patients who had undergone DBS. The survey showed moderate correlation with existing HRQL measures such as the SF-36. More substantial correlation was not expected due to the fact that the QLS-DBS scale is distinct conceptually and in content from more function-based HRQL scales.

DETERMINANTS OF QUALITY OF LIFE IN PARKINSON'S DISEASE

Because PD is characterized by a mixture of motor and nonmotor features of PD, it can impact on HRQL in a number of ways. Not surprisingly, severity of motor impairment has been shown to be a strong and consistent determinant of HRQL in cross-sectional studies of PD patients (25–29). The other factor that has most consistently been associated with HRQL is depression (25,26,29–31). In some studies, depression is more strongly associated with HRQL than motor disability.

There is controversy regarding the impact of motor complications on HRQL. This issue is relevant to surgical therapies for PD, since one of the main effects of surgery is to reduce the severity of dyskinesias and motor fluctuations. Several studies have shown a deleterious effect of motor complications on

HRQL (32,33). However, other studies have not confirmed these findings (28,34). Measurement problems may be partly responsible for this lack of consensus. For example, the presence of dyskinesias is highly correlated with advantageous factors such as a positive response to dopaminergic medications, and the opposing impact of these factors may be difficult to separate.

Other features that have been shown to be related to HRQL include psychosis and dementia (26,28) as well as impaired sleep and fatigue (35,36). Younger patients have been shown to have greater relative differences in HRQL compared to age-matched controls than older patients (37). One study found that patients receiving care at a PD specialty center had better HRQL than those receiving care at a community neurology clinic (38). Many of these factors are relevant when considering the possible impacts of surgery for PD on HRQL.

QUALITY-OF-LIFE OUTCOMES FOLLOWING STEREOTACTIC SURGERY FOR PARKINSON'S DISEASE

Pallidotomy and Pallidal Stimulation

A number of studies have examined the impact of pallidotomy and pallidal stimulation on HRQL. Although the heterogeneity of these studies makes comparisons difficult, they have generally shown improvements on both generic and disease-specific measures of HRQL over a period of three months to one year of follow-up. Results comparing right-sided to left-sided unilateral procedures have generally been comparable. Somewhat surprisingly, there have not been major differences in HRQL outcomes between unilateral versus bilateral procedures or for pallidal stimulation compared to pallidotomy (39). There is also limited evidence linking improvement in clinical symptoms as measured by the unified Parkinson's disease rating scale (UPDRS) with changes in HRQL. A list of studies that could be identified by a MEDLINE search supplemented with hand-searching of reference lists from available articles is shown in Table 2.

In these studies, the pattern of improvement in HRQL domains has emphasized changes in motor function. For example, Straits-Troster (40) found greatest improvement in the mobility and ADL domains following unilateral pallidotomy, and Gray et al. (41) found the significant improvement only in the ADL domains. Martinez-Martin et al. (42) also found improvements in the mobility and ADL domains and in the emotional well-being bodily pain domains. In spite of the effect that pallidotomy may have on speech, no study evaluating pallidotomy or pallidal stimulation reported a decline in the communication domain of the PDQ-39. Using an alternative HRQL instrument, De Bie (39) reported 32 patients with unilateral PVP and five with bilateral PVP. Evaluations were performed for 6 and 12 months after surgery. PDQL was significantly improved by approximately 20% six months after surgery and 15% 12 months after surgery.

The vast majority of studies of HRQL following pallidal procedures report outcomes at three or six months. In one exception, Zimmerman (43) reported

Table 2 Studies Examining Impact of Globus Pallidus Surgery on Health-Related Quality of Life

Study	Number of subjects	Duration of follow-up (months)	HRQL scales used	Comments
Carr (59)	22	2	SF-36	Improvement in SF-36 social function and bodily pain domains.
DeBie (39)	32	12	PDQL	14% improvement in PDQL score at 12 months.
Esselink (58)	13	6	PDQL	6% improvement in PDQL scores.
Gray (41)	53	3	SF-36, PDQ-39	Significant improvement in SF-36 physical score for unilateral and bilateral pallidotomy groups.
Martinez-Martin (42)	11	4	PDQ-39	Improvements in mobility, ADL, emotional well-being, and bodily pain domains of PDQ-39.
Scott (46)	20	3–4	SF-36, PDQ-39	Improvements in mobility, ADL, and bodily discomfort domains.
Straits-Troster (40)	23	3	PDQ-39, SIP	Improvement in ADL and mobility domains of PDQ-39, and physical and psychosocial subscores of SIP.
Zimmerman (43)	52	24	PDQ-39	Nonsignificant change in PDQ-39 summary index at 24 months.

Abbreviations: ADL, activities of daily living; HRQL, Health-related quality of life; PDQ, Parkinson's disease questionnaire; PDQL, Parkinson's disease quality of life.

HRQL outcomes on 27 patients who underwent either unilateral or bilateral PVP. They found improvements of approximately 40% in the PDQ-39 summary index at six months, but that effect diminished to an approximately 12% improvement over baseline at two years follow-up and was no longer statistically significant.

Although generic HRQL instruments are generally thought to be less sensitive to change than disease-specific measures, a number of studies found that pallidotomy lead to significant changes in generic measures of HRQL. However, the pattern of improvement on generic instruments is somewhat more variable than with disease-specific instruments. Vingerhoets et al. (44) reported on 20 patients who underwent unilateral pallidal stimulation. There was a 33% improvement in the physical domain of the SIP and a 38% improvement in the psychosocial domain at three months. Gray et al. (41) found improvements in the physical function, role-physical energy, and pain dimensions of the SF-36 for the unilateral cases, and improvements in the social function, energy/vitality, and general health perceptions domains for the bilateral patients. By contrast, Carr et al. (45) found significant improvements only in the social function (19%) and bodily pain 62% domains of the SF-36. Scott (46) reported on 20 patients with PD who underwent either bilateral or unilateral PVP. SF-36 scores improved significantly at three months on physical function, social function, energy-vitality, and bodily pain.

Subthalamic Nucleus Stimulation

Growing bodies of studies have examined the effect of bilateral STN stimulation on HRQL. As is the case with the reports on pallidal procedures, there is also substantial variability in duration of clinical follow-up and outcome measures, making comparisons between studies difficult. Most studies have used the PDQ-39 as the primary measure of HRQL. In the largest study, LaGrange et al. (47) found improvements in all domains of the PDQL in 60 patients followed for 12 months. One study (48) emphasized that only physical components of the PDQ-39 improved following STN stimulation. However, other studies have found that the emotional, stigma, and bodily discomfort domains also improve (49,50–52). One additional study (53) found improvements in all PDQ-39 domains except emotional well-being, social support, and communication. Several studies have found worsening in the PDQ-39 communication domain following STN stimulation (49,54). A list of these studies is shown in Table 3.

Three studies have evaluated the impact of STN stimulation on HRQL beyond one year. In two studies, gains in HRQL observed at one year were maintained after two years of follow-up (50,55). In the other, the gains in HRQL observed six months after surgery had declined somewhat at a mean of 33 months of follow-up (49). The exceptions were the bodily pain and stigma domain that showed substantial improvements over baseline, even at long-term follow-up. For individual patients, the best predictor of a good long-term

Table 3 Studies Examining the Impact of Subthalamic Nuclei Stimulation on Health-Related Quality of Life

Study	Number of subjects	Duration of follow-up	HRQL scales used	Comments
Erola (54)	29	12	NHP, PDQ-39	Improvement in ADL, emotional, stigma, bodily discomfort domains of PDQ-39. Worsening of communication.
Drapier (60)	27	12	SF-36, PDQ-39	Improvement in physical function and physical role domains of SF-36. Improvement in mobility, ADL, stigma, and bodily discomfort domains of PDQ-39.
Fraix (61)	95	6	PDQL	Significant improvement in all PDQL domains.
Esselink (58)	20	6	PDQL	23% improvement in PDQL summary score.
Just and Ostergard (53)	11	6	PDQ-39	Improvement in mobility, ADL, stigma, and bodily discomfort domains
LaGrange (47)	60	12	PDQL	Improvement in all domains of the PDQL.
Lezcano (62)	14	24	PDQ-39	Improvements in mobility, ADL, emotional well-being, stigma, communication, and bodily pain domains.
Lyons and Pahwa (63)	59	24	PDQ-39	Improvement at 24 months in mobility, ADL, stigma, and bodily discomfort domains.
Martinez-Martin (51)	17	6	PDQ-39	Improvement in the mobility, ADL, emotional well-being, stigma, and bodily discomfort domains
Patel (52)	16	12	PDQ-39	Improvement in ADL and stigma domains.
Siderowf (49)	18	36	SF-36, PDQ-39	Improvement in mobility, ADL, emotional well-being, stigma, and bodily discomfort. Significant worsening in communication.
Troster (64)	26	3	PDQ-39	30% improvement in PDQ-39 summary index strongly related to change in depression scores.
Spottke (65)	16	6	SIP	Improvement in physical and psychosocial SIP subscores.

Abbreviations: ADL, activities of daily living; HRQL, Health-related quality of life; NHP, Nottingham health profile; PDQ, Parkinson's disease questionnaire; PDQL, Parkinson's disease quality of life; SIP, sickness impact profile; STN, subthalamic nuclei.

HRQL response to surgery is a good initial response within the first 6 to 12 months.

As with pallidotomy, the link between clinical improvement in motor function or dyskinesia and change in HRQL has been modest with STN stimulation. Improvements in motor function in the medication "off" state appear to correlate with change in HRQL. Interestingly, studies have not documented a clear relationship between dyskinesia reduction and change in HRQL (49) in spite of the major effect that surgery has on this complication of medical therapy. It is likely that the nearly universal improvement in dyskinesia that occurs following surgery limits the statistical power to find a relationship between dyskinesia and improvements in HRQL. An alternative explanation is that improvement in nonmotor features of PD drives changes in HRQL. Troster et al. (56) found a strong relationship between overall HRQL and improvement in depression. However, LaGrange et al. (57) found no relationship between improvement in depression (which did improve significantly after surgery) and HRQL.

One study that reported HRQL outcomes randomized patients to either unilateral pallidotomy or bilateral STN stimulation (58). In this study, 13 subjects had pallidotomy and 20 had STN stimulation. Both groups showed overall improvement on the PDQL summary score. Although some outcome measures, including "off" medication UPDRS scores and dyskinesia scores favored STN stimulation, there were no significant differences between treatment groups on the PDQL.

CONCLUSION

Because surgical therapy for PD predominantly targets the symptoms of the disease, patient-reported outcomes such as HRQL are an important gage of the effectiveness of these procedures. There is a growing literature that suggests procedures that target both the globus pallidus and the STN improve many domains of HRQL, including some that may be more related to nonmotor features of PD. These studies clearly suggest a benefit of surgery over periods of approximately one year. Additional studies are still needed to address longer-term effects of surgery on HRQL and to determine if there are differences between HRQL outcomes for patients that receive pallidal as compared to STN procedures.

REFERENCES

1. Barron MS, Vitek JL, Bakay RAE, et al. Treatment of advanced Parkinson's disease by posterior GPi pallidotomy: 1-year results of a pilot study. Ann Neurol 1996; 40:355–366.
2. Limousin P, Krack P, Pollak P, et al. Electrical stimulation of the subthalamic nucleus in advanced Parkinson's disease. New Engl J Med 1998; 339(16):1105–1111.

3. Kumar R, Lozano AM, Kim YJ, et al. Double–blind evaluation of subthalamic nucleus deep brain stimulation in advanced Parkinson's disease. Neurology 1998; 51(3):850–855.

4. Simuni T, Jaggi JL, Mulholland H, et al. Bilateral stimulation of the subthalamic nucleus in patients with Parkinson disease: a study of efficacy and safety. J Neurosurg 2002; 96(4):666–672.

5. The Deep-Brain Stimulation for Parkinson's Disease Study Group. Deep-brain stimulation of the subthalamic nucleus or the pars interna of the globus pallidus in Parkinson's disease. N Engl J Med 2001; 345:956–963.

6. Moro E, Scerrati M, Romito LM, Roselli R, Tonali P, Albanese A. Chronic subthalamic nucleus stimulation reduces medication requirements in Parkinson's disease. Neurology 1999; 53(1):85–90.

7. Fine J, Duff J, Chen R, Hutchinson W, Lozano AM, Lang AE. Long-term follow-up of unilateral pallidotomy in advanced Parkinson's disease. N Engl J Med 2000; 342:1708–1714.

8. Kleiner-Fisman G, Fisman DN, Sime E, Saint-Cyr JA, Lozano AM, Lang AE. Long-term follow up of bilateral deep brain stimulation of the subthalamic nucleus in patients with advanced Parkinson disease. J Neurosurg 2003; 99(3):489–495.

9. Krack P, Batir A, Van Blercom N, et al. Five-year follow-up of bilateral stimulation of the subthalamic nucleus in advanced Parkinson's disease [see comment]. N Engl J Med 2003; 349(20):1925–1934.

10. Vickrey BG. Getting oriented to patient oriented outcomes. Neurology 1999; 53:662–663.

11. World Health Organization. International Classification of Functioning and Disability: ICIDH-2. Stationery Office Books, November 1999.

12. Guyatt GH, Bombardier C, Tugwell PX. Measuring disease-specific quality of life in clinical trials. CMAJ 1986; 134:889–895.

13. Doward LC, McKenna SP. Defining Patient-Reported Outcomes. Value in Health 2004; 7(supp 1):S4–S8.

14. Ware JE, Jr, Sherbourne CD. The MOS 36-item short-form health survey (SF-36). I. Conceptual framework and item selection. Med Care 1992; 30(6):473–483.

15. Bergner M, Bobbitt RA, Carter WB, Gilson BS. The Sickness Impact Profile: Development and final revision of a health status measure. Med Care 1981; 19:787–805.

16. Hunt SM, McKenna SP, McEwen J, Williams J, Papp E. The Nottingham Health Profile: subjective health status and medical consultations. Soc Sci Med—Part A, Medical Sociology 1981; 15(3 Pt 1):221–229.

17. Peto V, Jenkinson C, Fitzpatrick R, Greenhall R. The development and validation of a short measure of functioning and well being for individuals with Parkinson's disease. Quality of Life Research 1995; 4(3):241–248.

18. deBoer AGEM, Wijker W, Speelman JD, De Haes HJ. Quality of life in patients with Parkinson's disease: development of a questionnaire. J Neurol Neurosurg Psychiatry 1996; 61:70–74.

19. Calne S, Schulzer M, Mak E, Guyette C, Rohs G, Hatchard S, et al. Validating a quality of life rating scale for idiopathic parkinsonism: Parkinson's Impact Scale (PIMS). Parkinsonism Relat Disord 1996; 2(2):55–61.

20. Schulzer M, Mak E, Calne SM. The psychometric properties of the Parkinson's Impact Scale (PIMS) as a measure of quality of life in Parkinson's disease. Parkinsonism Relat Disord 2003; 9(5):291–294.

21. Welsh M, McDermott MP, Holloway RG, et al. Development and testing of the Parkinson's disease quality of life scale. Mov Disord 2003; 18:637–645.
22. Noyes K, Dick AW, Holloway RG, Parkinson Study Group. Pramipexole versus levodopa in patients with early Parkinson's disease: effect on generic and disease-specific quality of life. Value in Health 2006; 9(1):28–38.
23. Biglan KM, Schwid S, Eberly S, et al. Rasagiline improves quality of life in patients with early Parkinson's disease. Mov Disord 2006; 21(5):616–623.
24. Kuehler A, Henrich G, Schroeder U, Conrad B, Herschbach P, Ceballos-Baumann A. A novel quality of life instrument for deep brain stimulation in movement disorders. J Neurol Neurosurg Psychiatry 2003; 74(8):1023–1030.
25. The Global Parkinson's Disease Survey Group. Factors inpacting on quality of life in Parkinson's disease: Results from an international survey. Mov Disord 2002; 17:60–67.
26. Schrag A, Jahanshahi M, Quinn N. What contributes to quality of life in patients with Parkinson's disease? J Neurol Neurosurg Psychiatry 2000; 69(3):308–312.
27. Marras C, Lang A, Krahn M, Tomlinson G, Naglie G, Parkinson Study Group. Quality of life in early Parkinson's disease: impact of dyskinesias and motor fluctuations. Mov Disord 2004; 19(1):22–28.
28. Siderowf A, Ravina B, Glick HA. Preference-based quality of life in patients with Parkinson's disease. Neurology 2002; 59:103–108.
29. Behari M, Srivastava AK, Pandey RM. Quality of life in patients with Parkinson's disease. Parkinsonism Relat Disord 2005; 11(4):221–226.
30. Fitzpatrick R, Peto V, Jenkinson C, Greenhall R, Hyman N. Health-related quality of life in Parkinson's disease: a study of outpatient clinic attenders. Mov Disord 1997; 12(6):916–922.
31. Weintraub D, Moberg PJ, Duda JE, Katz IR, Stern MB. Effect of psychiatric and other nonmotor symptoms on disability in Parkinson's disease. J Am Geriatr Soc 2004; 52(5):784–788.
32. Pechevis M, Clarke CE, Vieregge P, et al. Effects of dyskinesias in Parkinson's disease on quality of life and health-related costs: a prospective European study. Eur J Neurol 2005; 12(12):956–963.
33. Chapuis S, Ouchchane L, Metz O, Gerbaud L, Durif F. Impact of the motor complications of Parkinson's disease on the quality of life. Mov Disord 1920; (2):224–230.
34. Marras C, Lang A, Krahn M, Tomlinson G, Naglie G, Parkinson Study Group. Quality of life in early Parkinson's disease: impact of dyskinesias and motor fluctuations. Mov Disord 1919; (1):22–28.
35. Scaravilli T, Gasparoli E, Rinaldi F, Polesello G, Bracco F. Health-related quality of life and sleep disorders in Parkinson's disease. Neurol Sci 2003; 24(3):209–210.
36. Herlofson K, Larsen JP. The influence of fatigue on health-related quality of life in patients with Parkinson's disease. Acta Neurologica Scandinavica 2003; 107(1):1–6.
37. Schrag A, Jahanshahi M, Quinn N. How does Parkinson's disease affect quality of life? A comparison with quality of life in the general population. Mov Disord 2000; 15(6):1112–1118.
38. Rochow SB, Blackwell AD, Brown VJ. Quality of life in Parkinson's disease: movement disorders clinic vs general medical clinic—a comparative study. Scottish Med J 2005; 50(1):18–20.
39. de Bie RM, Schuurman PR, Bosch DA, et al. Outcome of unilateral pallidotomy in advanced Parkinson's disease: cohort study of 32 patients. J Neurol Neurosurg Psychiatry 2001; 71(3):375–382.

40. Straits-Troster K, Fields JA, Wilkinson SB, et al. Health-related quality of life in Parkinson's disease after pallidotomy and deep brain stimulation. Brain Cogn 2000; 42(3):399–416.
41. Gray A, McNamara I, Aziz T, et al. Quality of life outcomes following surgical treatment of Parkinson's disease. Mov Disord 2002; 17(1):68–75.
42. Martinez-Martin P, Valldeoriola F, Molinuevo JL, Nobbe FA, Rumia J, Tolosa E. Pallidotomy and quality of life in patients with Parkinson's disease: an early study. Mov Disord 2000; 15(1):65–70.
43. Zimmerman GJ, D'Antonio LL, Iacono RP. Health related quality of life in patients with Parkinson's disease two years following posteroventral pallidotomy. Acta Neurochirurgica 2004; 146(12):1293–1299, discussion 1299.
44. Vingerhoets G, Lannoo E, van der LC, et al. Changes in quality of life following unilateral pallidal stimulation in Parkinson's disease. J Psychosom Res 1999; 46(3): 247–255.
45. Carr JAR, Honey CR, Sinden M, Phillips AG, Martzke JS. A waitlist control-group study of cognitive, mood, and quality of life outcome after posteroventral pallidotomy in Parkinson disease. J Neurosurg 2003; 99(1):78–88.
46. Scott R, Gregory R, Hines N, et al. Neuropsychological, neurological and functional outcome following pallidotomy for Parkinson's disease. A consecutive series of eight simultaneous bilateral and twelve unilateral procedures. Brain 1998; 121(Pt 4): 659–675.
47. Lagrange E, Krack P, Moro E, et al. Bilateral subthalamic nucleus stimulation improves health-related quality of life in PD. Neurology 2002; 59(12):1976–1978.
48. Drapier S, Raoul S, Drapier D, et al. Only physical aspects of quality of life are significantly improved by bilateral subthalamic stimulation in Parkinson's disease. J Neurol 2005; 252:583–588.
49. Siderowf A, Jaggi JL, Xie S, et al. Long-term effects of bilateral sub-thalamic nucleus stimulation on health-related quality of life in advanced Parkinson's disease. Mov Disord 2006; 21(6):746–753.
50. Lezcano E, Gomez-Esteban JC, Zarranz JJ, et al. Improvement in quality of life in patients with advanced Parkinson's disease following bilateral deep brain stimulation in subthalamic nucleus. Eur J Neurol 2004; 11:451–454.
51. Martinez-Martin P, Valldeoriola F, Tolosa E, et al. Bilateral subthalamic nucleus stimulation and quality of life in advanced Parkinson's disease. Mov Disord 2002; 17(2):372–377.
52. Patel NK, Plaha P, O'Sullivan K, McCarter R, Heywood P, Gill SS. MRI directed bilateral stimulation of the subthalamic nucleus in patients with Parkinson's disease. J Neurol Neurosurg Psychiatry 2003; 74(12):1631–1637.
53. Just H, Ostergaard K. Health-related quality of life in patients with advanced Parkinson's disease treated with deep brain stimulation of the subthalamic nuclei. Mov Disord 2002; 17(3):539–545.
54. Erola T, Karinen P, Heikkinen E, et al. Bilateral subthalamic nucleus stimulation improves health-related quality of life in Parkinsonian patients. Parkinsonism Relat Disord 2005; 11(2):89–94.
55. Lyons KE, Pahwa R. Long-term benefits in quality of life provided by bilateral subthalamic stimulation in patients with Parkinson disease. J Neurosurg 2005; 103(2):252–255.

56. Troster AI, Fields JA, Wilkinson S, Pahwa R, Koller WC, Lyons KE. Effect of motor improvement on quality of life following subthalamic stimulation is mediated by changes in depressive symptomatology. Stereotact Funct Neurosurg 2003; 80: 43–47.

57. Lagrange E, Krack P, Moro E, et al. Bilateral subthalamic nucleus stimulation improves health-related quality of life in PD. Neurology 2002; 59(12):1976–1978.

58. Esselink RA, de Bie RM, de Haan RJ, et al. Unilateral pallidotomy versus bilateral subthalamic nucleus stimulation in PD: a randomized trial. Neurology 2004; 62(2):201–207.

59. Carr JA, Honey CR, Sinden M, Phillips AG, Martzke JS. A waitlist control-group study of cognitive, mood, and quality of life outcome after posteroventral pallidotomy in Parkinson disease. J Neurosurg 2003; 99(1):78–88.

60. Drapier S, Raoul S, Drapier D, et al. Only physical aspects of quality of life are significantly improved by bilateral subthalamic stimulation in Parkinson's disease. J Neurol 2005; 252(5):583–588.

61. Fraix V, Houeto JL, Lagrange C, et al. Clinical and economic results of bilateral subthalamic nucleus stimulation in Parkinson's disease. J Neurol Neurosurg Psychiatry 2006; 77(4):443–449.

62. Lezcano E, Gomez-Esteban JC, Zarranz JJ, et al. Improvement in quality of life in patients with advanced Parkinson's disease following bilateral deep-brain stimulation in subthalamic nucleus. Eur J Neurol 2004; 11(7):451–454.

63. Lyons KE, Pahwa R. Long-term benefits in quality of life provided by bilateral subthalamic stimulation in patients with Parkinson disease. J Neurosurg 2005; 103(2):252–255.

64. Troster AI, Fields JA, Wilkinson S, Pahwa R, Koller WC, Lyons KE. Effect of motor improvement on quality of life following subthalamic stimulation is mediated by changes in depressive symptomatology. Stereotact Funct Neurosurg 2003; 80:43–47.

65. Spottke EA, Volkmann J, Lorenz D, et al. Evaluation of healthcare utilization and health status of patients with Parkinson's disease treated with deep brain stimulation of the subthalamic nucleus. J Neurol 2002; 249(6):759–766.

18

Conducting Clinical Trials of Deep Brain Stimulation in Parkinson's Disease

Frances M. Weaver

Midwest Center for Health Services Research and Policy Studies and Research, Spinal Cord Injury Quality Enhancement Research Initiative, Hines VA Hospital, and Department of Neurology and Institute for Healthcare Studies, Northwestern University, Chicago, Illinois, U.S.A.

Kenneth A. Follett

Department of Neurosurgery, University of Nebraska Medical Center, Omaha, Nebraska, U.S.A.

Domenic J. Reda and Kwan Hur

Cooperative Studies Program Coordinating Center, Hines VA Hospital, Hines, Illinois, U.S.A.

INTRODUCTION

The twenty-first century has ushered in a growing emphasis on the use of evidence-based medicine (EBM) in health care. Sackett et al. (1) have defined EBM as the "conscientious, explicit, and judicious use of current best evidence in making decisions about the care of individual patients." The recognition that there is wide variation in medical practice and that clinical decisions regarding treatment are often unsupported by research evidence has served as the basis for promoting EBM. EBM provides clinicians with a systematic and efficient way to assess the evidence to determine what is the best treatment for their patients (2). Several individuals have proposed grading systems for weighing the evidence based on study design, sample size, outcomes assessed, and threats to the validity of the findings. Large randomized controlled trials are

299

typically graded as level I evidence, whereas smaller randomized trials are considered level II, nonrandomized studies with concurrent control or comparison groups are rated as level III, nonrandomized trials with historical controls are categorized as level IV, and case series with no controls are considered level V evidence (3). In many cases, there is no evidence and guideline recommendations are then based on expert consensus. Although EBM is not and should not be restricted to the results of large randomized trials, these trials provide information about the effectiveness of an intervention that have a low risk of error in their conclusions.

In the field of Parkinson's disease (PD), there are many examples of large clinical trials for pharmacological management of disease that would be considered level I evidence for decision making (4,5). Yet, in the field of neurosurgery, the randomized controlled clinical trial is a rare occurrence. In a recent meta-analysis of published studies of deep brain stimulation (DBS) for PD (6), only one small randomized clinical trial was reported. The other 44 studies were all designed as pretest, post-test, quasi-experimental studies (most would be considered level IV studies).

There are many possible reasons for the lack of large clinical trials of neurosurgical interventions in PD. These include cost of the intervention, cost of conducting the trial, recruitment issues, and the difficulty of standardizing the intervention. Further, the field of neurosurgery changes very rapidly with new techniques and strategies presented in rapid succession. Whereas, pallidotomy was the accepted intervention in the mid to late 1990s, by 2000, most centers had switched to nonablative DBS surgery (7). Furthermore, many, if not most neurologists and surgeons have already decided that the best site of surgery for DBS is the subthalamic nucleus (STN) (8). Again, this change has been based primarily on anecdotal evidence, personal observations, and personal opinions of surgeons and neurologists and on studies that would be considered level III or lower as to strength of the evidence. However, a recent meta-analysis of DBS by site of implantation, as well as recent publications of the long term outcomes of DBS of the STN and globus pallium interna (GPi) suggest that STN may not be superior to GPi when outcomes such as activities of daily living (ADL) and adverse events such as depression, cognitive decline, and disturbances of speech, gait, and balance are considered (6,9,10).

STATISTICAL ISSUES IN DESIGNING CONTROLLED CLINICAL TRIALS

Randomization

In the controlled clinical trial, randomization refers to assigning subjects to the experimental (intervention) group or to the control (placebo) group using a chance mechanism in order to create comparable groups. If it is done properly, randomization eliminates systematic bias in the allocation of subjects and produces comparable groups on the average in baseline characteristics of the subjects at the time of randomization. Comparability of the groups at the time of treatment assignment is essential in making valid statements about the difference between treatments for the study subjects (i.e., if difference exists, it is solely due to treatment not selection bias).

There are different ways to randomize subjects into treatment groups. A simple way of randomizing subjects would be flipping a coin, rolling a die, or using a random number table. The process of randomization can inadvertently produce extreme allocation schemes, such as getting 10 heads in a row and produce baseline imbalances by chance. To reduce the likelihood of this occurring, putting constraints on the randomization to achieve equal group sizes, known as block randomization and/or assuring balance on important prognostic factors by stratifying the randomization on these factors (e.g., age, sex, or severity of disease) are common. In multicenter trials, it is common to stratify the randomization by participating center. To assure the integrity of the randomization process, the randomization codes should not be made available to the participating center until a patient has been determined to be eligible for the study.

Control Group

Parallel group controlled trials can be broadly classified as either placebo controlled or active controlled trials. In a placebo controlled trial, the group that does not receive the active treatment receives a placebo (e.g., a sugar pill), if it is a study evaluating a medication, or a sham intervention if it is a study evaluating a device or procedure (e.g., electrodes are implanted but the stimulator is not turned on). This class of studies also includes those in which the control group receives no treatment. Active control trials compare two treatments. For example, in studies of DBS, one might compare surgery to medical therapy, or compare the site of surgery (e.g., STN vs. GPi). One must consider the ethical issues involved in randomizing subjects to study arms. If a particular type of intervention has been shown to be effective, in many situations randomizing subjects to placebo would not be ethical. Factors such as the severity of the disease being studied and the duration of treatment need to be considered. However, if the purpose of the study is to determine effectiveness for an intervention in a disease where no treatments have been proven to be effective, a comparison to a placebo or sham situation would be appropriate.

Blinding

Blinding or masking in controlled trials means that all study participants (investigators, subjects, and sometimes those who collect and analyze the study data) have no knowledge of group assignment of the study subjects. Blinding is one of the most important design techniques in clinical trials for reducing bias that arises if the knowledge of a subject's group assignment may influence the assessment of the outcome measures. Blinding is particularly important when some subjectivity is involved in the assessment of outcome measures, such as assessing motor function score using the Unified Parkinson's Disease Rating Scale (UPDRS) (11) in PD trials. It is less important for objective criteria, such as death from any cause, when there is little possibility for ascertainment bias. Blinding is a standard procedure for most randomized clinical trials of medications. Trials of surgical interventions are often difficult to blind. In these cases, a separate evaluator, blinded to the treatment assignment, or an independent evaluator may be used to measure the patient's responses.

A single-blinded trial occurs when the study subjects are unaware of group assignment but investigators and data analysts (or a committee monitoring the trial) are aware of which treatment the study subject has been assigned. A double-blinded trial is designed so that both study subjects and investigators are unaware of group assignment. A triple-blinded trial is when the study subjects, investigators, and data analysts (or committee monitoring the trial) are unaware of the identity of group assignment.

Difficulties can arise in achieving the double-blinded or triple-blinded trials. Treatment may be of a completely different nature such as surgical versus medical therapy; drugs may have different formulation (e.g., use of capsules vs. tablets) and reformulation for comparability is either difficult or is not allowed; or the frequency or pattern of drug administration of the treatments may differ. Nevertheless, great efforts should be made to overcome these difficulties to ensure blinding. For example, in the case of surgery for PD, covering the head of the patient with a cap can hide whether a patient had surgery, and observers can be blinded to site of surgical target (e.g., GPi vs. STN). Unblinding of the treatment assignment should be considered only when it is necessary for the care of subjects. Any unblinding should be documented and included in a report of the study results at the end of the trial.

Sample Size

Determining the number of subjects, sample size calculation, to be entered into the study is an essential part of clinical trial planning. The number of subjects in a trial should always be sufficient enough to provide a reliable answer to the questions being addressed. The sample size is usually determined by the primary objective of the trial and the type of primary outcome of interest determines the statistical method used for calculation (i.e., continuous data such as the UPDRS motor score, proportional data such as mortality or infection rate, and survival data such as survival or remission at five years).

Some of the items to be specified in determining the appropriate sample size include: (*i*) the null hypothesis (e.g., there is no efficacy difference between the two drugs on average) and alternative hypothesis (e.g., the two drugs have different effects on average), (*ii*) the probability of rejecting the null hypothesis when the null hypothesis is true (the Type I error or alpha level), (*iii*) the probability of failing to reject when the null hypothesis is not true (the Type II error or beta level), (*iv*) the magnitude of clinically important differences between the groups, and (*v*) the expected variability in responses across patients. An alpha level of 0.05 or less is generally accepted for most trials. The smaller the alpha level, the larger the sample size required. The power of the study measures the ability of the test to reject the null hypothesis when it is actually false. In other words, the power is defined as the probability of not committing a Type II error [1 − the probability of Type II error or 1 − beta (β)]. Power ranges from minimum of zero to maximum of one. If the power of a study is low and the study finds no difference between treatment groups, the study results will be questionable (the study might have been too small to detect any differences). By convention, a power of 80% or more is acceptable which means that a study has an 80% chance of finding statistically significant differences between experimental and control groups when a true difference exists. The higher the power level, the larger the sample size required.

Calculation of sample size requires some information on the mean and variance for continuous data, response or incidence rates for dichotomous outcomes, and event rates within a specified time for survival, or time to event, outcomes. When estimating these values, a literature search or pilot study may be needed to obtain initial estimates. Estimates of the dropout rate, that is, the percentage of patients for whom outcome data is not expected to be available, should also be considered in the final sample size calculation. The estimate of potential dropouts is typically used to inflate the sample size after the sample is determined based on adequate power. The method used to calculate the sample size should be included in the protocol with any estimates and assumptions used in the calculations. Clinically meaningful differences to be detected also should be included in the protocol. In addition, a sensitivity analysis should be provided which shows the impact that alteration of assumptions to estimate the sample size would have on the power of the study.

Meta-analysis is a statistical procedure for combining data from various independent studies in order to come up with an overall conclusion in addressing research questions. Often times, a meta-analysis approach is useful for initial estimation of the primary outcome measures for the sample size calculation by means of combining the summary statistics (mean, standard deviation, event rates, etc.) from individual studies. To ensure comparability of the primary outcome measure, a careful review of the definition of outcome measure and the method of ascertainment is important.

DEFINING THE INTERVENTION AND THE STUDY POPULATION

Fundamental to any clinical trial is the need to identify a problem worthy of study. The question to be addressed should be of sufficient importance in terms of size of the population affected, cost of intervention to be studied, and/or the impact of the problem on the medical community (including patients and their families, physicians, payers, healthcare institutions, and facilities) or society.

The magnitude of PD on all of these fronts, and the potential impact and cost of DBS for PD, render DBS for PD worthy of study.

Inclusion and exclusion criteria should establish a well-defined study population, minimizing uncertainty about patient selection and eligibility and promoting appropriate uniformity of the study population. The study population should reflect the larger population of patients who might be affected by the study intervention or the results of the study. Selection of the study population should allow for results of the study to be generalized across gender, age, and ethnic backgrounds of people affected by the disorder. Proper inclusion and exclusion criteria also promote the safety of study subjects by identifying medical indications and contraindications for enrollment.

The intervention selected for study, as noted above, should be of sufficient clinical import to warrant conduct of the trial. Caution should be used to select an intervention that is expected to be durable such that it will not become obsolete prior to or shortly after conclusion of the study. For example, in the early to mid-1990s, a clinical study of pallidotomy for the treatment of PD might have been justified. By the late 1990s, it was becoming apparent that DBS was likely to supplant ablative surgical procedures as the surgical treatment of choice for PD, and a study of pallidotomy at that time likely would have provided outcomes data that were of relatively little clinical impact. Clinical trials can take a great deal of time to plan, fund, and implement, and special attention must be directed toward choosing a topic that will still be relevant at the conclusion of the study.

As an example, with these factors in mind, a randomized controlled trial (VA CSP 468) sponsored by the Department of Veterans Affairs, the National Institute of Neurological Disorders and Stroke, and Medtronic, Inc., was developed to address clinically important, timely, and relevant questions pertaining to DBS for PD (7). To meet these goals, the trial includes a comparison of best medical therapy to surgical intervention (a comparison that had not been performed in any previous large scale randomized clinical study of surgery for PD at the time of planning yet which is of fundamental importance in determining the role of surgery in the management of PD) and addresses the surgically relevant and clinically important question of whether DBS in one of two typical DBS targets (STN or GPi) provides better clinical outcomes. Care was taken to ensure, as best as possible, that the topic of the study would still be clinically relevant at the conclusion of the study.

Inclusion and exclusion criteria for CSP 468 were selected to be clinically relevant, reflecting "best clinical practice" at the time the protocol was developed, thereby facilitating the recruitment of subjects, and to provide a well defined study population that could be generalized to the larger population of potential candidates for DBS.

Inclusion criteria include:

(1)   Idiopathic PD
(2)   Hoehn and Yahr stage 2 or worse when off medications

(3)   L-dopa responsive with clearly defined "on" periods

(4)   Persistent disabling symptoms (e.g., on troubling dyskinesias, or disabling "off" periods at least three hours per day) despite medication therapy. Patients will have been treated with variable doses of levodopa and dopamine agonists (at a minimum) and will have had an adequate trial of other adjunctive medications

(5)   Stable on medical therapy for at least one month prior to study enrollment

(6)   Age > 21

(7)   Available and willing to be followed-up according to study protocol

Exclusion criteria include:

(1)   "Parkinson's plus" syndromes, secondary, or atypical Parkinson's syndromes (e.g., progressive supranuclear palsy, striato-nigral degeneration, multiple system atrophy, poststroke, post-traumatic, or postencephalitic Parkinson's)

(2)   Previous PD surgery

(3)   Medical contraindications to surgery or neurostimulation (e.g., uncontrolled hypertension, advanced coronary artery disease, other implanted stimulation or electronically-controlled devices including cardiac demand pacemaker, aneurysm clips, cochlear implants, or spinal cord stimulator)

(4)   Contraindication to magnetic resonance imaging (MRI) (e.g., indwelling metal fragments or implants that might be affected by MRI)

(5)   Active alcohol or drug abuse

(6)   Score on Mini-Mental Status examination of 24 or lower, or other neuropsychological dysfunction (e.g., dementia) that would contraindicate surgery or active participation in the study

(7)   Intracranial abnormalities that would contraindicate surgery (e.g., stroke, tumor, vascular abnormality affecting the target area)

(8)   Pregnancy

(9)   Concurrent participation in another research protocol

MEASURING OUTCOMES IN DEEP BRAIN STIMULATION FOR PARKINSON'S DISEASE

The primary goals of surgical intervention in persons with PD are to improve physical functioning and reduce PD symptoms following surgery. More recently, studies have also included the goal of improving quality of life (7,12–14). In a clinical trial, these outcomes are compared between the intervention and control groups to determine whether the intervention (in this case, surgery) was effective. Usually, the investigators will identify a primary outcome and several secondary outcomes. A baseline assessment of these measures is obtained prior to the intervention and then again at one or more times following the intervention (i.e., surgery). Appropriate duration of follow-up can be difficult to establish in clinical trials. Short-term outcomes may differ from long-term outcomes, and length of follow-up may have direct relevance to specific outcome measures (e.g., cost effectiveness may require longer rather than shorter duration of follow-up). Adequate duration of follow-up is particularly important in DBS trials, since study participants are likely to keep their stimulators for the remainder of their lives. Most studies of DBS of the STN and GPi have limited their follow-up to 6 to 12 months (6). More recently, a few studies have reported longer-term follow-up for as much as five years (9,10,15).

The outcome that is most apparent or easiest to measure is not necessarily the outcome of greatest importance to the study subjects. Ease and accuracy of measurement is important, but the primary outcome should be clinically relevant to the patient. For instance, in CSP 468 the primary outcome for the best medical therapy versus DBS phase of the study is time spent in the "on" state without troublesome dyskinesias. This outcome is measurable (using patient motor diaries) and, importantly, is an outcome of major functional significance to the patients. The primary outcome measure for the comparison of DBS targets is motor function (based on UPDRS motor subscale). The selection of this endpoint allows easy comparison to other studies of DBS for PD, most of which have used motor function as the primary outcome. Other outcomes often measured following DBS include ADL, dyskinesias, quality of life, medications, time spent in a good "on" state, cognitive status, neuropsychological functioning, adverse events, health care use, and costs. ADL may be as if not more important for persons with PD and should be included in an assessment of interventions. Each of outcomes identified above is discussed subsequently in the context of DBS in PD. In selecting a panel of outcomes measures, effort should be directed toward minimizing undue burden on the study subjects, for example, prolonged or uncomfortable testing.

Motor Function

The most common outcome that is reported in studies of DBS is patient motor function. The vast majority of studies reporting on function use the motor subscale of the UPDRS (11). The UPDRS is used widely in both clinical practice to monitor disease progression and in research to assess the effects of various medical and surgical interventions for PD. The UPDRS has four sections in which a total of 42 disease characteristics are assessed. The first section on mentation, behavior, and mood has four items assessing intellectual impairment, thought disorder, depression, and motivation (score may range from 0 to 16). Part II focuses on ADL including walking, writing, dressing, and speech; there are 13 items (score may range from 0 to 52). The third section assesses motor skills including facial expression and speech, tremors, rigidity, posture, gait, and bradykinesia. There are 14 items in the motor skills section (score may range from 0 to 104). The last section relates to complications of therapy and includes four items related to dyskinesias, four for clinical fluctuations of symptoms, and three items for other complications (nausea/vomiting, sleep disturbances, low blood pressure) (score may range from 0 to 23). A total of 195 points are possible, with 195 representing total (worst) disability and zero representing no disability. Assessment of the reliability and validity of the UPDRS revealed that it is multidimensional, reliable, and valid (16).

Assessment of motor function using the UPDRS is typically done in two states, an "off medication" state, and an "on medication" state. Most studies have asked patients to stop taking all PD medications by midnight on the night before the assessment is scheduled. This is defined as the "off" medication state. However, the length of time required for thorough medication washout may vary from individual to individual, and it is difficult to establish a single duration of time for which study subjects must refrain from medications in order to reach the "off" state. This confounding factor has been addressed in the Core Assessment Program for Intracerebral Transplantation (CAPIT) protocol (17), which describes a "practically defined off state." The practically defined off state is achieved when a patient has been off medication for at least 12 hours, and assessment is performed at least one hour after arising in the morning to eliminate a possible "sleep benefit." Following the off assessment, patients are asked to take their PD medications and undergo repeat assessment in approximately one hour, at which time they are typically in the "on" medication state. However, patients may require either additional time and/or additional medication before they are in a fully functional "on" state. It is important to assess patients in their full "on" state in order to determine highest functioning. In DBS trials, investigators may also include an assessment of the patient with the pulse generator or stimulator turned off, with and without medications. A typical sequence might include assessment in the morning after medications were stopped the night before, with the stimulator activated, then the stimulator is turned off and patients reassessed off medications and off stimulation approximately one hour later, and then a third assessment occurs an hour after patients take their medications and the stimulator is turned back on. As with variation in onset and washout of medication effects, it is recognized that washout of DBS effects following discontinuation of therapy or attainment of peak benefit following reinstitution of therapy may take longer in some individuals than others, and some judgment is required on the part of the patient and the evaluator as to whether the patient is in a full off or on state at the time of each assessment. Investigators have varied the time between assessments, but patient burden and stress should always be a consideration when multiple assessments are being conducted.

Other more general functional status assessments include the Hoehn and Yahr Rating Scale, Schwab and England Rating Scale, and a timed "stand–walk–sit" motor test. The Hoehn and Yahr Rating Scale (18) is a means of staging the degree and severity of PD. There are five stages ranging from stage 1 (i.e., mild symptoms, signs and symptoms on one side only, symptoms inconvenient but not disabling, usually tremor in one limb only, friends have noticed changes in posture, locomotion, and facial expression) to stage 5 (i.e., requires constant nursing care, cannot stand or walk, invalid, cachectic stage). The Schwab and England Activities of Daily Living rating system can be assigned by a rater or by the patient (19). The rating scale ranges from 100% in which the PD individual is completely independent and able to do all chores without slowness, difficulty, or impairment to 0% in which the PD individual is bedridden and vegetative functions such as swallowing, bladder, and bowel function are not working. The ratings are assigned in 10% increments. The third test, the timed "stand–walk–sit" test is a component of the CAPIT (17). It is used frequently for the assessment of patients with PD. It is considered a measure of postural and gait control. In this test, the amount of time required for the patient to arise from a chair (with seat 18 inches above floor), walk 23 feet, turn, walk back to the chair, and sit is measured in seconds.

Another way in which motor function has been assessed is through the use of motor diaries. Clinicians and researchers often use patient self-report diaries to assess patients' experiences. In the PD field, diaries have been used frequently to monitor fluctuations in motor functioning throughout the day. Patients are asked to complete the diaries in real time to avoid recall bias. To monitor motor functioning, patients are typically asked to complete motor diaries for at least two consecutive days at a time. The PD motor diary created by Hauser et al. (20) includes five categories: asleep, off, on without dyskinesia, on with nontroublesome dyskinesia, and on with troublesome dyskinesia. The patient (or caregiver) is asked to record in the diary every 30 minutes by marking which of the five categories best reflects the patient's predominant functioning for the prior 30 minutes. Good time is defined as the sum of 30-minute increments in which the patient was either on without dyskinesia or on with nontroublesome dyskinesia; where as the bad time is the sum of the off periods and on with troublesome dyskinesias periods. These numbers can be converted to the percent of the waking day spent in good "on" time as "on" time plus "on time with nontroublesome dyskinesias" divided by 24 hours minus "asleep" time times 100% (20).

$$\frac{\text{Hours of on time} + \text{Hours of on time with nontroublesome dyskinesias}}{24\ \text{Hours} - \text{Hours asleep}} \times 100\%$$

The majority of patients can complete these diaries without missing or duplicative information, particularly if the number of days they are asked to report their motor functioning is limited. The most recent trend in patient diaries is the use of electronic diaries (21). Patients report their functioning using a personal digital assistant (PDA) type device. This information can then be downloaded into a computer program that will automatically calculate on and off times.

Activities of Daily Living

ADL may be as important, if not more so, to assess in studies of surgery for PD as motor function (6,22). ADL include basic activities of life such as walking, dressing, eating, bathing, control of bodily functions, and ability to use the bathroom. Other activities, defined as independent activities of living include such things as being able to use the telephone, to pay bills, to do work around the house, and so on. ADLs are typically assessed using Part II of the UPDRS, but there are several other scales available. However, for comparison purposes, most PD researchers have relied on the UPDRS Part II. In addition to mobility issues, persons with PD are concerned about issues related to swallowing, handwriting, speech, and decision making. In fact, patients who undergo DBS may give greater weight to improvement in ADLs than to mobility (23).

Quality of Life

There have been several instruments developed to assess disease-specific quality of life for persons with PD. These include: the PD quality of life (PDQL) scale (24), the "Fragebogen Parkinson Lebens Qualität" (Parkinson Quality of Life scale, PLQ) (25), the Parkinson's Impact Scale (PIMS) (26), and the PD question-naire-39 item version (PDQ-39) (27). Marinus et al. (28) reviewed the psycho-metric properties of each of these scales and recommended the PDQ-39 for most situations; it is the scale used most frequently in surgical trials of DBS. Eight dimensions are assessed in the PDQ-39 including mobility, activities of daily living, emotional well-being, stigma, social support, cognition, communi-cation, and bodily discomfort. Each dimension is transformed to a scale that has a range from zero (best score; no problems) to 100 (worst possible score). Internal consistency of the eight dimensions is acceptable for all scales (Cronbach's alpha ranged from 0.94 for mobility to 0.69 for social support). Test–retest reliability was high for all scales (range $r = 0.80$ to $r = 0.94$).

A baseline assessment of general health-related quality of life, using an instrument such as the Medical Outcomes Study Short Form 36 (SF-36) (29) can provide additional useful information. Although such instruments are gener-ally insensitive to measure subtle treatment-related changes in a disease or symp-toms, the baseline measurement can be used to describe the study population. This is useful in describing the general burden of the disease on the study population in relation to other populations and to assess the generalizability of the study.

Medication Use

Pharmacologic therapy is the mainstay of treatment in individuals whose PD symptoms require treatment. The effect of surgical interventions on medication therapy is an important outcome of trials of surgery for PD. Many studies have reported that medication adjustments occur following DBS. In particular, most studies of STN DBS report the ability to reduce the dose or even stop use of some PD medications, where as studies of GPi DBS typically do not report reductions in medication (6). To facilitate comparison of pre- and postintervention medication use across subjects and across studies, some investigators have devised strategies for converting a large variety of PD medications to "levodopa-equivalents" (30). These conversion formulas were updated recently to take into account the newer PD medications available (7). Table 1 provides the recommended conversions for determining levodopa equivalents.

Cognitive/Neuropsychological Functioning

Of significant importance to any study of surgery in PD is the effect of surgery on cognitive and psychological functioning. Dementia and cognitive impairment are common in PD, with cognitive impairment demonstrated even in the first year or two after PD onset (31). Executive and attentional impairment is typical, but learning deficits can also occur early. The relative risk of developing dementia in PD is five times higher than in the general population (32) and may occur in 30% of persons with PD (33). Studies of the impact of DBS on PD have reported both improvement and permanent and significant worsening of cognitive function (15,34,35) but due to the limited quality of the existing research, the true impact of DBS on mood and cognitive changes is not known (36).

Studies of DBS often include a battery of neuropsychological tests that are given at baseline prior to surgery and then repeated after DBS. These assessments typically include an evaluation of dementia and cognitive function, as well as frontal-executive and complex attention functions, visuoperceptual functions, verbal fluency, working memory, and recall (34,37). Many studies have used both the Mattis Dementia Rating Scale (DRS) (38) and the mini-mental status exam (MMSE) (39). Individuals scoring 24 or lower on the MMSE are considered cognitively impaired and have been excluded from participation in most studies of DBS. The DRS has been shown to be sensitive to cognitive deficits in PD (40).

Table 1 Equivalents for 100 mg of Standard Levodopa

Brand name	Generic	Equivalents
Sinemet CR®	CR levodopa	125 mg
Parlodel®	Bromocriptine	10 mg
Permax®	Pergolide	1 mg
Mirapex®	Pramipexole	1 mg
Requip®	Ropinirole	4 mg[a]

[a]Pawha (2003) used 3 mg.
Note: Investigators should not include carbidopa, tolcapone, or entacapone in estimates of levodopa equivalents since these work in conjunction with levodopa and not alone.

Table 2 Randomized Clinical Trials of Deep Brain Stimulation for Parkinson's Disease

Study	Intervention	Control or comparison	Sample	Primary outcome	Other outcomes	Data collection points	Eligibility criteria
Public Health Service 5 MO 1 RR000334 (Portland) (Anderson et al. 2005)	Bilateral DBS-STN	Bilateral DBS-GPi Best medical management (6 mo)[a]	23	UPDRS on and off medications	Dyskinesia Neurological status Medication dosage	B, 3, 6, 12 mo	Ages 20–80 Idiopathic PD (Hoehn and Yahr of III or IV off meds) Prominent bradykinesia and rigidity MMSE ≥ 24 Beck Depression score ≤20 No intracranial abnormalities No prior PD or CNS surgery Stable does of PD meds for at least one month
DBS for PD trial (Atlanta and Cleveland) NINDS NCT00053625	Unilateral DBS-STN	Unilateral DBS-GPi	132	Motor function	Neuropsychological functioning Quality of life	Not available	Ages 30–75 Clinical diagnosis of idiopathic PD Hoehn and Yahr ≥III in off meds Intractable, disabling motor fluctuations, dyskinesias or freezing Unsatisfactory response to maximal meds or prior surgery Stable on PD meds for at least 30 days Cognitively able to sign consent No dementia or psychiatric disorder No significant medical comorbidities
Cognition and mood in PD, STN versus GPi DBS "COMPARe" (Florida)	Unilateral DBS-STN	Unilateral DBS-GPi Control (no DBS)	52 10	Mood state	UDPRS cognition	6 mo	Not available
PD SURG (England)	Immediate DBS or lesioning of STN or GPi	Delay of surgery for at least one year; medical therapy	400–600	PDQ-39	Quality of life (ED-5Q) MMSE UPDRS Neuropsychological evaluation Caregiver well-being (SF-36) Direct medical costs	B, 1, 3, 5, 7, and 9 yr	PD diagnosed by UK Brain Bank Criteria PD not controlled by current medical therapy Fit for surgical intervention Not demented Surgery is not definitely required within one year Can provide written informed consent

(Continued)

Table 2 Randomized Clinical Trials of Deep Brain Stimulation for Parkinson's Disease (*Continued*)

Study	Intervention	Control or comparison	Sample	Primary outcome	Other outcomes	Data collection points	Eligibility criteria
The effect of DBS compared with best medical treatment on the life quality in PD: A randomized controlled multi-center study (Germany)	DBS-STN	Best medical treatment	154	PDQ-39 UPDRS-motor (off meds)	Dyskinesia Handicap SF-36 Depression Apathy Neuropsychological status	6 mo	Idiopathic PD <75 yrs old PD symptoms or dyskinesias that limit ADLs No dementia or serious psychiatric illness No contraindications to surgery
Effect of DBS on depression and quality of life in Parkinson's patients NCT00179101	DBS	Patients evaluated and approved for DBS but do not complete surgery	42	Depression	Quality of life	Not available	Ages 50–85 years Idiopathic PD Have received neuropsychological testing (for possible DBS) Exclude if: not approved for DBS based on neuropsych tests, and those who received DBS less than one year ago
DBS in early stage PD (phase 1 trial) NCT00282152	Bilateral STN DBS	Medical therapy	30	Safety/tolerability	Medication use Time to "off" state	B, 6, 12, 18, and 24 mo	Ages 50–75 Idiopathic PD Response to dopaminergic therapy Hoehn and Yahr = 2 in off state No contraindications to surgery Levodpa or dopamine agonist therapy for two or less years, Normal MRI Exclude if: dementia, major psychiatric disorder, previous brain surgery or injury, evidence of existing dyskinesias or motor fluctuations

Study	Intervention	N	Outcomes	Visits	Inclusion criteria
CSP #468 A comparison of best medical therapy and DBS of STN and globus pallidus for the treatment of PD (United States)	Bilateral DBS–STN Bilateral DBS–GPi Best medical therapy	316	On time (motor diary) – 6 months UPDRS motor score off – 2 years UPDRS subscales Hoehn and Yahr Schwab and England Timed stand–walk–sit–test Medication dosage SF-36 PDQ-39 Quality of well-being Neuropsychological evaluation Adverse events Health care use	B, 3, 6, 12, 18, 24, 36 mo	Idiopathic PD Hoehn and Yahr ≥ II off meds L-dopa responsive with clear on periods Persistent disabling symptoms (off periods and/or troublesome dyskinesias ≥ three hours per day) Stable on PD meds for at least one month Age ≥ 21 No previous PD surgery No medial contraindications to surgery MMSE score > 24, no dementia No active drug/alcohol use No intracranial abnormalities Not pregnant

[a]Only two patients had been randomized to this arm at the time this study was stopped due to the start of CSP #468.

Abbreviations: DBS, deep brain stimulation; GPi, globus pallidum interna; MMSE, mini-mental status exam; MRI, magnetic resonance imaging; NINDS, National Institute of Neurological Disorders and Stroke; PD, Parkinson's disease; PDQ, Parkinson's disease questionnaire; STN, subthalamic nucleus; UPDRS, Unified Parkinson's Disease Rating Scale.

The battery of neuropsychological tests that have been used in studies of PD and surgery can require two hours or more to complete (7). Therefore, it is important to be sensitive to study participant burden. The neuropsychological testing should be scheduled on a different day from the other assessments if possible to limit burden and fatigue. Researchers need to be aware that "learning" and "practice" effects may occur with repeated administration of a given test, and this may skew outcomes data. When possible, tests should be selected to minimize this effect. For example, the Hopkins Verbal Learning Test offers the availability of six equivalent lists of alternative items that can be used for repeat assessments, minimizing practice effects (41). There is not sufficient room here to review the battery of tests that can be used in assessments of PD subjects, and the reader should refer to published articles of neuropsychological assessments in PD and consult with knowledgeable neuropsychologists as to what tests would be appropriate.

Adverse Events

Hariz (42) has identified three categories of adverse events in DBS. These events are related to the surgical procedure, the hardware, and the effects of stimulation. Complications of surgery are direct medical/surgical complications such as seizure, hemorrhage, infection, and pulmonary embolism. Complications related to the equipment or hardware include skin erosion, electrode migration, fracture of the leads, and generator failure. These complications often require additional surgery to remove, revise, repair, or replace some or all of the equipment. Complications may occur due to stimulation. Adverse motor and sensory effects, confusion, depression, gait and speech disturbances, personality, mood and cognitive changes, and weight gain are some of the adverse events that have resulted from DBS. These complications can often be mitigated or eliminated if the target of stimulation or the stimulation parameters are adjusted.

It is important to track the occurrence of adverse events in studies of DBS, because the beneficial outcomes of an intervention may be more than offset by adverse outcomes. Although many of the existing studies of DBS in PD report adverse events, investigators often use different terminology for the same event, use different definitions for events, and fail to report time to event (e.g., shortly after surgery or many months later) which makes comparisons across studies extremely difficult. In clinical trials, definitions of adverse events and key temporal relationships to the intervention should be established at the outset of the study (e.g., surgical mortality might be defined as any study subject death occurring within 30 days of surgery, whereas death occurring at a later time point might not be related categorically to the surgical intervention).

The Food and Drug Administration (FDA) makes a distinction between adverse events and serious adverse events. An adverse event is an untoward sign or symptom that occurs during the course of participation in the study. Adverse events are typically rated on severity, frequency, and relatedness to the study intervention. In studies of DBS, relatedness classifications are further ascribed to the disease, surgery, or device. In rigorous clinical trials, all adverse changes in study subjects' conditions may be recorded regardless whether the adverse event is related to the intervention or to the study.

Serious adverse events are a subset of adverse events that include death, life-threatening events, new or prolonged hospitalization, or institutionalization. Serious adverse events require expedited reporting and review procedures by the study site's institutional review board and the study sponsor. Serious adverse events that are severe and unexpected, that is, not previously reported, generally require a safety report be filed with the FDA.

Health Care Use and Costs

Costs are based on the resources required to provide the intervention and follow-up. These resources include the cost of the DBS equipment, the cost of the hospitalization, operating room, surgical team, DBS programming time, any adverse events requiring intervention, medications, follow-up visits, and ongoing health care needs (e.g., emergency room, nursing home care). The estimated health care costs of a PD patient are over US $6000 annually, with medications alone costing as much as US $4500 annually (43,44). Moreover, total costs of treating PD in the United States have been estimated at US $24 billion annually (43,45). A few studies have tried to estimate the costs of DBS surgery in PD. McIntosh et al. (46) estimated the costs of bilateral STN DBS over a five-year period. They estimated costs of preoperative assessment, surgery, and postoperative management to be approximately £32,526 or US $52,220 in 2002 prices; and found that almost 70% of costs were attributable to initial costs of equipment; of which approximately half of these costs were for initial surgery and the other half were for follow-up management, replacement and complications. This did not include any direct costs incurred by patients, informal care or productivity costs, or patient assessment of effectiveness.

DBS is a costly intervention. The cost of the devices (electrodes, extension wires, pulse generator) alone for bilateral intervention is approximately US $20,000 (2003, dollars) (7). The charge to the patient or insurance carrier may be much greater. The procedure to implant the electrodes requires radiographic imaging and six to eight hours of operating room time with a neurosurgical team may be required for bilateral electrode implantation. The placement of the battery pack(s) requires additional operating room time, whether done at the same time as lead implant or at a later date. Recurring costs include the visits needed to program and modify the stimulation parameters and adjust medications to maximize motor function while minimizing side effects of therapy. There may be additional costs associated with postoperative recuperation following DBS surgery, such as need for skilled nursing or rehabilitation therapy following surgery. Other costs relate to ongoing needs of PD management, including physician visits, medications (which may be decreased, increased, or remain unchanged depending on response to DBS), and ancillary healthcare services.

Particularly in trials that involve costly interventions, it is important to obtain information not only about the effectiveness of each treatment, but also the costs of providing each intervention. If one treatment is determined to be both more effective and less costly, then that treatment is said to be the "dominant" (i.e., the preferred) treatment. If two treatments are equally effective, the cost-effectiveness analysis essentially becomes a cost-minimization analysis that reveals which treatment strategy provides the same effectiveness at a lower cost. However, if one treatment is both more effective and more costly, then the trade-off between costs and effectiveness should be examined.

A cost-effectiveness analysis is a method for assessing the relative impacts of expenditures on different health care treatments. A Panel on Cost-Effectiveness in Health and Medicine, convened by the US Public Health Service, has published detailed guidelines for the conduct and presentation of such studies (47). The costs included in the analysis will depend on the perspective of the analysis. When thinking about the costs of treatments for PD, we could consider the costs from the perspective of health care provider (costs for physicians, medical facilities, and pharmaceuticals), the patient (lost work time and cost of travel to get to the physician's office or hospital), or the costs to society (costs to patients, physicians, and anyone else in society). The Panel on Cost-Effectiveness advocates that costs be estimated from the societal perspective. The advantage of conducting the cost analysis from this perspective is that it takes into account all the costs stemming from the treatment choice. Quality-adjusted life year (QALY) is the recommended measure of effectiveness (47). QALYs capture both changes in quality of life and mortality that may result from one treatment relative to another. QALYs provide a broad measure of effectiveness that will allow the cost-effectiveness of a treatment to be compared with the cost-effectiveness of a variety of other treatments and health care interventions. It is important to note that there need not be differences in mortality for QALYs to differ between the two treatment groups.

Other Outcomes

There are many other aspects of the life of a person with PD that can be affected either positively or adversely as a result of DBS and these may also be assessed. They include sleep quality, pain, satisfaction with care, gait and balance, speech, swallowing, and sexual functioning. Due to space constraints and the fact that these outcomes are not regularly reported in published DBS studies, these outcomes will not be discussed in this chapter.

Measurement Issues

The frequency and extent of measurements and assessments obtained from patients with PD need to be carefully considered. If a patient perceives the assessment to be burdensome, then the quality of the measurements will be diminished and can become unreliable. In addition, the likelihood of a patient becoming non-compliant with follow-up or withdrawing consent from participation is increased.

Since most analysis of treatment responses will compare the patient's measurements at baseline to those at a later point in time after treatment has begun, standardization of factors that may influence the patient's response, such as time of day, amount, and timing of medication, is important. It is essential to have the same person performing the assessment at each study visit to eliminate imprecision due to differences between raters. Evaluators should also be retrained periodically to minimize shifts in ratings over time.

Certain assessments may be subject to practice effects if given repeatedly. As noted earlier, when possible, different versions of the instrument should be administered over time. To avoid systematic biases in the sequence of administering the different versions, a randomized sequence of test versions should be determined at the first evaluation.

Intention to Treat

It is also important to maintain the integrity of the randomized groups throughout the study. Thus, study designs should consider the potential impact on the patient's willingness to remain in the study for the planned duration. Studies with substantial drop-out rates cannot rely on the benefits of randomization to certify the validity of the treatment comparisons. Many studies have established that patients withdrawn early from the trial differ from those who remain in the study. Thus, study design strategies that intentionally drop poorly responding patients or increase the likelihood of certain types of patients withdrawing early introduce bias and diminish the randomized nature of the treatment groups. Because of this, an analysis of results based on the comparison of treatment strategies, that is, intention to treat, rather than actual treatment received, has highest validity.

RECENT/ONGOING TRIALS OF DEEP BRAIN STIMULATION IN PARKINSON'S DISEASE

In this last section, we provide examples of recently completed and ongoing randomized clinical trials of DBS in PD (see Table 2). The first randomized trial of STN versus GPi stimulation (48) was published in 1999 and included 10 patients who completed 12 months of follow-up (six STN and four GPi). Enrollment criteria included: idiopathic diagnosis of PD, Hoehn and Yahr score greater than or equal to 3 off medications, disabling motor symptoms, unsatisfactory response to medications, on a stable dose of PD medications for at least one month, cognitively intact with no medical or psychiatric comorbidities. Patients and evaluating clinicians were blinded to the site of stimulation. The primary outcome was UPDRS motor score off medications. The outcomes examined included levodopa dose, motor symptoms, ADL, and complications. Motor function improved in both groups; 39% for GPi and 44% for STN (p = 0.71). Although it is the first published randomized trial of site of DBS stimulation, it is limited by the small sample size and that it was conducted at a single site. This group recently published a follow-up to this study in which their sample size was increased to 20 subjects (49). Their findings were similar to their earlier finding. There are several studies currently ongoing that also address these issues.

A multi-site study recently completed in Germany included 154 patients with PD randomized to either STN DBS or best medical therapy (14). Follow-up was for six months with primary outcomes including quality of life and motor function (PDQ-39 and UPDRS-motor). Pairwise comparisons found significantly greater improvements from baseline to six months for quality of life and motor function in those patients who underwent bilateral STN DBS than those who were treated with medication. In fact, there was little change from baseline in the medication group at six months. Serious adverse events were higher in the DBS group than the medication group (13% v. 4%; $p < 0.04$).

The PD SURG trial is a multi-center study being conducted in the United Kingdom (50). It involves the randomization of subjects with PD that is not controlled by current medical therapy to either surgery or medical therapy. Within the surgical arm, patients may undergo bilateral STN surgery or unilateral or bilateral pallidal surgery by either stimulation or lesioning. The choice of surgical site and type will be determined at the site dependent on equipment, expertise, and clinical judgment. Patients in the best medical therapy arm will have a delay of surgery for PD for at least one year. The goal of this study is to conduct a large simple randomized trial that is indicative of real life experiences. Investigators hope to enroll between 400 and 600 patients, with the primary outcome being quality of life (PDQ-39). Follow-up will continue for nine years. Although this study will provide valuable information about medical therapy versus surgery, since the surgical arm includes a number of different procedures that are not randomized or controlled, it will not be possible to conduct a direct comparison of lesioning versus stimulation, nor of site of surgical intervention. The results of the study will be limited primarily to a comparison of best medical therapy to some type of surgical intervention without specifying the surgical intervention. However, the delay to surgery for the medical therapy arm might provide information regarding a possible neuroprotective effect of surgical intervention by demonstrating change in the rate of progression of PD in the early surgery versus delayed surgery group.

A study funded by National Institute of Neurological Disorders and Stroke (NINDS) compares unilateral DBS of the STN and the GPi in a randomized trial (51). The study will evaluate the effect of DBS in the GPi and STN on motor, neuropsychological and psychiatric function, and quality of life in patients with PD in 132 subjects. Two other key issues will be addressed: whether there are differences between unilateral GPi-DBS and STN-DBS and which patients are the best candidates for bilateral DBS.

Another study supported by NINDS, the COMPARe study, is a randomized trial of 52 patients with PD (13). The primary outcome, change in mood status, will be compared between STN and GPi DBS patients. A parallel group of 10

PD patients will serve as a no surgery control group. These same investigators are also conducting a study of mood and STN DBS, where outcomes are being compared between unilateral and bilateral STN DBS patients with PD refractory to medication (52).

Two clinical trials have been recently funded through Vanderbilt University. One is a study of DBS in early stage PD (53). This study will recruit subjects are at stage II Hoehn and Yahr off medications. This stage I trial will enroll 30 patients, half of whom will undergo bilateral STN DBS and the other half will continue with medical therapy. The primary goal is to address safety, tolerability, and time to 'off' state at 6, 12, 18, and 24 months. A second study will assess depression and quality of life in persons with PD who undergo DBS (54). They will be compared to a group of individuals with PD who were approved for DBS but did not undergo surgery. The enrollment target is 42 subjects. Unlike the other studies reviewed in this section, this study is not a randomized controlled trial. However, the primary outcome, depression, has not been a primary outcome for other trials.

The largest randomized clinical trial of DBS for PD ever mounted is currently ongoing with the goal of enrolling 316 patients with PD (7). This study (VA CSP 468) is funded by the Department of Veterans Affairs Cooperative Studies Program, the NINDS, and Medtronic, Inc. Patients with PD are first randomized to either immediate surgery or to six months of best medical therapy. Those randomized to surgery are then randomized to site of stimulation: STN or GPi. Patients in the medical therapy arm undergo randomization to site of surgery at six months. The primary outcome for the comparison of medical therapy to DBS is time in the "on state without troublesome dyskinesias" based on patient motor diaries. The primary outcome for the STN/GPi comparison is UPDRS motor function, on stimulation/off medication at two years. Other outcomes include quality of life, activities of daily living, medication usage, neuropsychological functioning, and adverse events. This study will address many of the questions regarding the outcomes of DBS by site, as well as provide information about what patients may do better with DBS at one site versus the other.

In total, these ongoing randomized trials will provide strong evidence as to how DBS for PD should proceed in the future.

REFERENCES

1. Sackett DL, Rosenberg WM, Gray JA, et al. Evidence based medicine: what it is and what it isn't. BMJ 1996; 312(7023):71–72.
2. Gray GE. Evidence-based medicine: an introduction for psychiatrists. J Psychiatr Pract 2002; 8(1):5–13.
3. Sackett DL. Rules of evidence and clinical recommendations on the use of antithrombotic agents. Chest 1989; 95(suppl 2):2S–4S.
4. Parkinson Study Group. A randomized placebo-controlled trial of rasagiline in levodopa-treated patients with Parkinson disease and motor fluctuations: the PRESTO study. Arch Neurol 2005; 62(2):241–248.

5. Schneider E. DATATOP-study: significance of its results in the treatment of Parkinson's disease. J Neural Transm Suppl 1995; 46:391–397.
6. Weaver F, Follett K, Hur K, et al. Deep brain stimulation in Parkinson disease: a metaanalysis of patient outcomes. J Neurosurg 2005; 103(6):956–967.
7. Follett K, Weaver F, Stern M, et al. VA Cooperative Study #468. A comparison of best medical therapy and deep brain stimulation of subthalamic nucleus and globus pallidus for the treatment of Parkinson's disease. Study Protocol. Cooperative Studies Program, Research & Development Service, Department of Veterans Affairs, Washington, D.C., October 1, 2001.
8. Vitek JL. Deep brain stimulation for Parkinson's disease. A critical re-evaluation of STN versus GPi DBS. Stereotact Funct Neurosurg 2002; 78(3–4):119–131.
9. Rodriguez-Oroz MC, Obeso JA, Lang AE, et al. Bilateral deep brain stimulation in Parkinson's disease: a multicentre study with 4 years follow-up. Brain 2005; 128:2240–2249.
10. Krack P, Batir A, Van Blercom N, et al. Five-year follow-up of bilateral stimulation of the subthalamic nucleus in advanced Parkinson's disease. N Engl J Med 2003; 349(20):1925–1934.
11. Fahn S, Elton RL, Members of the UPDRS Development Committee. Unified Parkinson's Disease Rating Scale. In: Fahn S, Marsden CD, Goldstein M, eds. Recent developments in Parkinson's disease, Vol. 2. Florham Park, NJ: Macmillan Health Care Information 1987:153–164.
12. Lyons KE, Pahwa R. Long-term benefits in quality of life provided by bilateral subthalamic stimulation in patients with Parkinson disease. J Neurosurg 2005; 103(2):252–255.
13. Okun M. Effects of deep brain stimulation on motor, mood, and cognitive symptoms in Parkinson's disease. University of Florida, Gainesville, FL. http://www.pdtrials.org/trial_detail_print.php?trial_id=333 (accessed January 2006).
14. Deuschl G. The effect of deep brain stimulation compared with best medical treatment on life quality in Parkinson's disease: a randomized controlled multi-center study. The 16th International Congress on Parkinsonism and Related Disorders. Berlin. June 8, 2005.
15. Schupbach WM, Chastan N, Welter ML, et al. Stimulation of the subthalamic nucleus in Parkinson's disease: a 5 year follow up. J Neurol Neurosurg Psychiatry 2005; 76(12):1640–1644.
16. Martinez-Martin P, Gil-Nagel A, Gracia LM, et al. Unified Parkinson's Disease Rating Scale characteristics and structure. The Cooperative Multicentric Group. Mov Disord 1994; 9(1):76–83.
17. Langston JW, Widner H, Goetz CG, et al. Core assessment program for intracerebral transplantations (CAPIT). Mov Disord 1992; 7(1):2–13.
18. Hoehn MM, Yahr MD. Parkinsonism: onset, progression and mortality. Neurology 1967; 17(5):427–442.
19. Schwab RS, England AC. Projection technique for evaluating surgery in Parkinson's disease. Third symposium on Parkinson's disease. Edinburgh: Gillingham and Donaldson, 1969.
20. Hauser RA, Deckers F, Lehert P. Parkinson's disease home diary: further validation and implications for clinical trials. Mov Disord 2004; 19(12):1409–1413.
21. Nyholm D, Kowalski J, Aquilonius SM. Wireless real-time electronic data capture for self-assessment of motor function and quality of life in Parkinson's disease. Mov Disord 2004; 19(4):446–451.

22. Lezcano E, Gomez-Esteban JC, Zarranz JJ, et al. Improvement in quality of life in patients with advanced Parkinson's disease following bilateral deep-brain stimulation in subthalamic nucleus. Eur J Neurol 2004; 11(7):451–454.
23. Parkinson Alliance. Focus 1 Report DBS/STN Patient Survey on Pre and Post Surgery Symptoms. January 2004.
24. De Boer AG, Wijker W, Speelman JD, et al. Quality of life in patients with Parkinson's disease: development of a questionnaire. J Neurol Neurosurg Psychiatry 1996; 61(1):70–74.
25. Van den Berg M. Leben mit Parkinson: Entwicklung und psychometrische Testung des Fragenbogens PLQ. Neurol Rehabil 1998; 4:221–226.
26. Calne S, Schulzer M, Mak E, et al. Validating a quality of life rating scale for idiopathic parkinsonism: Parkinson's impact scale. Parkinsonism Relat Disord 1996; 2:55–61.
27. Peto V, Jenkinson C, Fitzpatrick R. PDQ-39: a review of the development, validation and application of a Parkinson's disease quality of life questionnaire and its associated measures. J Neurol 1998; 245(suppl 1):S10–S14.
28. Marinus J, Ramaker C, van Hilten JJ, et al. Health related quality of life in Parkinson's disease: a systematic review of disease specific instruments. J Neurol Neurosurg Psychiatry 2002; 72(2):241–248.
29. Ware JE, Sherbourne CD. The MOS 36-item short-form health survey (SF-36). I. Conceptual framework and item selection. Med Care 1992; 30(6):473–483.
30. Pahwa R, Wilkinson SB, Overman J, et al. Bilateral subthalamic stimulation in patients with Parkinson disease: long-term follow up. J Neurosurg 2003; 99(1):71–77.
31. Ehrt U, Aarsland D. Psychiatric aspects of Parkinson's disease. Curr Opin Psychiatry 2005; 18(3):335–341.
32. Hobson P, Meara J. Risk and incidence of dementia in a cohort of older subjects with Parkinson's disease in the United Kingdom. Mov Disord 2004; 19(9):1043–1049.
33. Lauterbach EC. The neuropsychiatry of Parkinson's disease. Minerva Med 2005; 96(3):155–173.
34. Fields JA, Troster AI, Wilkinson SB, et al. Cognitive outcome following staged bilateral pallidal stimulation for the treatment of Parkinson's disease. Clin Neurol Neurosurg 1999; 101(3):182–188.
35. Fields JA, Troster AI. Cognitive outcomes after deep brain stimulation for Parkinson's disease: a review of initial studies and recommendations for future research. Brain Cogn 2000; 42(2):268–293.
36. Rodriguez RL, Miller K, Bowers D, et al. Mood and cognitive changes with deep brain stimulation. What we know and where we should go. Minerva Med 2005; 96(3):125–144.
37. Taylor AE, Saint-Cyr JA. The neuropsychology of Parkinson's disease. Brain Cogn 1995; 28(3):281–296.
38. Mattis S. Dementia Rating Scale: Professional Manual. Psychological Assessment Resources Inc, Odessa, Florida, 1973.
39. Folstein MF, Folstein SE, McHugh PR. "Mini-mental state." A practical method for grading the cognitive state of patients for the clinician. J Psychiatr Res 1975; 12(3):189–198.
40. Brown G, Rahill A, Gorell J, et al. Validity of the Dementia Rating Scale in assessing cognitive function in Parkinson's disease. J Geriatr Psychiatry Neurol 1999; 12(4):180–188.

41. Trepanier LL, Saint-Cyr JA, Lozano AM, et al. Neuropsychological consequences of posteroventral pallidotomy for the treatment of Parkinson's disease. Neurology 1998; 51(1):207–215.
42. Hariz MI. Complications of deep brain stimulation surgery. Mov Disord 2002; 17(suppl 3):S162–S166.
43. LePen C, Wait S, Moutard-Martin F, et al. Cost of illness and disease severity in a cohort of French patients with Parkinson's disease. Pharmacoeconomics 1999; 16(1):59–69.
44. Tomaszewski KJ, Holloway RG. Deep brain stimulation in the treatment of Parkinson's disease: a cost-effectiveness analysis. Neurology 2001; 57(4):663–671.
45. Whetten-Goldstein K, Sloan F, Kulas E, et al. The burden of Parkinson's disease on society, family, and the individual. J Am Geriatr Soc 1997; 45(7):844–849.
46. McIntosh E, Gray A, Aziz T. Estimating the costs of surgical innovations: the case for subthalamic nucleus stimulation in the treatment of advanced Parkinson's disease. Mov Disord 2003; 18(9):993–999.
47. Gold MR, Russell LB, Seigel JE, Weinstein MC. Cost-effectiveness in Health and Medicine. New York: Oxford University Press, 1996.
48. Burchiel KJ, Anderson VC, Favre J, et al. Comparison of pallidal and subthalamic nucleus deep brain stimulation for advanced Parkinson's disease: results of a randomized, blinded pilot study. Neurosurgery 1999; 45(6):1375–1382.
49. Anderson VC, Burchiel KJ, Hogarth P, et al. Pallidal vs subthalamic nucleus deep brain stimulation in Parkinson disease. Arch Neurol 2005; 62(4):554–560.
50. PD SURG Trial—A large randomised assessment of the relative cost-effectiveness of surgery for Parkinson's disease. Protocol Version 2 (November 21, 2001). Birmingham Clinical Trials Unit, University of Birmingham.
51. Vitek JL, DeLong MR. Deep brain stimulation for Parkinson's disease trial. http://www.clinicaltrials.gov/ct/show/NCT00053625 (accessed March 2006).
52. Okun M. The MOST study: Mood and STN DBS. University of Florida, Gainesville, FL. http://www.pdtrials.org/trial_detail_print.php?trial_id=332 (accessed January 2006).
53. Charles PD. DBS in early stage Parkinson's disease. http://www.clinicaltrials.gov/ct/show/NCT00282152 (accessed March 2006).
54. Schadt CR, Charles PD. Effect of deep brain stimulation on depression and quality of life in Parkinson's patients. http://www.clinicaltrials.gov/ct/show/NCT00179101 (accessed March 2006).

―――――――――――――― **19** ――――――――――――――

Ethical Issues in Deep Brain Stimulation

Paul Root Wolpe

Departments of Psychiatry, Medical Ethics, and Sociology and Center for Bioethics, University of Pennsylvania, Philadelphia, Pennsylvania, U.S.A.

Paul J. Ford

Departments of Bioethics and Neurology, The Cleveland Clinic, Cleveland, Ohio, U.S.A.

Michael Harhay

Center for Bioethics, University of Pennsylvania, Philadelphia, Pennsylvania, U.S.A.

INTRODUCTION

Deep brain stimulation (DBS) is a fairly recent surgical therapy for the treatment of Parkinson's disease (PD), having first won Food and Drug Administration (FDA) approval in 1997 [for use in the thalamus; approval for use in the subthalamic nucleus (STN) came in 2001]. As a surgical procedure involving the brain, DBS requires the ethical oversight that is applied to any surgery and the additional scrutiny due to a novel procedure that affects brain function. In addition, DBS is used most often on patients who are elderly, in whom other treatments have failed or ceased to be effective, who may be cognitively or affectively impaired, and who may have comorbidities.

Though specific numbers are elusive, DBS is clearly growing both in terms of its increasing use for movement disorders and the recent expansion of DBS to psychiatric disorders (1). Despite its growing popularity, placebo controlled or comparative studies on the effectiveness and safety of DBS are lacking.

Complicating the spread of DBS is that the procedure, like many invasive neurotechnologies, has an image problem among the public (2). The public is wary of novel devices that involve altering brain processes, and they have some historical justification for their caution (see next section). The resistance of some lay psychiatric groups to the use of DBS for depression and other psychiatric syndromes has complicated the public reception of DBS. The role of industry in pushing the technology has also come under scrutiny. The neural stimulation market, which exceeds half a billion dollars and is growing 20% a year, has begun to publicly speculate on the use of neural stimulation for everything from eating disorders to addiction (3). Concerns have been raised that the industry will rush products to market and push them with heavy sales forces, mimicking some of the worst practices of the pharmaceutical industry. The worries seemed compounded when Daniel Schultz, Director of the Center for Devices and Radiological Health at the FDA, overruled a review committee and approved the vagus nerve stimulator for depression, despite equivocal data of its effectiveness and the unanimous opinion of his scientific staff not to grant approval (4). Concern about the FDA's oversight of implants and other medical devices has led Senator Charles Grassley of Iowa to begin a review of FDA practices.

Currently, there is no consensus regarding the appropriate screening procedures for patients being considered for DBS, the proper makeup or training of the medical team, the need for establishing multidisciplinary functional neurosurgery committees, or guidelines for much of the medical management (5). For these reasons, it is important in this early phase of the use of the technology to assure that DBS is performed with proper ethical and regulatory oversight. In this chapter, we will review some of the most challenging aspects of DBS. After a short historical perspective, we will examine both clinical and research ethics issues in the use and spread of the procedure.

HISTORICAL PERSPECTIVES

New medical technologies do not exist in a vacuum, but are instead the latest products of traditions going back thousands of years. To understand some of the concerns expressed about DBS, it is important to have some perspective on the history of neurosurgery for behavioral and psychiatric disorders. The excesses and enthusiasms that led to preventable suffering and death at the hands of neurosurgeons, even within the last century, lead some to pause when they see a new procedure that generates the excitement of DBS, particularly when it so quickly is advocated for psychiatric as well as neuromotor disorders (6).

Surgery on the head and brain may well be among the most ancient practiced medical arts in general. Trephaning traces back to late Neolithic times, over 12,000 years ago, and given the healing of bone discovered in these cases, the success rate was surprisingly high. Surgeries on the head continued virtually uninterrupted from ancient times to the present in a variety of societies, even absent the modern techniques of sterilization. Despite the long history of such surgeries, they were primarily epidural, and it was not until the late 19th century that advances in antisepsis, anesthesia, and an understanding of brain function and cerebral localization allowed for the first modern neurosurgeries to be performed (7).

While the purpose for much of prehistorical cranial surgery is unknown, in modern times neurosurgery was developed to a large degree to treat psychiatric disorders. The first modern psychosurgery was performed by Gottlieb Burckhardt (8), who between 1888 and the spring of 1890 performed the first cited cortical excisions on six of his chronic schizophrenic patients. Burkhardt's innovation was not well received in his native Switzerland, and he eventually abandoned it. Psychosurgery was performed irregularly thereafter until the 1930s when the famous Portuguese neurologist Egas Moniz suggested that ablation of the frontal cortex in humans might mitigate psychiatric disease (9). Moniz and his associate Almeida Lima at the University of Lisbon went on to perform a systematic series of prefrontal leucotomies. Moniz's technique was transformed into the transorbital frontal lobotomy and popularized by Walter Freeman and James Watts, whose overexuberance led, by the 1960s, to a legacy of coerced psychosurgery, ice pick lobotomies, Freeman's "lobotomobile," and ultimately to over 40,000 psychosurgical procedures performed without oversight or proper scientific assessment (10).

If the activities of Freeman led to a general wariness of psychosurgery, the neurophysiological and behavioral experiments of the American (and Soviet) Cold War governments using drugs and other mind control techniques fueled additional fears of interventions in the brain. The famous experiment of Jose Delgado, whose neural implant arrested a charging bull, added brain stimulation to the public consciousness of emerging understandings of the brain. Delgado's prediction of a society controlled by neurotechnology lead to experimental programs such as the one at Tulane (11), a controversial program that came under intense scrutiny after media reports of experiments such as the 1972 attempt to alter the sexual orientation of a male homosexual via neural stimulation while he had intercourse with a female prostitute (12). Popular media portrayals, such as Jack Nicholson's in *One Flew Over the Cuckoo's Nest*, further undermined public confidence in the neuropsychiatric system in the United States. As Joseph Fins writes, "Those eras of psychosurgery ended with widespread condemnation, congressional calls for a ban, and a vow that history should never repeat itself." (6. p.303)

Modern neurosurgery bears little resemblance to those (hopefully) bygone eras. In place is much more stringent oversight, Institutional Review Board (IRB) review, and perhaps most importantly, the troubling memory of previous excesses to keep neurological care vigilant. DBS itself is not a form of psychosurgery but rather a form of neuromodulation (though so was the work of Delgado), and the scientific underpinnings of the procedure are far more sophisticated than those that drove lobotomies, for example. Although surgical treatment for PD began by lesioning different functional targets within the basal ganglia (13), DBS, which is the functional equivalent to lesioning, is controllable and reversible, and allows for scientific studies in a way that ablation could not (9). Still, the public remains wary of all neurosurgical interventions to modify human behavior. The turn to use of DBS for psychiatric disorders (1) particularly has raised concerns that are clearly influenced by the history of psychosurgery (a term that has been abandoned due to its associations). As the neurologist and ethicist Joseph Fins writes about ethical questions surrounding the increasing use of DBS: "Can today's investigators avoid the moral blindness of their predecessors? Will society tolerate this new foray into somatic therapy and seek to regulate it as legitimate science, or will a lingering memory of psychosurgery be so overwhelming as to make this impossible?" (6. p.303).

Historical precedents must be considered, but they need not determine the course of a seemingly valuable procedure like DBS. Still, therapies exist in a social context; novel techniques such as DBS must struggle for public acceptance with the troubling legacy of psychosurgery in the United States.

DEEP BRAIN STIMULATION AND CLINICAL CARE

Concern about the ethics of the clinician–patient relationship in the Western world traces back to the ancient world. Almost all medical ethics since that time has been based on the recognition of the power imbalance of the doctor and patient. Patients come to physicians suffering and vulnerable, and with a knowledge deficit about the procedures and treatments to be considered. Physicians not only have superior knowledge, they also often have incentives, financial, and otherwise (e.g., filling hospital beds, gaining experience, or increasing prestige), that can have subtle but pernicious influences on their recommendations. In the case of a novel procedure for a debilitating illness, all those elements come into play, along with the interests of the biomedical industry seeking to increase the use of its products. For these reasons, the ethical course is to err always on the side of patient protection.

Side Effects and Risks

Ethical assessment of a therapy involves an examination of its risks and benefits, and a review of the degree to which that ratio is considered in treatment recommendations and communicated adequately to patients. In treatments of debilitating conditions such as PD, risk may increase because the potential for benefit is so great. However, the risk/benefit assessment must not be taken for granted, but kept under continuous review. Monitoring outcomes and side effects as the therapy diffuses geographically and medically, is an important part of diligent review. In the case of DBS, that oversight could be improved. The literature on the surgical and postoperative effects of DBS is in need of greater synthesis, and a national or international registry would facilitate better assessment of the therapy's progress.

In general, the efficacy of DBS for PD is adequate to justify its use, and in many cases improvement is dramatic (14–17). A growing body of research suggests that DBS for PD is generally safe and that the benefits of motor improvements come at the relatively low cost of minimal cognitive morbidity. Improvements from DBS have consistently been observed in the cardinal PD symptoms and dyskinesia and in activities of daily living, as well as improvement from baseline across the Unified Parkinson's Disease Rating Scale (UPDRS-III). DBS has also facilitated lowering daily dosages of levodopa. Improvement is generally shown in the patient's baseline rigidity, hypertonous, bradykinesia, tremor, and axial symptoms, including speech, gait, posture, and postural stability (18).

DBS also can lead to a number of complications and side effects. Homodynamic complications include arterial hypertension, bradycardia, arterial hypotension, and tachycardia, while more serious complications reported include pneumocephalus, hematoma, air embolism, epileptic seizure, anisocoria, and dyspnea and/or airway obstruction (19,20). Adverse events included cognitive decline, speech difficulty, decline in verbal fluency, balance instability, gait disorders, and depression. Localized hemorrhaging, infection, and seizure (21–23) have also been reported. Hemorrhage from incursion of blood vessels during the procedure remains a concern.

Problems have also been reported with device function, often due to poor medical management. Patients report failure of the device to function as indicated and poor outcome. Hardware dysfunction includes breakage of the electrode lead in vivo, systemic or localized infection, battery or connector problems, battery failure, electrode breakages and erosions, short or open circuits, foreign body reactions, and lead migrations to name a few (24–28). Many failures require additional surgeries.

Okun et al. (5) reviewed 41 cases of DBS failure during a two-year period. Reasons identified for failure include problems in patient selection, lead placement, and programming. Many problems stemmed from initial misdiagnosis and mismanagement. Forty-six percent of the subjects in the study had misplaced leads, 37% had been inadequately programmed, and 17% had no or poor access to follow-up care. Over a quarter had not seen a movement disorder specialist before surgery.

Neuropsychological disturbances are mild and usually transient and include bouts of mania, visual hallucinations (29), and cognitive impairment. Permanent cognitive complications appear to be rare (30,31). A recent literature review of 1398 patients who underwent bilateral STN DBS found cognitive problems in 41%, depression in 8%, and (hypo)mania in 4% of the subjects. Anxiety disorders were observed in less than 2%, and personality changes, hypersexuality, apathy, anxiety, and aggressiveness were observed in less than 0.5% of the group studied. About half of the patients did not experience behavioral changes (32). One study found that, despite clinical motor benefits at three to six months postoperative, significant declines were noted in working memory, speed of mental processing, bimanual motor speed and coordination, set switching, phonemic fluency, long-term consolidation of verbal material, and the encoding of visuospatial material, especially in older patients (33). Patients also report weight gain and excessive eating (34), increased bladder activity (35), and restless legs syndrome (36). Other reports raise some concerns, such as reports of impairments in accuracy in decoding facial expression, STN function, and processing olfactory information in PD patients (37,38). The settings of amplitude and frequency have a major influence on the intelligibility of speech (39). Similarly, modifying individual stimulation parameter, while still maintaining motor symptom efficacy, may mitigate adverse cognitive/behavioral responses (40) and affective responses (41). Mood changes may be greater in STN DBS than in globus pallidus internus (GPi) (42).

One report of concern is the possibility of an increased risk of suicide in after use of DBS for movement disorders. A study by Burkhard et al. (43) found a suicide rate of 4.3% (6 of 140 patients) in patients receiving DBS. Suicide was not correlated with successful motor outcome postsurgery, but was instead correlated with a previous history of severe depression and multiple DBS surgeries. The authors conclude that patients with a pre-existing high suicide risk be excluded from surgery. Certainly, in any case, the increased risk, especially if confirmed in other studies, should be communicated to patients in the informed consent process.

Many of the complications of DBS can be lessened or eliminated through proper diagnosis and assessment, careful placement and programming of devices, and adequate follow-up visits and monitoring. While exact figures are not available, the literature suggests significant numbers of patients are not receiving the standard of care in DBS surgery and medical management. The optimal management approach for surgically related neuropsychiatric problems is unknown at present (44). All patients receiving DBS should have a multidisciplinary treatment team, both pre- and postoperatively. It is also important that further neurobehavioral research be pursued to address things, such as the long-term effects of DBS, risk factors for cognitive and affective dysfunctions, and comparison of DBS with ablation as well as other desirable variables (45). Careful records should be kept to facilitate multicenter and international data gathering. The establishment of a national or international registry is highly desirable.

Patient Selection

The selection of patients for DBS surgery presents a number of ethical and clinical challenges (46). While there has been a tendency in some quarters to assume that, with full informed consent, patients have great latitude to decide whether they want the surgery, taking that standard to its extreme places on non-expert patients certain types of decisions that are more appropriately made by the surgeon. Informed consent becomes pertinent only after the patient has been deemed a suitable candidate for the procedure.

Determination of proper inclusion and exclusion criteria for the surgery depends on a number of factors, such as the certainty of diagnosis, the status of the patient, and the role of comorbidities. For instance, mood disorders and cognitive deficits are among comorbidities that many medical teams put forth as contraindications for DBS candidacy for PD patients. For mood disorders, a common programmatic description of a contraindication would be "severe depression and remarkable anxiety present (47)." A similar sentiment is often expressed regarding dementia and changes in executive function as contraindications. There is no good data that demonstrate poor motor outcomes for patients with these comorbidities or data demonstrating an exacerbation of patient problems in these realms. The absence of data does not support the exclusion or inclusion of patient's with these conditions. Rather, the ethical challenge lies in setting appropriate exclusion criteria through balancing known, or reasonably expected, harms against potential motor benefits. This includes recognizing the role the behaviors such as past suicidal ideations might play in future patient behavior. These considerations should be raised in selecting a patient so that the limits of professional obligations to "do no harm" can be explicitly discussed by the medical care team. If surgery is deemed to be within professional boundaries, the patient needs to be made aware of the lack of data and the potential for a diminished quality of life even if motor function improves.

Uncertainty in the primary diagnosis presents even trickier ethical problems. The diagnosis of idiopathic PD is arrived at clinically, since an objective diagnosis can only be made at autopsy. Although there are spectrums of diseases that share similar symptomatology with idiopathic Parkinson's disease, they do not uniformly respond to DBS therapy. Given these facts, a value judgment must be made whether to err in offering therapy too broadly or too narrowly. The decision becomes both a clinical and an ethical problem, since the goal in clinical care is to maximize the potential to help those who suffer while minimizing the potential for harm. In the one case, a patient is subjected to harm with little chance of benefit. In the other, patients are kept from receiving a beneficial therapy.

The problem of uncertain diagnosis is more than a gray area in diagnosis. Professional disagreements can create significant moral distress. For instance, if the DBS team disagrees with the diagnosis of a referring physician, professional ethics and, at times, business ethics intersect with clinical ethics. To challenge a referral source about a diagnosis—particularly a diagnosis that has a great degree of subjectivity—runs the risk of offending and alienating the patient's primary neurologist. Further, the DBS program may see fewer referrals from that neurologist if offense is taken, which is both bad for the DBS program and, perhaps, for the referring neurologist's patients if the neurologist fails to refer appropriate patients for DBS. At the present time, when there are a limited number of practices doing DBS, the reputation of the physicians and the practice itself is a valuable commodity not to be lightly put in jeopardy. Although these are very practical and important concerns, it is generally agreed upon that the fiduciary responsibility to the patient for whom the physician is currently treating must be weighed more heavily than concerns for the physician's own practice and concerns about groups of patients.

The above discussion assumes that the patient's movement disorder has a completely organic basis. The ethical balancing in uncertain cases becomes more complex when a psychogenic component is suspected for the movement disorder. How strong a suspicion needs to be present in order to be a contraindication for DBS therapy? Unlike epilepsy monitoring that has a good rate of detection for pseudo seizures, psychogenic symptoms like dystonia or tremor have no definitive objective tests. Perhaps the best test for these symptoms involves a placebo test of drugs that have shown some efficacy in symptom reduction for the patient. As long as the patient agrees to a blinded-placebo trial this could be ethically permissible to undertake. It is apparent, when discussing these various kinds of uncertainty, that a careful balancing of truthfulness, transparency, protecting from harm, and professional standards is important when considering patient selection for DBS.

A final consideration of patient selection involves evaluation and negotiations about postoperative care. Patients need to be discharged to a safe setting during the period of time needed to adjust programming to minimize the potential harms from falling. Often this is judged by the strength of patients' social support. Although a patient with poor support should not be discriminated against, it is ethically reasonable for the medical team to require a plan of care for safety and supervision to be in place prior to agreeing to place DBS. Further, in order to gain maximal benefit and minimize the harms, patients need to commit to follow-up with a programming specialist. Again, making this a condition of acceptance can be ethically justified on the basis of avoiding harm. Finally, in preoperative evaluation there needs to be explicit discussion concerning patients' goals and the potential need for stimulator adjustment, if the medical team deems it to be creating more harm than benefit. The patients should also have the ability to turn off the device themselves.

Multidisciplinary Neurosurgery Committees

Increasingly, multidisciplinary teams in major institutions have been constituted to review the candidacy of complex patients under evaluation for functional neurosurgical procedures (48). Because, as we have seen, functional neurosurgery has the potential to alter essential features of a patient's personhood, including mood, personality, and cognitive abilities, such multidisciplinary committees merit special consideration not as applicable to non-neurological committees. Functional neurosurgical patients present some unique challenges. For example, in DBS placement the patient is typically awake, which can lead to unique challenges such as anxiety, or cognitive deficits that might significantly impact intraoperative procedures. It may even lead to the unique problem of a patient revoking consent to surgery intraoperatively (see the informed consent section). Functional neurosurgical patients can also provide unique management challenges following surgery. DBS for PD is palliative and aimed at improving the patient's quality of life and reducing motor symptoms. Managing stimulation settings and medications in patients with ongoing neurodegenerative disorders with potentially significant neuropsychiatric symptoms can be challenging and is greatly facilitated by a committed multidisciplinary team (48).

In addition to their role in clinical care and patient selection, the professional time used to resolve conflicts and discuss emergent problems in these committees provides the opportunity for the development of careful practice guidelines informed by both science and values (48). Because neurosurgical interventions can result in nonreversible damage to brain structures and given the potential impact of the proposed neurosurgical procedure on the brain, including the neural underpinnings of mood, personality, and cognitive abilities, the consensus building and checks and balances of such committees seems warranted.

Informed Consent

Informed consent has become a cornerstone of accepted physician–patient relations and proper clinical care. The elements of informed consent include information, understanding, consent, and authorization; all four must be satisfied before the informed consent is considered valid. Patients should be given information that is complete and adequate for decision making, should demonstrate an understanding of the information given, should consent freely and without coercion from the medical team, and finally the patient, or authorized surrogate, should give official authorization for the procedure (49).

The basic elements of informed consent are constant in most major medical procedures. Physicians have the responsibility to assure that the patient is informed of their (*i*) diagnosis, (*ii*) the procedures involved in the surgery and its probable outcome, (*iii*) expected benefit, (*iv*) transient complications and the therapeutic remedies available, (*v*) other possible and probable complications, (*vi*) the likelihood of permanent results and complications (including such things as scarring), (*vii*) other foreseeable risks, and (*viii*) alternatives to the procedure (50). Informing a patient and responding to concerns should be a constant process in the medical encounter, not limited to the "official" informed consent moment, when the patient authorizes the procedure by signing the paperwork.

As with all procedures, it is important to employ a robust consent process in DBS that is respectful of patient values. Patients should have enough cognitive capacity to understand the information provide about the therapy, appreciate the implications, judge the costs, be able to question adequately and communicate a choice, and freely choose to participate in collaboration with health care providers. A procedure may still be undertaken even if the patient does not have an ideal understanding. However, it is always advisable to involve others in decision making in these instances in order to have a balanced approach to respecting each individual patient. Not only can family members be useful to this end, but also employing a team approach among healthcare providers can be beneficial (48).

The consent process continues throughout surgery and beyond. Part of the accepted standard is the principle that consent can be withdrawn at any time, even after surgery is planned and within safety limits underway. Although the use of any implantable device highlights the need for continuous informed consent, since the device becomes part of the persons "regular" body, DBS implantation provides at least one unique challenge. The fact that DBS leads are placed during an awake craniotomy makes the idea of continuous consent trickier. DBS for PD is a quality of life therapy and not a life-saving intervention. This aspect distinguishes DBS placement from awake craniotomies performed for brain tumor where the participation of the patient is not necessary for the accomplishment of the primary life saving goal of the surgery. In DBS placement, the patient must actively participate during the micro-electric recording phase, which is directly related to the primary goal of maximizing potential motor function. A surgical team may be confronted by a patient who, after being awake several hours in an operating room, requests discontinuation of the surgery. The team would be faced with the difficult situation of having started an operation and having put the patient at some risk, yet being asked to discontinue with little chance of benefit for the patient. In this situation, there is an obligation to act in the patient's best interest, with "interest" being defined by the patient's goals. It is the obligation of the medical team to advise and perhaps even to strongly encourage the patient to continue surgery if the team still believes benefit is likely. If the remainder of the surgery could be undertaken safely and the physician believes that the continued surgery is an important aspect of the patient's previously articulated goals, and that the suffering would not be undue, then therapeutic privilege could be used to justify continuation independent of decision-making capacity. However, if a patient has significant decision-making capacity, then generally the patient is allowed the revocation if it is informed and well articulated. Of course, there is always a requirement to discontinue any procedure in a safe manner. The patient does not have an ethical right to force the surgeon to put the patient at unnecessary risk. The best way to handle intraoperative revocation of consent is to put in place good processes beforehand in order to avoid its occurrence.

RESEARCH ISSUES

Many difficult methodological issues plague DBS research, most notably the difficulty in disentangling the multiple variables influencing comparisons between patients before and after surgery (51). Yet surgeons and patients need to make decisions about their care, and well-conducted scientific studies are necessary to decide between surgical and medical options, as well as between competing surgical approaches.

Freeman et al. (52), noting that it is unethical for surgeons and patients to be required to make surgical decisions with insufficient scientific information, interviewed 48 North American surgical researchers studying PD about trial designs. A separate study looked at other stakeholders, such as representatives from academic centers, device manufacturers, federal and state agencies, patient advocacy groups, and third party payers. Among other findings, participants concluded that surgical placebo-controlled trials for DBS were ethically and practically infeasible, that device manufacturers have fewer incentives to fund trials than their pharmaceutical counterparts, and that the United States has inadequate infrastructure for conducting clinical trials, necessitating novel funding mechanisms. The result is that medical devices are routinely diffused without adequate data registry, standardization, or compelling data.

It is important, when developing and testing novel surgical procedures, to assure patient safety through adequate feasibility studies, task force oversight, full IRB review, audit, morbidity, and mortality conferences, and tracker studies (53). Surgeons are sometimes slow to make the distinction between surgical innovation and research protocols, and therefore, at times, do not call into play all the protections due a person about to become a subject in an experimental procedure, rather than a patient undergoing standard of care. While the regulations that control research may, at times, seem burdensome to the surgeon, they are there to protect both the subject and the surgeon.

A few basic ethical principles and values related to research ethics have been articulated by physicians, bioethicists, legislatures, and the courts over the last 40 years. Respect for the self determination and dignity of all subjects in research; the need for free, informed consent; the importance of protecting subject confidentiality; equity in the selection of subjects and the distribution of any risk associated with research; and the rights of subjects to withdraw their participation at any time without penalty are the foundations of contemporary research ethics. Researchers should recognize that significant subpopulations of the subjects undergoing neurosurgical procedures are best classified as vulnerable populations, and require increased vigilance to provide adequate informed consent and subject protection. Modern bioethics has emphasized the importance of recognizing that human subjects' research is a privilege. Researchers should remember that through the generosity of subjects, their careers and income are enhanced. They, therefore, owe a duty to their subjects to follow the highest standards of integrity and accountability (54).

Informed Consent in Research

As suggested in the above discussion of informed consent for DBS treatment, the standard for consent changes when the intervention, or portion of the intervention, has a research component. Special consent is required from the patient/subject and informed consent processes need research oversight committees (in the United States these are referred to as IRBs). Since the generalizable knowledge portion of research studies are not intended to benefit the particular subject, research ethics stresses the rights of the subject and the need for voluntary participation as key ethical principles. To that end, process of consent to enter a research study is somewhat arduous compared to the ease with which a subject may withdraw from research.

The three primary ethical challenges in informed consent for DBS research involve coercion, revocation of consent, and decisional capacity. Currently the treatment modality of STN stimulation for movement disorders is well understood and accepted as a standard of care. Hence, most research involves either a small portion of the implantation procedure (e.g., new instrumentation, techniques, or ancillary medications) or follow-up studies (e.g., psychosocial research, variations of stimulator settings, or imaging). In these types of research the patient receives therapy and participates in the research all at the same time. As with all clinical research with a therapeutic component, patients may either believe they are required to participate in the research in order to receive the therapy, or may feel so indebted to clinicians that they subjugate their self-interest and personal desires to loyalty to clinicians. Clinician researchers must make every effort to emphasize the voluntaries of the research portion, disconnect the discussion of treatment and research in some way, and be clear about the available alternatives.

In STN stimulation for movement disorders, the patient should be well informed about the aspects of the procedure being studied, to know in which portions of the procedure consent may be easily revoked, and in which portions revoking consent may be more difficult because it is primarily intended as treatment. If a patient/subject intraoperatively requests the procedure to stop, nontherapeutic research portions should be discontinued as quickly and safely as possible without pressure from the researcher. For example, if the patient is undergoing DBS lead placement and has agreed to intraoperative neuropsychological testing during standard electrode mapping, the patient can withdraw from the neuropsychology portion easily and in a manner that should not affect the continuance of the therapeutic portion. A separate discussion would be needed about the discontinuation of the therapeutic procedure itself.

It should also be noted that a higher standard of decision-making capacity applies for consent to research than that for therapy. Given the cognitive impact of late stage PD, patients who may be allowed to participate in the decision about their treatment may not be in an appropriate position to give informed consent for research. Although it is ethically important to include all populations in research, subjects with diminished capacity require special protections. These issues need to be addressed carefully by research oversight committees.

When research is intended to extend the indications for DBS to other illnesses, then more standard research ethics applied. In early trials where a population may be desperate because of the refractory nature of their disease, then potential coercion becomes particularly important to recognize and attempt to ameliorate. The entire process from initial review through surgery and follow-up should follow careful research protocols with appropriate institutional review.

Sham Surgery

The acceptability of sham and placebo surgeries in PD and other neurological conditions has been widely debated in the clinical ethics literature (though much of the controversy has focussed on transplantation of fetal tissue rather than DBS). Though, in general, such surgeries are safe (55) and a large majority of PD clinical researchers in one study believe that sham surgery is better than unblended controls for assessing the efficacy of the surgery (56), many have also written in opposition to the technique (57–59), and another study mentioned above by Freeman et al. (52) found that a majority of researchers thought placebo trials for DB were ethically and practically infeasible. While placebo surgery may increase the confidence in a procedure, and there are situations where placebo surgery may have a place, in the case of neurosurgery, other methodologies may provide adequate reliability (58,59). For that reason, and particularly in cases employing placebo craniotomy, alternative protocols should be used whenever possible in DBS research.

CONCLUSION

DBS for the relief of symptoms of movement disorders such as PD is a valuable addition to the treatment options for this devastating disease. The overriding principle in providing clinical care, however, must be the assessment of the treatment and its risks and benefits in the context of the value system of the patients and their support system (60). In order to protect patients, and to maintain the confidence of the general public in support of the treatment, DBS must be administered and studied with the highest level of ethical oversight and care.

REFERENCES

1. Kopell BH, Greenberg B, Rezai AR. Deep brain stimulation for psychiatric disorders. J Clin Neurophysiol 2004; 21(1):51–67.
2. Cavuoto J. Neural engineering's image problem. IEEE Spectrum 2004; 32–37.
3. Slater L. Who holds the clicker?. Mother Jones November/December 2005. http://www.motherjones.com/news/feature/2005/11/who_holds_clicker.html (last accessed May 23, 2006).
4. Harris G. Device won approval though F.D.A. staff objected. New York Times, 17 February 2006.
5. Okun MS, Tagliati M, Pourfar M, et al. Management of referred deep brain stimulation failures, a retrospective analysis from 2 movement disorders centers. Arch Neurol 2005; 62(8):1250–1255.

6. Fins JJ. 2003. From psychosurgery to neuromodulation and palliation: history's lessons for the ethical conduct and regulation of neuropsychiatric research. Neurosurg Clin N Am 2003; 14(2):303–319, ix–x.
7. Apuzzo ML, Liu CY. The genesis of neurosurgery and the evolution of the neurosurgical operative environmentL Part 1—concepts for future development, 2003 and beyond. Neurosurgery 2003; 52(1):20–33.
8. Stone JL. Dr. Gottlieb Burckhardt. The pioneer of psychosurgery. J Hist Neurosci 2001; 10(1):79–92.
9. Mashour GA, Walker EE, Martuza RL. Psychosurgery: past, present, and future. Brain Res Brain Res Rev 2005; 48(3):409–419.
10. El-Hai J. The Lobotomist: A Maverick Medical Genius and His Tragic Quest to Rid the World of Mental Illness. New York: John Wiley & Sons, Inc., 2005.
11. Baumeister A. The tulane electrical brain stimulation program, a historical case study in medical ethics. J Hist Neurosci 2000; 9(3):262–278.
12. Horgan J. The Forgotten Era of the Brain. Scientific American 2005; 66–74.
13. Breit S, Schulz JB, Benabid AL. Deep brain stimulation. Cell Tissue Res 2004; 318(1):275–288.
14. Rodriguez-Oroz MC, Obeso JA, Lang AE, et al. Bilateral deep brain stimulation in Parkinson's disease: a multicentre study with 4 years follow-up. Brain 2005; 128(Pt 10):2240–2249.
15. Erola T, Heikkinen ER, Haapaniemi T, et al. Efficacy of bilateral subthalamic nucleus (STN) stimulation in Parkinson's disease. Acta Neurochir 2006; 148(4):389–394.
16. Miyawaki E, Perlmutter JS, Troster AI, et al. The behavioral complications of pallidal stimulation: a case report. Brain Cogn 2000; 42(3):417–434.
17. Goodman RR, Kim B, McClelland S III, et al. Operative techniques and morbidity with subthalamic nucleus deep brain stimulation in 100 consecutive patients with advanced Parkinson's disease. J Neurol Neurosurg Psychiatry 2006; 77(1):12–17.
18. Anderson VC, Burchiel KJ, Hogarth P, et al. Pallidal vs subthalamic nucleus deep brain stimulation in Parkinson disease. Arch Neurol 2005; 62(4):554–560.
19. Santos P, Valero R, Arguis MJ, et al. Preoperative adverse events during stereotactic microelectrode-guided deep brain surgery in Parkinson's disease. Rev Esp Anestesiol Reanim 2004; 51(9):523–530.
20. Landi A, Parolin M, Piolti R, et al. Deep brain stimulation for the treatment of Parkinson's disease: the experience of the Neurosurgical Department in Monza. Neurol Sci 2003; 24(suppl 1):S43–S44.
21. Terao T, Takahashi H, Yokochi F, et al. Hemorrhagic complication of stereotactic surgery in patients with movement disorders. J Neurosurg 2003; 98(6):1241–1246.
22. Binder DK, Rau G, Starr PA. Hemorrhagic complications of microelectrode-guided deep brain stimulation. Stereotact Funct Neurosurg 2003; 80(1–4):28–31.
23. Constantoyannis C, Berk C, Honey CR, et al. Reducing hardware-related complications of deep brain stimulation. Can J Neurol Sci 2005; 32(2):194–200.
24. Benabid AL, Chabardes S, Seigneuret E. Deep-brain stimulation in Parkinson's disease: long-term efficacy and safety—What happened this year? Curr Op Neurol 2005; 18(6):623–630.
25. Oh MY, Abosch A, Kim SH, et al. Long-term hardware-related complications of deep brain stimulation. Neurosurgery 2002; 50(6):1268–1274.
26. Terao T, Okiyama R, Takahashi H, et al. Comparison and examination of stereotactic surgical complications in movement disorders. No Shinkei Geka 2003; 31(6):629–636.

27. Lyons KE, Pahwa R. Deep brain stimulation and essential tremor. J Clin Neurophysiol 2004; 21(1):2–5.
28. Beric A, Kelly PJ, Rezai A, et al. Complications of deep brain stimulation surgery. Stereotact Funct Neurosurg 2001; 77(1–4):73–78.
29. Terao T, Okiyama R, Takahashi H, et al. Comparison and examination of stereotactic surgical complications in movement disorders. No Shinkei Geka 2003; 31(6):629–636.
30. Salvador-Aguiar C, Menendez-Guisasola L, Blazquez-Estrada M, et al. Psychiatric symptoms of Parkinson's disease following deep brain stimulation surgery on the subthalamic nucleus. Revista de Neurologia 2004; 39(7):651–655.
31. Funkiewiez A, Ardouin C, Caputo E, et al. Long term effects of bilateral subthalamic nucleus stimulation on cognitive function, mood, and behaviour in Parkinson's disease. J Neurol Neurosurg Psychiatry 2004; 75(6):834–839.
32. Temel Y, Kessels A, Tan S, et al. Behavioural changes after bilateral subthalamic stimulation in advanced Parkinson disease: a systematic review. Parkinsonism Relat Disord 2006; In press.
33. Saint-Cyr JA, Trépanier LL, Kumar R, Lozano AM, Lang AE. Neuropsychological consequences of chronic bilateral stimulation of the subthalamic nucleus in Parkinson's disease. Brain 2000; 123(10):2091–2108.
34. Barichella M, Marczewska AM, Mariani C, et al. Body weight gain rate in patients with Parkinson's disease and deep brain stimulation. Mov Disord 2003; 18(11):1337–1340.
35. Seif C, Herzog J, van der Horst C, et al. Effect of subthalamic deep brain stimulation on the function of the urinary bladder. Ann Neurol 2004; 55(1):118–120.
36. Kedia S, Moro E, Tagliati M, et al. Emergence of restless legs syndrome during subthalamic stimulation for Parkinson disease. Neurology 2004; 63(12):2410–2412.
37. Dujardin K, Blairy S, Defebvre L, et al. Subthalamic nucleus stimulation induces deficits in decoding emotional facial expressions in Parkinson's disease. J Neurol Neurosurg Psychiatry 2004; 75(2):202–208.
38. Hummel T, Jahnke U, Sommer U, et al. Olfactory function in patients with idiopathic Parkinson's disease: effects of deep brain stimulation in the subthalamic nucleus. J Neural Transm 2005; 112(5):669–676.
39. Tornqvist AL, Schalen L, Rehncrona S. Effects of different electrical parameter settings on the intelligibility of speech in patients with Parkinson's disease treated with subthalamic deep brain stimulation. Mov Disord 2005; 20(4):416–423.
40. Francel P, Ryder K, Wetmore J, et al. Deep brain stimulation for Parkinson's disease: association between stimulation parameters and cognitive performance. Stereotact Funct Neurosurg 2004; 82(4):191–193.
41. Okun MS, Green J, Saben R, et al. Mood changes with deep brain stimulation of STN and GPi: results of a pilot study. J Neurol Neurosurg Psychiatry 2003; 74(11):1584–1586.
42. Vitek JL. Deep brain stimulation for Parkinson's disease. A critical re-evaluation of STN versus GPi DBS. Stereotact Funct Neurosurg 2002; 78(3–4):119–131.
43. Burkhard PR, Vingerhoets FJ, Berney A, et al. Suicide after successful deep brain stimulation for movement disorders. Neurology 2004; 63(11):2170–2172.
44. Burn DJ, Troster AI. Neuropsychiatric complications of medical and surgical therapies for Parkinson's disease. J Geriatr Psychiatry Neurol 2004; 17(3):172–180.
45. Fields JA, Troster AI. Cognitive outcomes after deep brain stimulation for Parkinson's disease: a review of initial studies and recommendations for future research. Brain Cogn 2000; 42(2):268–293.

46. Deuschl G, Bain P. Deep brain stimulation for tremor: patient selection and evaluation. Mov Disord 2002; 17(suppl 3):S102–S111.
47. Lopiano L, Rizzone M, Bergamasco B, et al. Deep brain stimulation of the subthalamic nucleus in PD: an analysis of the exclusion causes. J Neurol Sci 2002; 195(2):167–170.
48. Ford PJ, Kubu CS. Stimulating debate: Ethics in a multidisciplinary functional neurosurgery committee. J Med Ethics 2005; 32(2):106–109.
49. Moreno J, Caplan AL, Wolpe PR. Updating protections for human subjects involved in research. JAMA 1998; 280(22):1951–1958.
50. Scarrow AM, Scarrow MR. Informed consent for the Neurosurgeon. Surg Neurol 2002; 57(1):63–69.
51. Van Horn G, Schiess M, Soukup V. Subthalamic Deep Brain Stimulation, Neurobehavioral Concerns. Arch Neurol 2001; 58(8):1205–1206.
52. Freeman TB, Vawter DE, Gervais KG, et al. The modern era of surgical trial designs: Perspectives of Parkinson's disease (PD) researchers. Exp Neurol 2006; 198(2): 568–569.
53. McKneally MF, Daar AS. Introducing new technologies: protecting subjects of surgical innovation and research. World J Surg 2003; 27(8):930–935.
54. Wolpe PR, Moreno J, Caplan AL. Ethical principles and history. In: Pincus HA, Lieberman JA, Ferris S, eds. Ethics in Psychiatric Research: A Resource Manual for Human Subjects Protection. Washington, D.C.: The American Psychiatric Association, 1999.
55. Frank S, Kieburtz K, Holloway R, et al. What is the risk of sham surgery in Parkinson disease clinical trials? A review of published reports. Neurology 2005; 65(7): 1101–1103.
56. Kim SY, Frank S, Holloway R, et al. Science and ethics of sham surgery: a survey of Parkinson disease clinical researchers. Arch Neurol 2005; 62(9):1357–1360.
57. Dekkers W, Boer G. Sham neurosurgery in patients with Parkinson's disease: is it morally acceptable? J Med Ethics 2001; 27(3):151–156.
58. Weijer C. I need a placebo like I need a hole in the head. J Law Med Ethics 2002; 30(1):69–72.
59. Macklin R. The ethical problems with sham surgery in clinical research. New Engl J Med 1999; 341(13):992–996.
60. Drizis TJ. Ethics in surgery. Eur Surg Res 2004; 36(suppl 1):88–89.

Index

Note to think abt context
The lifstyle of patient
e.g. undertaker